ACUPUNCTURE IN MEDICINE

A METAPHOR FOR THERAPEUTIC TRANSACTIONS IN HISTORY TO THE PRESENT

MOOLAMANIL THOMAS

authorHOUSE®

AuthorHouse™ UK Ltd.
1663 Liberty Drive
Bloomington, IN 47403 USA
www.authorhouse.co.uk
Phone: 0800.197.4150

Published by AuthorHouse   06/20/2014

ISBN: 978-1-4969-7574-4 (sc)
ISBN: 978-1-4969-7576-8 (hc)
ISBN: 978-1-4969-7575-1 (e)

CONTENTS

INTRODUCTION

Acupuncture is a specific therapeutic function which had its origins and progressed within a historical context, systematised in an epistemology relating to that history. We cannot ignore that context while arriving at the possibility of its development in clinical medicine. Clinical scientists visualise problems for a specific discipline and attempt solutions by its stipulated methods. But in this instance we attempt these methods to solve problems associated with a discipline that is from the past with its own therapeutic methods of practice. Should these be ignored for finding relevance to its therapeutic function, or are they necessarily irrelevant because seen to be so by the methods fashioned for present therapeutic products? To consider acupuncture as a function within scientific medicine and to survey it in relationship to the Science of Pain without its background to the knowledge as was transmitted in history or even a nodding acquaintance with the more specific epistemology of Traditional Chinese Medicine (TCM) can be done only by denuding acupuncture of a prospective and testable potential. The neurophysiology of Pain demonstrates a pronounced inhibitory response that can be activated endogenously by the organism from different environmental inputs. The acupuncture needle inserted into peripheral tissues of an organism is one such input, albeit, therapist controlled. A tradition which discovered that function some millennia ago, developed and phrased it in a therapeutic system for a wide range of ailments, is now rephrased by neuroscience and its clinicians, without making much allowance for its past.

Metaphysical theories that sustained acupuncture are not within this brief except to illustrate and discuss (Ch. III) a few of its concepts as empirical possibilities. There are many renderings of Chinese Acupuncture traditions in English. At least two pay close attention in translation to the metaphysical concepts rendered in the Chinese language[i], and Porkett[ii], states its functional principles by adhering closely to semantics.

My acquaintance with Traditional Acupuncture suggests that some of its practical applications were based in an empiricism which could be investigated by clinical trial (Ch. IV). Researching acupuncture within scientific medicine is to necessarily contend with a tradition based in metaphysics. This has problems due to incompatibilities to their respective epistemologies. However the clinician/scientist assumes that regulations of method to obtain therapeutic validation should apply per se to any therapeutic modality, even those that have been with us from the past. Questions relating to the method for ascertaining the validity of traditional therapeutics need more answers.

The opportunity was fortuitous that brought me to TCM in China to the Beijing School for Traditional Medicine and a few months of sustained contact with the traditional teachings of acupuncture. The period was hardly sufficient for me to claim a deep knowledge of acupuncture and further, a scepticism of my medical background stood in the way of being a whole-hearted novice. We were told at the commencement of the course to put aside any baggage of modern medical science we might be carrying in order to understand traditional Chinese medical theory within its epistemology[1]. The lectures on theory were delivered by esteemed academics of that School, and later applied to patients at a hospital clinic under the supervision of its doctor of TCM who was, within that tradition, unmistakably an inspired clinician. Based on physical, including variant pulse and tongue examination followed by due deliberation and discussion, a traditional diagnosis of disease was treated with appropriate acupuncture point selections within those theories.

Non medically qualified participants in the course were from a Traditional school for Acupuncture in Los Angeles, and there were as well doctors of Medicine from Iran, Africa, Europe and South America and physiotherapists from Scandinavia. The Californian therapists were the most impressed by the rational presentation of traditional theory. They had an impressive prior fluency to discussing proto-scientific theories. Many months later a visit to their school of Traditional Medicine in Los Angeles was an experience in the exegesis of TCM, but as a later Western interpretation of Chinese Medical thought it appeared to be losing out to the empirical content and continuous systematisation of the Chinese[2].

---

[1]   Is there a semblance here to the application of science to traditional therapies?

[2]   The pragmatism and the practice within the Chinese School of Traditional Medicine at Beijing were already attempting corrections, the trends to the later Phase

However, the doctors were generally naive to this content, willing listeners, though most were sceptical. It was the daily clinical routine with patients at the hospital which gained us the most from the course.

At the Beijing School, I found that their Teachers and Scholars were dismissive of medical Science. The attitudes of the professional rank and file within either of today's active health delivery systems is mutual, both stressing exclusivity and a conviction in the superiority of their own separate systems of learning. I must admit to not becoming a votary of acupuncture in the setting of TCM. But nor can present methods for clinical study be relied upon as a certain means to assessing worth. Prior to the Chinese experience my attitude was that of the many colleagues, that traditional therapeutics have little to offer, even may be hazardous to patients, and its teachings have no relevance, in this day and age.[3]

I have since been impressed by the variety of expression and opinions about acupuncture by teachers, colleagues and collaborators, views that

---

Energetics. There, obviously, were considerable faults to meteorological assessments of 1500 years ago which was the basis of computational charts of energy flows (see Porkett p 105-6 and my later chapter)

[3] My first experience to the use of acupuncture was with a friend and patient of mine at New Delhi in the late '70s. He was a constitutional lawyer at the Supreme Court as well as an old time member of the Communist party, one amongst an elitist group of sympathisers then called 'The Friends of China'. Following one of his visits there he decided to start an acupuncture clinic with the help of a young medical licentiate. I was taken to visit this clinic and was appalled at the neglect of hygiene generally and sterilisation in particular in using needles—a wipe with spirit had obvious shortcomings which I mentioned to my friend. These opinions were summarily dismissed. Months later he had asked me to see his wife who had an upper respiratory infection. She was ill, but he too appeared quite unwell and in the next bed. He was jaundiced but said he expected to be better, treating himself with drinks of cane sugar juice (recommended locally), and asked me to confine my attentions to the wife A few days later he asked for me to visit him. The man was grossly jaundiced and quite unwell. I asked, on a sudden suspicion, if by any chance he had used acupuncture. He had, he said, been using it for a backache for months, and with benefit he added! I shipped him off to hospital since his jaundice required special care and further investigations. He was diagnosed with serum B hepatitis. From the hospital, a few days later he called and said his nephew was also ill with jaundice. The answer over the phone to my by now routine question to him was that this boy was being treated for a depression with acupuncture. He too was shipped off to the hospital, Uncle and nephew then sharing a room and diagnosis!. Both, however, recovered in time.

are debated, often hypothesised and researched; in sharp contrast to my initial exposure to acupuncture, straight from the horse's mouth, so to speak, from the Academic Chinese Traditionalist whose singular position maintains that dissent or another viewpoint was due to inadequate knowledge which needed improvement and correction. In this context one is also up against positions held by the practitioner/scientist in medicine with strongly held notions about the discipline of science and who often forgets that even those are held within socio-historical influences and the regulatory compulsions of his discipline. Attitudes do colour issues but debate is always possible. The progressive resolution to the subject of acupuncture in science in the final analysis is a testable proposition, although there are impossibilities about the metaphysics of traditional acupuncture which cannot be conveyed for scientific evaluation. *Although in clinical trials the practices of acupuncture, or recent versions, are evaluated certain obvious empirical propositions that are evident in traditional theory, even as expressed in an original epistemology convey in interpretation to controlled studies.* Neurophysiological research in basic experimental work demonstrates increased thresholds to pain, while experimental and clinical studies show that pain inhibition can be achieved by acupuncture needle stimuli in variant applications. Clinical responses relating to inflammatory, immune related and circulatory patient pathology continue to be widely investigated in clinical trials using acupuncture, and experimental work demonstrates responses at molecular levels in many biological species[ii].

Acupuncture in the present culture of Medicine.

For knowledge to develop into science, the revolutionary advance of a new investigatory paradigm is essential; the scientist is convinced that previous developments and knowledge lacking that authenticity may be no longer viewed as functional science, but appreciated for their history. This position applies to the many physical sciences but past and present therapeutic knowledge is established as functional when the ailment shows responses in human biology. The responses, objective or stated patient perceptions, are the measure of any therapeutic system. Additional to the alleviation or reduction of signs and symptoms from therapeutic inputs, substances or procedure, there is the evidence of conditioned responses which can reduce pain or ameliorate a subject's physical or mental distress and which had a therapeutic role in tribal societies from pre-historic time (Ch. II). There remain today demonstrations of similar responses in the cultural lore of societies as they recall a tribal past[4]. It is the potential of a biological trait which in pre-history was used for therapeutic purposes, and a continuity of the response is furnished by the 'placebo' in the present medical culture. Medical research poses the response as a nullity, a therapeutic artefact in order to differentiate from a virtual therapeutic source. The amelioration or cure for disease are available in the records of history, for easing pain, recognising symptoms of ill health or reducing fevers. We have the extant tomes of therapeutics and pharmacopoeias from world sources (Ch. II). In the final analyses it is the response, either perceived and/or demonstrated in biological parameters of measurement, which has sustained therapeutic systems. The medical scientist accepts that position, provided there is consistent experimental evidence. For therapeutics a determination is made not only by science but in social choices as well, a factor that does not feature for other sciences. Experimental laboratory demonstrations, accepted or rejected by the small community in the practice of the latter disciplines, are the absolute benchmark of the functional value of the other physical sciences.

It was a repeated experience of the 19th century scientist as he was confronted by the various disciplines in other cultural contexts to consign the painstaking knowledge gathered over centuries to an irrelevance. Chapter I consider a few colonial compulsions which required new disciplinary institutions to promote their interests, and amongst them the health needs of the coloniser had to be catered to in the emerging disciplines of medicine. But, it also emphasised a predicament, further cultivated in undertones of race towards the native and his knowledge. Countries with a pronounced Colonial past, when today required to consider those therapeutic traditions of the Orient are still unable to do so with an objectivity sufficient to supplant attitudes. The British approach to the social relevance of traditional medicine is quite unlike that in Sweden where a subject like acupuncture is taken up in methods for objective study and use and concerned Swedish administrative organisations coordinate with scientific institutions in determining their value for research and to educate and train medical auxiliaries to the use acupuncture for their society.

---

[4]   The dancers in bare feet over hot coals, firewalking, in India and the Katharagama, Sri Lankan body skewering rituals.

The term 'alternative' medicine is a self-imposed hurdle in countries where these traditions have arrived, the impression being that like acupuncture they must remain outside the prevailing medical culture. While the epistemology will not assimilate, traditional applications may arrive in the practice of medicine as the evidences unfold. Presently its many practices are in the public domain without sufficient evidence substantiating a specific value from the treatment. Investigating them for evidence of therapeutic value, side effects and hazards in their use is not merely a research necessity but a social imperative. That position recognises the need to proceed from acupuncture as an 'alternative' therapeutic modality to exploring its diverse possibilities and defining the indications for its use for pathological categories or, if possible, for the complex patient pathology seen in clinics. If acupuncture can be established as useful for a particular pathological problem or a possible way to manage a chronic problem, at least for a while, in lieu of surgery, or provide immediate and spectacular relief for either prodromal aura or an attack of migraine, or likewise, for the intense muscular spasm, the acute pain and distress of trismus or lumbago, then it is not an alternative therapeutic mode but becomes part of a physician's treatment armamentarium for specific indications.

Historical interactions relating to medical knowledge (Ch. I, II)

The epistemic passage of knowledge, therapeutics in this instance, has a fairly long history from tradition to Science. The chapters that relate to history are an acknowledgement of what medicine as science owes to that history; the general acquisition of knowledge through the ages, from many sources and traditions to their more systematic cultural applications. In sifting an application like traditional acupuncture through the sieve of clinical research the relevance of historical processes may help us to appreciate that the evidence we seek may not come about by a direct transposition to the epistemology of science, and beyond that, the looming social issue of therapeutic systems which are still widely used, despite the presence of Medicine and its science.

Science is apparent within societies when special groups test empirical knowledge by application or by the strictures of method and then systematise that knowledge in a theoretical structure. The displacement of populations in violent local strife, war and migrations brought them into foreign cultures, but for groups with special talents it was also a contact with those of a similar bent, and the exchanges inevitably enhanced the content of specialised knowledge. But knowledge systems also get debilitated in the short run in conflict, although hardly ever to extinction. More often than not they survive and quality is enhanced in newer inputs and fresh ideas from other peoples. The gains to civilisations and the quality of their achievements are reasonably obvious, but not usually attributed to foreign incursion, nor to the inevitable addition to the variety of biological attributes by mixing ethnic stock. Inevitably cognitive processes have the imprint of the mix, allowing a fresh look at older systems, whether of the arts or other forms of knowledge.

There is a marked tendency, on the contrary, for achievement to rest in Civilisations and be identified by: geographical spaces—Europe, China; ethnicity—the Incan, Aryan; religion—the Islamic or the Hindu, and so on. The tendency in history for culture and knowledge in their narration to be insulated within an identity bound culture offers greater appreciation for studies of literature and art. But, civilisational identity can also obscure the contribution either from the influx of other peoples or as achievements enhanced in the wealth of exchange. Civilisations gather momentum from the upheavals of war and from admixture, the considerable biological exchange across vast land spaces through history offering innumerable shades which are lost in identity. Migration was a process from antiquity, the movements of people and apparent in the borrowing, acquisitions and advances to the content of forms of knowledge, even while they developed distinctive cultural markings.

There is well-known evidence of movement, the trade route from the Chinese mainland across to the substantial civilisations of what is now N.W Afghanistan into West Asia, the routes of the Old Silk Road. But not merely a trade route, it was responsible for much exchange to stock; through nearly four millennia, the prior exchange was of the Europoid with peoples of the distant Far East, from what is now Xingjian in China; in later centuries the reverse flow was along the centres of the antique civilisations of Bactria and Sogdiana, transforming essentially into the Persian. By then peoples identified as Mongoloid or Caucasian and Europoid had in a considerable mix, attained physical features that were shared, now confirmed as genetic exchange from DNA studies of surviving mummies[iii]. We have evidence of the mix to population but are yet to appreciate the full exchange between civilisations of culture and the transactions providing recognisable features between knowledge systems.

Knowledge develops in the absorption of extraneous peoples and in adaptation for the differing social needs, local problems, or in the older culture of an existing society. The present discussion lays stress on the medicine of West Asia and Persia, the transmission of the knowledge and achievements from their mediaeval civilisations and its influence and impact on Europe, despite all the turbulence of confrontation. It is unreal to read the period for Europe as the Dark Ages[iv] considering the scholarship conveyed by Arab and Jewish physicians aiding and working with scholars in Europe's centres of learning. Lifetimes were expended in compiling and translating the not inconsiderable knowledge of the times sustained and developed largely in the Persian and Arab world. Large land areas of Europe were dominated by Arab or Moor who instituted centres of learning, and created cities with their unique architectural imprint. Medicine flourished from that contact followed by innovative institutionalised facilities for teaching students and treating patients.

The difficulty for historians in the past was not the dearth of knowledge or its applications which is suggested in Europe's Dark Age but that in accepting its quality and its extent also required a concession to their origins. The age was one of achievement in technology, mathematics and medicine, largely outside an European space as we know it now. Discovery relating to therapeutics, in seepage across the worlds, revive, and the restitution has enhanced its content. Transformed knowledge in the past obscured its origins. It may be difficult to relate particular discovery to preceding ones until we seek that evidence in the past since acknowledgements to precedence was not required. An example in medicine is of small pox and its prophylaxis. There were methods of delivering an attenuated virus throughout the centuries. Variolation and inoculation in its variety of practices may be recalled before Jenner. Another, the commonplace attribution of a blood circulation to the pioneer of the 17th century, William Harvey, also requires examination for influences, if not precedence; there have been statements in China in antiquity and, much later, the definitive demonstration of a separate pulmonary circulation by Ibn Nafiz, in West Asia in the 13th century[v]. The availability of that knowledge to workers like Cesalpino who later still followed with discovery of a venous circulation and the valves of veins are hardly referred to in Harvey's substantial discovery. The process of continuities to discovery, the knowledge that went before was likely to have been available to William Harvey before he stated the physiology of the Blood Circulation in the De Motu Cordis. Considering a period he spent in Italy, tutored by the eminent Fabricus, this may not be speculation. The period, 'the Dark Ages' of Europe was suggested in the backward look at history from a later period of her 'Enlightenment' and colonial dominance. The ravages of prolonged internecine wars, religious fratricide and devastating famine, the final collapse of the Crusades against the Saracen and the period of Moorish dominance over much of Mediterranean Europe, and then the cowering at the ceaseless thrust of the Ottoman to her East—those times were, indeed, bleak, but not 'dark' for the lack of intellectual lamps. Past the turbulence, seeping into Europe was the considerable knowledge from the East shaping her intellectual history. European history as a disciplinary exercise in the heyday of Europe's later world dominance had a distinct predilection for the readings slanted to her conquests and Power. To the European historian of those times it was not Europe's medieval crusades, her own barbaric incursions ostensibly to safeguard Christendom from the infidel, but Europe's Colonial might and mercantile gains that leave its mark on standard narratives. Rather than acknowledge the debts she owes to others for her knowledge base, narration stressed debility as the preferred condition in the history of pre-mediaeval Europe. Transmission of knowledge and accretion occurred before the Renaissance. If readings confine the history of Medicine and European science as merely extending from Europe's Greek forbears, it shows an insularity which obscures the immensity of the addition to that knowledge. Newer medical disciplines evolved form that contribution and influenced Renaissance medicine. *But its evolution from Greek sources was not in Europe but West Asia.* In antiquity the exchanges between Egypt and Greece, knowledge relating to mathematics and astronomy was transmitted from the former to the latter, and was barely acknowledged[vi]; but by around the 7th century CE much of the recorded knowledge in Greece itself was lost possibly following an Arab onslaught. However, the works from Hippocrates (460-451 BCE) to Galen (170-189 CE) were available for scholars in Rome, Alexandria and Constantinople. In Alexandria, that learning was sequestered having been subject to Roman aggression and internal turmoil. Knowledge also passed in antiquity between many civilisations in the further East, China and much of the therapeutic systems of India across to West Asia with considerable enhancement in the two way exchange. But it was the medieval Civilisation of Persia where medicine made the greatest progress and many qualitative improvements that flowered in related disciplines.

It was a Syrio-Arab community, the Nestorians, and their translations of ancient learning into Syriac, a derived language from the Aramaic that preserved and developed Greek knowledge in the centuries that followed. Greek knowledge had already been conveyed in Latin, and was available to the community at Alexandria. They rendered the Latin into Syriac, a language into which Latin translated with particular felicity. It was these scholars, who carried the knowledge of the Hellenes as they fled Alexandria from persecution and found refuge in Byzantium. Their patriarch Nestorius had founded his Church at Constantinople but his theological interpretations came into conflict with Rome and its Church. High theology, interpretations of the nature of Christ, a principle of the Roman Catholic Church was disputed and the result was the Edict of Ephesus which pronounced the patriarch and the community heretics; expulsions and migration followed, initially to Edessa in Syria. As exponents of a theological position which was suppressed they were bound to propagate their 'heresy' with missionary zeal and conveyed it far into the East, to India and China. There were theological consequences to Christianity in the East and to South Indian Christian denominations in particular but for this discussion the importance are the pursuits of Nestorians relating to medicine and its practice. These scholar missionaries had transmitted medical knowledge which had a bearing on the future development of medicine across the globe. Their incessant travail was the gain toward an universal future for medicine.

Again, after Edessa, the respite was brief and not until they had reached Persia around CE 500 where medical institutions were already flourishing, did they finally find a welcome and repose[vii]. The Sassinian dynasty's encouragement of these Syrian scholars helped bring in translation knowledge of the ancient medicine of Greece to Persian medicine. There were also remarkable conclaves and exchanges between physicians and scholars from Greece in the West and to the East, from India and China. It gained for Persian medicine universality in synthesis of their medical practices, later reworked to great sophistication and reaching a far wider civilisational space. Under Shapur I, 271 CE, an eminent ruler, Gundeshapur had already become an academic and medical power house with its ancient University, older than Bologna or the al-Azhar in Egypt. Syriac and Arabic scholarship flourished and the scholarship of the Nestorians, encouraged by Kobad a later Sassanian ruler, qualitatively improved medicine in the institutions for healing patients and teaching students. Much of their improved medical facilities were due to the work of their own renowned physicians but medical scholarship of Persia was with contributions from original Greek, Syriac and Arabic sources and recourse through extensive translations of Sanskrit medical texts and other sources into Pahlavi[viii]. We now know more of that medicine, but the extent of the influence of Islam on European culture and medicine is a comparatively neglected, though an increasingly investigated field. The various disciplines, including medicine, during this period of Persian renaissance are being explored, and the many Islamic libraries of Cairo, Damascus, Baghdad, and Suraj Kund near New Delhi, and also Spain's Escorial, should all be fruitful sources for investigations with particular reference to transmission and influences.

Post Renaissance European science is now accessible by application of an universal culture of mathematics, and medicine has developed within that science. But the new culture of medicine is indebted to the traditions founded in West Asia and later in the development of knowledge in regions under Islamic influence. It evolved from the ancient Greek, and in a pre-Renaissance history of the, often turbulent, relationship between Mediterranean Europe and West Asia. The extent of transmission into Europe was quite considerable from the civilisations of West Asia; to them and then into Mediterranean Europe, almost certainly, farther from China, through the Asiatic civilisations centred around Bactria. The extent of the two-way traffic, material and information, to and from these lands across the ancient Silk Road in antiquity, is as yet not entirely appreciated. The scientific revolution relegated traditional medical systems and past medical epistemologies as of little value, and then further demoted them in the more recent history of colonialism with its racial overtones. In that period the study and passage of knowledge in and from past civilisations were of little consequence, and even less were the therapeutic systems to medical history and its science. Deconstruction has reached history, while the general trend is for increased specialist interest in traditional therapeutics, but with hardly any reference to the continuities of exchange and their historical context.

Medical history implies more than just an acquaintance with names and a nod in the direction of singular discovery. The Industrial Revolution was an impulse for the progress of the sciences and, for medicine, the social context in the ensuing problems of rapid urbanisation and altered social conditions. Industrialisation changed social relationships and brought unprecedented pressures on society and living conditions. In the wake of the large migrations from the countryside came the new urban conglomerations built around the factories and their appalling physical conditions. Folk unable to change from the habits of village life, now found themselves in overcrowded, dismal, smog-hazed industrial and mining towns, living in unparalleled pollution of air, earth and water.

The energies of medical practitioner/scientists were stimulated by the need for a newer approach in science, and its innovative methods for finding evidence for ill health related to the environment. Discovery followed as the beginnings of the epidemiological sciences put in place important sanitary and public health measures from the evidence that cholera was a water-borne disease. The consequent and effective control of that disease commenced quite simply by ensuring a strict separation of sewage from drinking water supplies, *preventing contamination.* From there on continued the further and consistent discoveries of the bacterial aetiology of diseases or the vectors for the transmission of others. The great killer diseases in the West for centuries, small-pox, cholera and plague, soon became diseases of the past until they surfaced again later with a different connotation, a scourge of the Tropics. Pathological classification now included Tropical Medicine, its previous decimating endemicity in Temperate Europe forgotten. Medical Science had arrived in the colonies.

The new paradigm of hypothesis and experimental evidence was in place. While influencing previous systems of medical thought and practice the impetus was social and community health. Using the changing paradigms of the discipline, concerned scientist/physicians, found evidence for initiating public health measures for the control of epidemics. It was a revolution of medicine in science that owed much to the social context, a ferment of the Industrial Revolution and the new disciplinary methods of the natural sciences that established medicine in science.

Traditional therapeutics and access to Primary Health Care

The history of Medicine, besides discovery and its great names, is also of exchange, borrowing, transmission and reinterpretation of knowledge from many sources. Within those substantial contributions one can discern in today's science and medicine recognisable insights, its primacy hardly acknowledged. The recourse to a few of its offerings in the present approach to acupuncture is not an academic exercise but a perspective, a reinforcement of value of the heritage to modern therapeutic programmes. Programmes and projects hardly acknowledge the salience of traditional therapeutics in the formulation of health delivery systems. Yet they are a presence.

Looking beyond my own discipline at acupuncture, has necessarily to be from a point of view formed in the study of medicine in India; later in the different clinical routines of surgical and general practice in England and India, the sojourn in China, and, finally research in neurophysiology and Pain in Sweden. It offers a perspective of issues with a degree of familiarity but no claim to scholasticism, in separate cultural and social milieus, issues which are not merely restricted to establishing the validity of a therapeutic tradition. In many countries the use of traditional medicine is widespread. There is extensive dependence on them for primary health care rather than the esoteric alternative availed of for a developed world. The problems they pose are not just an issue of validity but of making the general public and practitioners aware of their possibilities, limitations and dangers within a more unified culture of medicine[5]. (Ch. IV)

---

5   The Role of Traditional and Alternative Health Systems
In Providing Health Care Options: Evidence from
Kerala

Deepa Sankar*
Health Policy Research Unit
Institute of Economic Growth
University Enclave
Delhi 110007, INDIA

Summary: In the context of growing interest and demand for traditional and alternative systems of medicines, this paper tries to understand the nature of the demand for these systems in the context of Kerala, South India where the traditional and alternative systems of medicines are preserved are institutionalised by the government and provided in large number by the private sector. Based on the utilisation of health services data collected through a primary survey in a district in the state, the analysis shows that the traditional and alternative systems of medicines are demanded and used according to the specificity of the need of the hour. *The analysis showed that people are not choosing the traditional or homeopathic systems as alternatives to modern medicines or as the last resort; rather, they have specific purpose for choosing them as patients distinguish certain systems of medicines as better suited for the treatment of specific diseases. It showed that systemslike Ayurveda and homeopathy*

Today, in a country like India, primary health care remains to a substantial degree with Traditional Medicine because there is insufficient institutional infrastructure for modern health delivery. The state of Kerala, (see footnote) is exceptional. In other States universal health care has not been achieved and health needs are served by various therapeutic cultures, state and private institutions for modern medicine and many forms of traditional therapeutics both authentic and questionable. The expenses for the most part are the responsibility of those in need. For the public the question of choice does not arise, due to their lack of education, deficiencies of infrastructure and inadequate trained manpower. The important question of scientific evidence for traditional therapy is not an administrative concern as it should be, especially when Traditional Medicine and innumerable 'other' practices using its epistemological terms are the only available health care for much of the populace. There is an economic drain due to improper or inadequate first line care and a strain on the services of secondary emergency and management centres. The wastage in economic terms would possibly be sufficient to initiate better supervised, collaborative efforts, including a basic medical educational discipline that exposes traditional practices to medical science. The needs are specified in the conclusions of many committees set up by a Central administration to examine health requirements of society. Basic medical education is thought to require an orientation to the context of society, but currently follows the norms laid out by a previous colonial administration over a century ago.

The most extensive use of traditional therapies remains in the lands of their origins where their disciplines are appreciated by the public as part of their culture, unlike the acceptance of Western societies. It possibly introduces another set of variables, patient responses dependent on their culture. Cultural appreciation of therapeutic rationale is an importance common to West and East. It is a support mechanism, the patient's hope for succour. In the West public interest in the esoteric is often without substantiating evidence or cultural affinity, but the Western public is increasingly uneasy with pharmaceuticals and aspects of modern medicine,

---

should be seen as 'complementary' rather than as 'alternative' to the modern medicines, indicating the need for integrating the different systems of medicines or collaboration and partnerships between systems of medicines for the better health care provision in the society. (my italics)

'Address for Correspondence

perceiving a remoteness and lack of empathy in medical personnel which affects patient/physician relationships. Complementary and Alternative Medicine in the context is an attraction because practitioners are accessible and communicative even if the explanations are not within a patient's cultural orientation.

Complementary and Alternative Medicine.

The Medical Establishment in Britain is aware of the gathering plethora of unconventional therapies and often, while looking askance at them for the lack of regulated evidence for its efficacy, acknowledges their increasing popularity. Thus, in an attempt at impartiality towards all therapeutic procedure on their scene it characterises all practices as Complementary and Alternative Medicine (CAM). It is non-committal, all-encompassing and non-discriminatory. But using the term side steps issues relating to public health and the need for informed definition to therapies that epistemologically are not of medical science.

High powered committees in Britain appointed to inquire into the role of these practices over the past few decades have generally grouped together under the umbrella of CAM a number of newer therapies without any link to the systematised disciplines of tradition. The distinctions in CAM say that some therapies 'complement' in reference to conventional medicine, while others presume to be complete therapies and hence 'alternative'. Traditional therapies may be, and often are, used as an alternative over a wide range of pathology. Their theories, however, formulate a pathology that is remote from the classification in medicine. Their pathological formulations have answers in traditional treatment and therapists, when they undertake to treat diabetes or tuberculosis, are a matter of grave concern since they do not understand the need to recourse the ancillary disciplines or biological parameters which are the norm not only to establish pathology but very essential to monitor the progress of these diseases. In present medical practice they are consistently used to determine medication, procedure, the relevant choice of therapy, and to assess the therapeutic response to illness. There is a need for better public information about the range of illness that CAM therapies may be used for. These therapies often feature in primary health care but limitations to CAM are ill defined. In the final analyses Medical Establishments and the Commissions of Inquiry offer only well intentioned advice when conceding public interest in the range of CAM therapies.

The disinclination to distinguish between the many therapies except broadly as CAM also shows a disinterest in the question of what would constitute traditional disciplines. Traditional Chinese Medicine (TCM), Ayurveda, Tibb or Unani (the last with its West Asian orientation) and a few others deserve recognition of their substantial development of empirical medical knowledge into Systems of Theory as compared to the numerous prevalent techniques of Healing presently on the scene. One reason why the CAM grouping is injudicious is that lack of definition withholds a possibility of informed choice for patients. In Britain, the Sixth Report of the The House of Lords, Session 1999-2000 on Science and Technology, was one of several Commissions of Inquiry instituted since 1986. While making considered contributions, they seemed unable to distinguish medical legacies, systems with a theoretical content sustained, at least in their cultures, from the later fly-by-night modes claiming therapeutic possibility. By any account one would even hesitate to group Homeopathy, constituted in an unsustainable empiricism along with Reflexology and Bach Flower Therapy. *In general the conclusions of the August Commissions of Inquiry are that beyond science lie the somewhat 'dusky' areas of clinical propositions which the practitioners of those therapies should as far as possible regulate by standardising methods of training and shedding light on its therapeutic value by research.*

A few CAM therapies based in variations of traditional theories, use metaphysical semantics without the empirical relevance to the theorising meant to sustain them. Others, like Osteopathy, are stated in the basic sciences of the day but are un-researched propositions. Ayurveda, Siddha. TCM and Unanni (Tibb) are undertakings that have come about through centuries of sustained evidence in empirical observation and study, have accumulated theories, sometimes stated with a striking inner logic and constructed in metaphysical reasoning. But today those certainties are certainly questionable in science. The functional effects of therapies can be unravelled in a way that only medical science can, but possibly not without a far greater appreciation of the systems of knowledge that have traditionally sustained their function. The routines and methodologies formulated for obtaining therapeutic evidence will not furnish evidence of worth unless adapted to the subject under investigation. Stated in metaphysical structure, acupuncture derives from the empirical, but traditional practice is within a complete system of theory.

Medical scientists, called to these inquiries, are unlikely to furnish evidence for these therapies. Most have opinions about CAM which, in the absence of evidence, reflect a scientist's point of view. Exponents of the therapies may themselves offer opinions about mechanisms and efficacies in their own terms, but incontrovertible scientific evidence for the therapies that feature in CAM are scanty. An establishment assuming responsibility and offering information about CAM must undertake to inform the public about their respective utility, and that requires a direction towards collaborative efforts in research. Some stable evidence for acupuncture is increasingly available in research from Europe and from China, while China and Japan, the source and home of certain traditional therapies that featured in these Inquiries are processing them in many ways. In India and China there are medical schools teaching their respective medical traditions, but China also has collaborative research centres inquiring into their Traditions. Going beyond national confines for the illumination of some CAM therapies may better serve the respective contexts of their use. It is the continuity with previous collaboration and the transmission of medical tradition envisioned in the context of Science that makes a globalised enterprise possible. The World Health Organisation is moving in that direction.

In the considerable but confounded information available there is the shrouded definition to CAM which the Cochrane Collaboration proposes as a generalisation. The suggestion is that many therapeutic propositions are available beyond the conventional medicine of the dominant culture. But past all the deliberations and 'Inquiries' the implication is that they do not quite demonstrate effective evidential mechanisms or biological responses of validity on patients following investigations.

Hazards for patient and the practitioner

Commissions of inquiry in recommending regulation on the subject of CAM, acknowledge a Medicine which is in practice beyond the pale of Science and operating in the public domain. (Ref. BMA Inquiry, 1983, 1986 and of the House of Lords). Scientific medicine and its practice is supervised under strict institutional regulation and its practitioners are registered to respective medical councils by constant monitoring of the systems of education. The General Medical Councils in Britain have certain statutory powers over their registered doctors, their practices and the institutions they work in. Many countries follow some form of statutory control over the delivery of health care, requiring registration of its personnel. However, the lack of appropriate and considered regulation over practitioners of CAM and the lack of distinction between traditional and other therapies do pose public health hazards. Practitioners of CAM have harmed patients, but so have physicians of modern medical practice who resort, for example, to untrained use of acupuncture insertions in seeking therapeutic effect (Ch. IV). It brings to the fore the question of legal liability, presently a hazy area. Practitioners of modern medicine have qualifications and their registration entitles them to the protection of the laws of medical jurisprudence; but can that protection extend to an untrained practice of a traditional therapeutic procedure? The practitioners of traditional therapeutics generally have no qualifications which entitle them to statutory recognition. In the event of mishaps to patients are they liable under civil laws of criminality? The registered practitioner of medicine has recourse to representation, protection and costs through their Medical Councils. In Britain a distinction must be drawn between the many medically qualified practitioners who practice acupuncture and those therapists who practice traditional therapeutics including acupuncture but do not possess any recognised qualification. The legal position of practitioners of CAM has to be addressed. CAM, as a general health utility requires its training procedures to be evaluated, qualifications scrutinised and its members licensed to practice Disability and worse may occasionally result from the use of any therapy. To the patient it is immaterial whether it occurs in modern practices or from CAM, but appropriate forums for inquiry should be constituted to sustain a legal practice for any valid system that is recognised as providing health care.

If that is understood, therapeutic knowledge may not be misinterpreted, or at least its function not diminished or discounted just because it was used in another culture within an epistemology not of modern science. At present we miss out on the background for therapies, discovered in past empirical utility which had provided benefit for patients. Whether of a former millennium or today, human biology, its mechanisms and behavioural responses are unlikely to have altered substantially, and a patient will valorise a procedure like acupuncture in roughly similar terms despite the intervening millennia, the varying cultures and minor difference to expectations from treatment that is brought about. Whether these statements are accepted or not, a therapeutic past could be acknowledged without veneration and its continuity of use for many populations of the world suggests that medical science is obliged to take greater note of that utility than is presently seen in its more convenient accommodations as CAM.

The Scandinavian experience to the promotion of acupuncture

Since the 17th century there has been a limited awareness of acupuncture in Europe through early Dutch Colonial contacts and the surgeons of their trading Company in Java. In the West interest was maintained by physicians who had stayed in Far Eastern enclaves and were curious about their therapies. However, it was the more drastic counter-irritation methods like cauterisation that found general favour amongst physicians well into the 20th century in Europe.

Nixon's historical visit in 1971 to China is a comparatively recent political event, demonstrating a thaw in their relations. Increased interest in acupuncture, especially in the USA and Scandinavia, followed. The fortuitous experience of an accompanying journalist who had an emergency appendicectomy and was treated with acupuncture for post-operative pain made for an enthusiastic journalistic account followed by rather disproportionate media interest[ix]. The considerable reportage on acupuncture with an exaggerated enthusiasm for what the Chinese were doing was naturally of interest to the public. In general the scientific community had not till then been enthused by acupuncture although it was a practice amongst the Far Eastern communities in many countries. The subject has since taken off as worthy of investigation.

Interest in Scandinavia was confined to a few Pain scientists and physicians in the early nineteen eighties. Basic experimental research and clinical studies in treating certain patient categories were encouraging and meanwhile the World Health Organisations recommended acupuncture for those in chronic pain. With that support on board a few of these scientists, with typical Swedish flair for organisation, obtained the support of the Socialstyrelsen (Medical Council) and set about the education and the trained practice of acupuncture for pain. Courses were designed for personnel in medicine, dentistry and rehabilitative ancillary disciplines, while simultaneously embarking on programmes for basic research and clinical trials at selected centres. It was a comprehensive approach to teaching the subject and training medical personnel, with local councils supporting the programmes for the accredited use of acupuncture. A trend was set, which was a matter of immense social importance in the field of health care, for introducing a traditional therapy into a modern system of health care.

Much basic work on pathophysiological pain was in progress in the Departments of the Karolinska Institute and Hospital, and by separate groups at the Universities of Gothenburg and Lund. A project for teaching a method for its Socialstyrelsen-recognised practice in that country was unhesitatingly promoted. The outcome may be another hybrid acupuncture practice, but patients have already benefited from its practice by a large number of trained ancillary medical staff. The science of Peripheral Sensory Stimulation (PSS) was the essential focus to the teaching, while Chinese precepts were not ignored. For example, traditional acupuncture points and meridians were used, while the points' location stressed their local morphology in surface anatomy, nerve and blood supply, the tissues penetrated or those in the vicinity, the indicators of likely hazards if the strict rules of Chinese measurements and penetration depths were not adhered to. Point location was stressed and localised in TCM's unique modular methods of measurement.

Lectures in the syllabus focussed on the physiology and molecular biology of PSS, but the practical sessions and clinical practice on patients, a major part of the courses, stressed some of the empirical insights of tradition. It was impressed on students that outcomes depended on varying stimulation techniques and an appreciation of individual clinical presentation of patient problems even within a single diagnostic category. In clinical practice and patient problems a few precepts of TCM were invaluable; point location, their effective combinations and the merit of varying stimulation techniques or procedure to clinical findings for particular patient problems, even restricted to pain and at each attendance. Many precepts I learnt at the Chinese hospital clinic from the vast experience of a traditionalist Teacher, a supreme empiricist in the clinic, and from teaching courses in the UK were invaluable for the teaching and safety of a clinical practice of acupuncture.

I am aware that the perspective of Swedish teaching can be criticised within the advocacy of rephrasing and abbreviating this ancient therapy with its massive theory. But in such rephrasing and transcribing of a sophisticated traditional therapeutic procedure we may begin to find answers to 'how acupuncture works' and attempt innovative improvements for a modern society. Greater empathy with methods of a medical tradition transcribed whenever possible to science has been the Swedish Teaching advocacy. The nuances and a better definition to the variety of its usage may provide an understanding of acupuncture in the present culture of medicine.

Traditional therapeutics and Science

To make something new out of knowledge from the past is to recover its history and develop its value. Acupuncture is a continuing practice within a therapeutic knowledge system and functions stated for its practice could be investigated in clinical studies. They require interpretation in medical science. Past the weavings of theory, much of the traditional practice of acupuncture is empirical: apparent in the therapist's acumen for observing patients, and his experience in using its functions is a message as to how steeped the practice is in empiricism which carries to any clinician. The evidence of utility was a gradual accretion over time, stated in a structure of knowledge. Some of its functions may reinterpret in the disciplinary principles of scientific medical practice.

A traditional Chinese medical concept is exemplified in the conduits or meridians of acupuncture drawn up from the idea of a circulation of energy the 'ching lo'. Blood in circulation, however, was conducted through separate channels of the *'ching mo'* systems. The evidence for a blood circulation was arrived at by traditional methods, but from which a definite calculation of a circulatory time was possible. That time calculated at 28.8 minutes for a complete revolution was mistaken but closer to the present reality of a circulation time than the 'even a day' as a possibility in the epochal record by William Harvey in his De Motu Cordis experiments[6]. Chinese experimentation methods were not explicit and lacked the quality of science, for example an essential of experimental work is its replicability which was possible in Harvey's methods. Although morphological attributes have not been forthcoming for the configuration of meridians, the *'ching lo'* conduits for 'energy' were drawn up from the primary empirical observations of effect following stimulation of groups of

---

[6]   Celestial Lancets. p 32. Full reference in endnote[1].

localised points and grafted on to metaphysical pegs in an elaborate theory of parallel circulatory system. The theory stressed that 'points' situated along specific conduits transporting energy when needled correctly affected the circulation of blood to correct pathological syndromes. Syndromes amongst others diagnosed by pulse readings.

The classical observation then is the empirical discovery of function, of the many hundreds of foramina (hsüeh), their very precise locations described on the body surface; in facile translation, the 'points' of acupuncture. Their functional utility, noted over centuries, grouped them into twelve conduits or Meridians. Meridians possibly followed nominal patterns of the familiar, much as Chinese interest in the skies joined stellar groups as recognisable constellations, and twelve fitted the theoretical systematisation. They extend the logic of Yin and Yang groups, with six named after hollow (Yin) organs, the urinary bladder for instance, and six after solid (Yang) organs, for example, the liver. Whether or not the meridians or the conduits are as functional as the 'points' are, they do in a few instances conform to the 'patterns' that later medical science demarcated for sensory nerves on the body surface, especially over the head and neck. So far the exercises by experimental methods to clarify the existence of meridians as morphological structures have been, not surprisingly, unsuccessful.

The functional effects of point stimulation, however, are in parts distinctly recognisable in the sketch of dermatomes, the surface markings of areas served by cutaneous afferents of spinal nerves. Stimulation effects of acupuncture points predate anatomical dermatomes by centuries, possibly millennia. Neurology and models of neural anatomy, unknown to metaphysics yet the patterns of dermatomes, convey a functional physiology now apparent in some meridians of acupuncture as, for example, the meridians of the Urinary and Gall Bladder. *Stimulation of points localised on them elicit biological responses, both somatic and reflex autonomic, on myotomes and sclerotomes (those human tissues and organs innervated from spinal nerves in their embryonic mesodermal origins).* That functionality of a 'point' where an apparent conformity of meridians and dermatomes is seen, is contained in the Chinese name of the organ which notably is of that sclerotome. Thus that localised laterally in the paraspinal muscles, at the level of thoracic spinuous process 5, is called Xinshu. Xin, for the heart, has its Back Shu point, Bladder 15. Or, again, Shenshu, Bladder 23, is localised at the level of lumbar 2 spine; Shen being the Chinese organ of the kidney.

The empirical character of the meridian is more apparent when the points along it are related to innervation and blood supply of the skin and tissues penetrated[x]. Stimulation effects relate closely to that relationship. A note of caution to organ correlations is that in TCM a Chinese organ does not convey as an anatomical structure.

But, with reservations, meridian configuration is drawn to a diagrammatic precision as much as the markings of Kellgren, Head and Sherrington in their dermatome maps. The latter have experimental evidence, and yet, dermatomes offering the degree of precise demarcations that they do, are a diagrammatic exaggeration. There is always considerable overlap and individual variation to sensory patterns of innervation by spinal nerves. Surface stimulation confirms it. The maps serve in many respects as useful guidelines for the clinician even as meridians and point localisation do, and even more as the surface landmarks for stimulation that an acupuncturist would invariably use. (**Ch. III** where details and figures of meridians and dermatomes are offered).

Acupuncture and Pain (Ch. V & VI)

The concept of Pain, growing into a multidisciplinary Science, was the spur for acupuncture's acceptance, particularly in Sweden. The epochal statements on mechanisms that contribute to pain, elaborated upon in papers by Melzack and Wall[xi], emphasised interactions between somatosensory afferent impulses and the inhibition of pain, and also pain inhibition as an inbuilt feature of neural sensory function. Melzack and Wall suggested that stimulation at peripheral sites that activated the specialised receptors and their neurons conveying sensations of touch, warmth, cold or pain to dorsal horn cells of the spinal cord, could block pain impulses from other sources as they reached those spinal cord cells. Later work has emphasised a nociceptive modulatory system separate from the interactions of different somatosensory afferents. That modulatory system may be activated at discrete levels of the midbrain to inhibit pain. Much of the substantiation for understanding pain inhibition in man is extrapolated from experimental studies. They have a direct bearing on acupuncture mechanisms.

Previous work on patients had demonstrated that maladaptive manifestations of pain may be conveyed along sensory pathways not necessarily earmarked for pain. Much useless and sometimes harmful surgery was based on the idea that the sensation of pain was conveyed by unique neural pathways. Such Cartesian simplification of pain conveyance was expressed even up to 1958. "Knowledge concerning the primary sensory systems is well established and a part of neurological orthodoxy. Each of these systems, from specific receptor through laterally situated lemniscal pathways to localised cortical receiving zone, is sensitive to a *single* (my italics) modality of sensation" (French, as quoted on p 173, next ref.). It led surgeons to the excision of painful neuromas to commence with, then going further to amputations. These brought more suffering, including 'phantom' pains. But surgeons, sometimes in unwarranted assurance, instead of taking a second look at the neurophysiology, were undeterred and went on to the higher reaches of the 'pathway to pain'— surgical section at spinal cord levels for the continuing and intractable pain of patients. The cure for pain was not to be found in an enunciated theory and the self-assurance of surgeons eager to undertake cures based on them. Critical reconsideration by others[xii] was seen in the crucial possibility that there were other neural pathways rather than a dedicated one for the transmission of a unique sensation, and these could continue to transmit pain impulses to central levels from the periphery. The major impact of the work of the many pioneers working on clinical pain and basic research was to widely disseminate the enterprise of a Pain Science amongst surgical and medical disciplines from the middle decades of the previous century, and basic research led to discoveries in the neurophysiology of pain and information to the morphology of nociceptive pathways. The previous simplicities were replaced by the unfolding complexity to the experience of mammalian and human pain (Ch. VI).

The thinking that pain is only a symptom of disease has substantially changed within decades. Pain has its own pathology attributable to the somatosensory system, chronic pain in particular has a plethora of pathophysiology which may progressively involve the autonomic nervous system but which has broader neurophysiological qualities of differentiation (see below). Following trauma or disease, pain can be maintained by maladaptation of the entire sensory system or by dysfunctional peripheral nerves. Certain intractable types of pain involve the sympathetic component of the autonomic system. These are known comprehensively as Complex Regional Pain Syndromes (CRPS), but the syndromes themselves have differing symptomatic manifestations amongst patients. Surgical and orthopaedic specialities should acquaint themselves with CRPS problems. For the surgeon it should be a reminder of the eagerness for surgical answers derived from unreliable basic science. The present shift is to the use of bio-mechanical applications. Replacement of arthritic joints by prosthesis is too eagerly practiced, although a specific patient problem should be the indication for prosthetic replacement. A traditional adherence to nonsurgical rehabilitative measures, with the possibility of using bio-mechanical appliances if and when these fail, allows the patient, by alternatives to management and less invasive forms of surgery, to retain the joint. Ablation is not merely the loss of function of an organ for mobility but as in amputations, when resecting a joint there is total loss of the neurones and peripheral neural connectivity, into the cortical field.

The context of market promotion has infiltrated the long standing problem of degenerative joints with ready answers of prosthetic replacement, and the surgeon ignores patient assessments in his clinical acumen. Corporates play a great role in their extensive promotions. The benefits of early replacement are immediately apparent and the procedure deemed a success by the surgeon. Unfortunately patients do turn up in Pain Clinics long after the surgical 'success'. Surgical specialties need to be specially aware of iatrogenic pain and its early recognition in long term follow-ups to prevent it[xiii]. However, one must keep in mind the immense benefits, from dedicated outfits of prosthetic improvements and by their use the enhancement to the quality of life following the mutilation of war, and from landmines causing civilian casualties.

The mechanisms underlying endogenous pain inhibition (Ch. V) by acupuncture, as research has so far unravelled them, suggests the basis for acupuncture for the treatment of pain. The neurophysiology of Pain is then discussed (Ch. VI) towards a further understanding of acupuncture and possibly some traditional theory in biological principles and practice. Acupuncture is possibly most widely used today on patients with chronic musculo-skeletal pain. The investigation of its claims is attempted in a stipulated methodology for finding evidence of therapeutic efficacy. From psychiatry to surgical intervention, through to physical therapies including acupuncture or the use of drugs, the evidence will not invariably be found or be reliable in routine RCT requirements. Considerable adaptations to methodology are required for acupuncture, and hands-on procedures to obtain the evidence for their efficacy. That endeavour on patients in pain resulted in six sequential studies (**Ch. VII**). The problem of responses to acupuncture while treating clinical pain must also be considered in the possible differentiation of pain. Some pioneer studies[xiv] had established basic differentiation between neuropathic, nociceptive and idiopathic in clinical pain pathology which appears to have a bearing on response to morphine and with acupuncture as well. The subject though controversial is from clinical trials not without evidential merit[xv].

Placebos and the Conditioned Response

We can see a trait in animals to an environmental threat which extends to human biology, where response mechanisms are generated to reduce pain or obviate its perception. For the animal it is an aid to survival either for 'flight' or 'fight' are only possible if pain, which normally enforces rest in order to heal, is reduced or held in abeyance. The factors that reinforce that response in the animal are those of attention, anxiety and fear. An imminent threat can sometimes be countered in the exaggeration of 'playing dead' as the animal can reduce both normal metabolic parameters and pain perception. This is a conditioned response, an evolutionary trait for species survival but a significant extension for humans in pain. Attention, anxiety, anticipation or expectation and distraction are cognitive factors which can alter, and usually reduce, the quality of human pain

In the context of prehistoric society, the response is availed of by those endowed with special powers within a culture. The rituals of magic, incantations, sacrifice etc. are the models used for the tribal subject to focus his anxiety and attention on. Conditioned responses to these model types have a long history referred way back to tribal beginnings, of healing or assuaging human ailments and reducing pain. The characteristic differences of tribal cultures impress a cultural mark on the individual in their totems and taboos. The interventionists who dealt with ailments in tribal societies used their knowledge often for therapeutic intent. Acute forms of dementia also manifest where strongly embedded belief systems regulate societies and the transgression of stern regulations may provoke intense guilt, fantasies and aberrant behaviour; the agency of a priest or a praying group may restore the afflicted person to normal. On occasion, the invocation could destroy a subject if, by ignoring taboos, he had caused or was presumed to have caused damage to the tribe. It was an early recognition of a power to manipulate the inherent traits of human beings as they became organised in definitive social culture.

The interaction between the therapist and patient has these historical continuities as differences in culture and its changing models of therapy, whether anthropomorphic, religious or scientific, extend the conditioned response of the patient toward therapeutic relief. The response supplements treatment in a specific context, from ancient herbal remedies, like the liverwort of a Paracelsian age, to the present use of pharmaceuticals, elective surgery, rehabilitation procedures or mere communication and counselling. Placebo is the generic term for the response in the present therapeutic and psychosocial culture: an inherited biological trait and, in the present cultural environment, an appropriately modified response. In prehistory the response was available through the intercession of an elder with the tribe's totem. In clinical research the placebo response in a control group of patients is meant to evaluate the effects on the patient group who receive the true ingredient of therapy. It has the connotation of an artefact as posed against genuine therapeutic value. The Placebo-controlled clinical trial denotes reliability to the evidence and acts as a regulation to the development of therapeutic products. The placebo has demonstrated its own neurobiological effectiveness for the patients, especially in pain and other pathological entities. Reliance on the placebo response for incontrovertible evidence of therapeutic efficiency, the sole attribution to the impact of a substance or a therapeutic mode tested against that control, has not been achieved[xvi].

With acupuncture and other therapies intensely dependent on agent mediation, the effect on the patient is not derived from a singular input. It is a misconception to consider the needle in tissue, the peripheral sensory stimulus, as *the* therapeutic ingredient. The pursuit over decades for a plausible placebo for acupuncture suggests an adherence by investigators to a paradigm of study rather than an exploration of the many possible factors that constitute its therapeutics. The method of investigating evidences of true drug potency created the trial methods, the placebo control reduced innumerable other variables to confirm that evidence. Finding evidence for effectiveness of therapies with a variety of inputs compared to drugs, must account for the comprehensive nature of those therapies. In other words, a procedure with multiple environmental inputs may each produce putative therapeutic effects and an additional placebo component to each. The therapist, his methods of manipulating needles, varying stimulation intensities, positions and depth of needle insertions, his communication with the patient while eliciting his reaction to the manipulation and his appreciation when deemed satisfactory; all these do not exhaust the totality of Acupuncture as a therapeutic procedure. The techniques are never quite the same from one therapist to the next and ideally they should be varied to the patient and according the TCM diagnosis on that individual. Investigation for evidence of such therapy cannot be reduced to protocols where 'blinding' asserts quality to the trial and 'placebos' for the needle believed to enhance that quality. Nor can outcome to treatment ignore the natural history of a patient complaint, or its regression to the mean in the progression of investigation. The importance of the inserted needle's effect is a major contribution, but does not constitute the sole content of the patient responses to acupuncture therapy.

The placebo, for determining therapeutic efficiency is science only in that it is a part of a paradigm, but if it is an imperative, a doctrinal entrenchment amounting to a certainty; it may hamper the progress we seek[xvii]. We cannot claim to have found, in the protocols for study of 'hands-on' therapies, sufficient evaluative certainty in the uncertain placebos designed for their study. Acupuncture cannot be defined merely as the sensory stimulus from a needle insertion. If that were so, the many 'sham' needle insertions in innumerable clinical studies, hitherto accepted as placebo, were in fact not the placebo for acupuncture but yet another form of acupuncture. The modes of acupuncture in clinical use have many regulations and specific requirements to stimulation. Some specific modes in use are mentioned within the text.

From records of the many clinical trials that are available, Acupuncture obtains another definition. The placebo defines it as sensory stimulation since an 'inert' needle may finally be available (Streitbeger). The history of that hunt for inertness in other areas of peripheral stimulation such as Transcutaneous Electrical Nerve Stimulation (TENS) began with bizarre study designs and the evidence derived must be dubious. Even the patient's perception of response contains uncertainties of subjectivity, memory and expectation. A volunteer patient to controlled trials of hands-on therapies within its informative setting has further strains placed on him in respect of the information required; his discernment of an experience of pain, for example, is a variable subjective determination and its cognition is certainly influenced by his culture. The trial circumstance is unreal to the extent that it is not the situation of the patient attending the clinic.

A possible Determinant of Variable Response

The question of patient responses to a placebo has been under critical review for a while[xviii] and criticism of it was sustained in recent experimental and narrative evidence[xix]. The placebo is further discussed as a part of the history of inhibiting pain in man. Evaluations of its use as a control must take into account the variety of human responses to pain. Chapter VIII offers an explanation of the mechanisms in the sensory system which imposes this variety to pain response amongst individuals, discussed as a possible function of the Mas Related Genes (MRG) and their properties. The features of Positive Selection Genes, which create novel receptor-ligand interactions result in *rapidly* alterable nociceptive properties and are available for some mammalian species, including the human. MRG is expressed at extracellular neuronal sites involved only with pain transmission their specific tissue affinities, differing from the more widely expressed genes of the opioid system. MRGs offer rapid diversity to nociceptive responses. That rapid amplification to pain response in evolution is invaluable for species exposed to environmental change and, for man, the changes and threats being ever present and cognisable, even though the comparatively short time span of his evolution, makes for a variable amplification to response. It allows individual diversity in the experience of pain within further cultural determinants; traits offering diversity are invaluable to species survival[xx].

Paradigms and the Problems of Acupuncture Research

Evidence is a scientific necessity for assessing therapeutic efficacy. The curative claims for acupuncture and other Traditions in Medicine are stated without that quality of evidence.

Experimental validation of therapeutic efficacy is a facet of the problem. With acupuncture it is substantially affected today within a range of high to poor quality clinical studies with protocols which usually attempt the methods for validating pharmaceuticals. Invariably a high value is attributed to very questionable placebo controls, especially those in a few meta-analytical studies. Conclusions reached by them go on to suggest acupuncture to be not more effective than its placebo. To extend methods of blinding and placebo controls may not be the definitive way to arrive at evidence for patient response to therapeutic procedures like acupuncture where hands have the skill for therapeutic effect or to communicate non-specific effects in the overall setting of treatment: or even to a modern discipline like psychiatry (Ch. I).

A paradigm constructed for a specific issue in science to establish evidence of the therapeutic value for drugs and pharmaceuticals, products that were developed in the pharmacological sciences, is now in general use and extended to the establishing of evidence of therapeutic value for the practices of acupuncture based in Chinese medicine of a previous age. That there is as yet only an uneasy resolution of the problem is not surprising[xxi]. Clinical studies sustained in that paradigm necessarily minimise variables in the protocol, which means attempting the reductive analyses of a traditional therapy whose theoretical system is a rationalisation of inductive principles to arrive at diagnosis in the *individual* patient. Although unaware of biology the epistemological rationalisation of TCM recognised the individual and his responses in the variety of natural states. Classical diagnosis relates to the individual which in turn determines the process of therapy, variations to the way the needle is handled, point selections, intensities of stimulation etc. The methods of clinical trials, on the other hand, are designed to obtain evidence by reducing complexity; categorised patient cohorts, standard treatment protocols and often, in the case of acupuncture, stipulations to needle use when the protocol demands that points for insertion of the needle are uniform which as acupuncture treatment would be an absurdity in the clinic. Further stipulations of minimum communication with the patient by interventionists or the assessor, and the latter blinded as to whether patients are in the treatment group or its control, and so on, are remote from the clinical reality of acupuncture. With acupuncture treatment for patients in pain, their variable responses are again reduced to simplified scales of measurement for ease of data gathering.

Protocols satisfy the paradigm designed for particular problem-solutions. The double blind, placebo controlled study was designed for evidence of therapeutic efficacy and safety, basically to allow the regulation by a Health Authority for *patents* sought for pharmacological products. Pharmaceutical agents have a dose-related therapeutic input and are presumed to have an endpoint to their site of action. Acupuncture is not a comparable therapeutic function, and its clinical practices need accommodation in protocols designed to investigate it. The issue of efficacy is not solved if acupuncture as a practice is constrained to satisfy the paradigm for another problem. Investigators require to reformulate hypotheses considering the clinical practices of the system of acupuncture, and attempt the appropriate paradigm to address them.

The best treatment practice of acupuncture, its clinical reality, is necessarily a point selection and stimulation technique tailored for the individual and her/his diagnosis and, further, dependent on the natural history and progress of an ailment with assessments made by examination at each session of treatment. Study protocols must convey the naturalism of the clinic as much as possible. References to a few published studies are made in a later chapter where some adaptation was attempted to correlate with a few epistemic concepts to treatment (Ch. VII). The studies were conducted on well recognised clinical conditions of Pain but they do not, in the numbers, scale or variable use to needle techniques, relate to the procedures of the clinic—even the attempted adaptation to the principle of naturalistic paradigms had not been achieved.

Patient populations of the clinic can be assessed individually for respective diagnoses, but categorised further, for example for disability, deformity or other signs. Responses to any form of treatment on those categories then offer a measured outcome. The controls should be found amongst the patient population attending the clinic. The therapist, whether acupuncturist or physician, should maintain his clinical routine, make decisions about the nature of treatment, as the clinic would, in the best interest of the patient. The assessments on patients are made by separate medical personnel, unaware of treatment details or locale. Within such an approach reductive analyses and controls are not ignored but the inductive principles of treatment could be retained. The paradigm is naturalistic to an extent that allows the therapist unrestricted function in his/her clinical routine. However, the study is feasible only if institutions organise extensive collaborations to provide large patient populations over long periods of time. The concept illustrates a possible paradigm change for investigating acupuncture and does not presume to be a novel proposition. It is not definitive, and to commence with will not provide robust results. A trial run in a changed paradigm for maintaining naturalism to research would serve as the base from which other hypotheses could be formulated for specific evidence.

Evidence may also be forthcoming in basic experimental work. Sophisticated experimental techniques offer substantial evidence of systemic effects. A notable series of studies suggests a mechanism in pain inhibition using stimuli at painful intensities—Diffuse Noxious Inhibitory Control (DNIC)[xxii]. This was a well demonstrated confirmation of a noxious stimulus inhibiting pain in animals. Acupuncture technique employs painful stimuli for certain TCM diagnoses. Needling of human periosteal tissues can elicit intense pain and used momentarily is clinical practice for a variety of pathology beyond and including pain (see Chapter by Dickenson, within next ref. and Ch. VI study). Even here, to be effective in patients, technique is an absolute requirement for therapy which develops in a practitioner's clinical acumen[xxiii].

Chinese Acupuncture arrived on the therapeutic scene a couple of millennia ago and science only a couple of centuries ago, but although many more forms of acupuncture treatment are in the public/patient/ physician domain, yet after decades of clinical research they are not deemed to have quite answered the question of efficacy in the evidence. My contention is that its pursuit is not related to the subject of acupuncture but of a model of acupuncture constructed to answer to the paradigm. This monograph is not a promotion for a traditional treatment mode. It is not required. Millions across vast swathes of the world, living in conditions of comparative economic deprivation, access health needs mostly through traditional therapies[xxiv].

Traditional Practice, Social Medicine. Caring and healing or commerce and cures.

Traditional Therapies (defined as systematic formulations), on their own cannot be posed as an answer to the needs of modern health care. However they do function in the sphere of health care amongst populations of many countries of the world who access these therapies for different reasons. While their therapists function largely in the private sector they do not have the same potential for profit or power as wielded by corporate enterprises in the field of Health. These maintain a high profile as the cutting edge of progress in medicine, and Private Institutions consider individual health or societal Health Care as they would any commercial product, subject to the regulations of the market and a commodity for managing financial gains. Institutions with that background provide the immense attraction of better remuneration for trained personnel, therapists and others, obvious in the far greater numbers that now serve a Private Health Sector. Physicians once fulfilled a social role, caring for while attempting to heal, those in ill-health; and while catering to the particular needs of an illness they were aware of family circumstances and so on. The larger question is not how worthwhile is the social role of medical personnel; it is largely dependent on the organisation of Health Care in a country. That was evident in recent decades when organised for the Welfare State, with Universal Health Care as an entitlement for its people. Within a decade of its institution the health of national populations reflected in health indices showed steep improvements and, importantly, the insecurities of ill-health no longer haunted the innumerable families of the working classes.

Trained manpower and skills are vital for any modern society to provide primary to tertiary levels of Health Care. They are established by government Health Authorities or by an increasingly visible private sector. In some countries, and India is an example, state of the art institutions exist, but access to them is uneven and dependent on social determinants; there is extreme unevenness to regional development and highly variable empowerment of populations, dependent on social hierarchies, financial and educational factors. For many the consequence is the meagre availability of health aid which partly explains why traditional systems of medicine and treatment modes with spurious links to the traditional are still widespread health supports. Yet traditional systems still have a hold on the upper classes also, even amongst doctors and scientists who will use them in acceptance of their metaphysical explanations. The well-to-do and an increasing tourist clientele subscribe to expensive private institutions which provide traditional techniques of meditation, and therapeutic rehabilitation, an ephemeral but subjectively satisfying process of 'rejuvenation'. Private Clinics engaged in the Traditional do not provide cheap or necessarily safe techniques of rehabilitation, but a cultural orientation and beliefs systems are strong determinants to choice in societies where science is a limited appreciation and tradition has its pronounced niche.

The culture of medicine is a continuum of values and principles derived from its social past into the medical practices of the day. Past tenets in the practice of medicine, either the unwritten codes or institutional regulation have, for society, instilled confidence in its function and in its practitioners. However, regulations may be breached in areas of scientific medicine, and the erosion of public confidence is notable as the ethos of practice changes. The increasing popularity of traditional therapeutics and the traditional practitioner, East or West, can partly be accounted for by the fact that they continue the heritage of a prestigious social asset in which their special knowledge and intuition constituted not just the physician's skills for healing, but their counsel and practical ways of sympathising with the families in trouble continued a tradition of being part of the fabric of the community.

Today that visibility of the physician is depicted more in its contrast. Corporate enterprise increasingly partners institutional medicine, affecting its science and practice. The values, unsurprisingly, seep into non-transparent remunerative arrangements between physician and the ancillary clinics which provide investigative support. There are obvious drawbacks to solutions that draw profit-oriented private enterprise into the universal entitlement for providing the means to health for society. It is certainly the reason for the routine, but often unnecessary, adherence to medical investigations for problems that could be decided entirely by the physician's examination. The traditional practitioner could be expensive but not of the order incurred in the routine patient attendance to a doctor's clinic in the private sector with their 'best practice' routines, the safeguard against litigation. Financial and political power is vested with powerful pharmaceutical and bio-technical industries. They promote medical advancement, but Corporate values are essentially profit motivated, and societal need provides just another way to realise it. Research has repeatedly been controverted to those ends. Association with industry and the enticements offered for marketing bio-technology and drugs are all too well known. Often newer drug formulations are not even relevant but still reach a market only to be withdrawn later, despite the fact that the drugs are in the market based on evidence of their efficacy. Debates are on and some regulations for research workers in place but much more is overdue. The public is becoming wary of medicine and the practitioner where their ethos is competitive free enterprise.

Recent debates in the U.S.A. to empower an administration seeking to provide universal health cover for its citizens demonstrated the range of vested interests, their liegemen in political power aligned to an industry in the business of medicine and public health; private insurance complexes have to be borne piggy-back on the State Exchequer if health care is to be a social right. The contradictions are glaringly apparent when health care, as a public need, is pitted against the possible dilution of the principles of Free Enterprise and Corporate power, and even a compromise involves formidable costs to implement universalised health care in the United States. A medical fraternity cannot be absolved of the need to pursue certain timeless philosophical precepts, the values for social ends, even as it moves away from the metaphysical limitations of its traditions towards the expanding horizon of medicine as a social science. Its professionals have demonstrated little hesitation in converting the temple of science into a marketplace.

There is this looming threat to the occupation of 'doctory' marked in the shift of creeds once expressed in the positivism of Auguste Comte in the 19th century for the social sciences. The well-being of society was to be in the hands of its responsible citizens. These were medical practitioners, technologists and managers, the new 'priests'; the former catering to the needs of the sick and ailing and the latter in their respective areas of social function. These were altruistic principles and they had posed selflessness for early industrial societies, but these had signally failed to achieve them. The guidelines served a world transformed to principles of scientific socialism riding high in Britain and the post-war world. A health welfare system forced the older altruism into place in the National Health Service (NHS) and its democratic vision was proved as a science in the outcome[xxv]. At the outset implemented against a very determined, almost general, opposition from the medical fraternity, these are now the guardians against the erosion of its principles. Apart from its immediate importance in universal health cover for a British public it served as the harbinger of the many models of socialised health amongst other nations. Today the concept which served Britain so well is still substantially in place despite rising costs and policies veering toward privatised medicine.

As yet nothing other than Health services with an universalised reach, with supportive non-profit organisations for drugs and medication regulated by the state, and government institutions for health care integrating traditional and modern therapeutics for primary care and expensive tertiary health care procedures, have brought tremendous improvements to the health indices of any society. European societies have achieved such care, and China along with a couple of South American nations are pointing the way for the rest. Individuals and families are more secure in the knowledge that illness will not result in insurmountable financial stress. The mid-20th century saw the commencement of the achievement of a monumental *enhancement to the culture of medicine*; a commodity to be paid for, often beyond the means of many, to that revolutionary concept—the public right to be maintained in health, and the transaction to be financed by a national exchequer and managed by national institutions.

The lack of funding and adequate institutions seen in countries like India highlight the abysmal educational quality and the health parameters of the population, where the failure of both is evident in a dependence on the virtues of Private enterprise in these fundamental fields of human welfare. Traditional therapeutics in these circumstances satisfies a popular need but in the present organisation do no more towards improving the health of this nation. Once again the Chinese and Vietnamese experience of integrated practice and education in the two medical cultures may be a worthwhile experimental direction towards systems of Universal Health Care.

Chapter 1

Rediscovering Traditional Knowledge in Scientific Disciplines.

An Indian Folk Tale

A.K. Ramanujan Indian poet, linguist, a notable translator and writer introduces his 'Folktales from India' with the story below.

"In a South Indian folktale—, one dark night an old woman was searching intently for something in the street. A passer-by asked her, "Have you lost something?"

She answered, "Yes, I have lost my keys. I have been looking for them all evening"

"Where did you lose them?" "I don't know. Maybe inside the house" "Then why are you looking for them here"? "Because it's dark in there. I don't have oil in my lamps. I can see much better here under the street lights."

Ramanujan goes on to say,
'Until recently many studies of Indian civilisation have been conducted on that principle: look for it under the light, in Sanskrit, in written texts, *in what we think are well-lit spaces of the culture, in places we already know.* There we have, of course, found precious things. Without carrying the parable too far, in a book like this we may say we are now moving indoors,

1

into the expressive culture of the household, to look for our keys. As often happens, we may not always find the keys we are looking for and may have to make new ones, but we will find all sorts of other things we never knew we had lost, or even ever had'. *(A K Ramanujan. Introduction. Folktales from India. Viking by Penguin Books India, 1993)*

Pursuing Acupuncture as medical science

As a general trend in present medical culture the conduct of most clinical trials and the explanations in neurophysiological research are without reference to the past practices of a therapeutic culture. Medical Science assumes the history of establishing a complete system of therapeutics to be an irrelevance for the present context. The culture of science has superseded past knowledge, providing amongst much else, the basis for explaining response to treatment. It is not for science to empathise with or appreciate the considerable culture that fashioned an epistemology for as vast a base of empirical content as Traditional Chinese Medicine (TCM) and the practice of acupuncture that is still with us in its many nuances. For the medical scientist in the earlier years research into it amounted to the insertion of a needle and, in causing pain, finding a therapeutic function for the organism. The 1936 self-infliction studies by Kellgren and Lewis revealed an approach to science which later expanded into wider fields of Peripheral Sensory Stimulation (PSS), in studies with evidence-based support for many variant techniques[i]. Science considers obsolete or ignores, with some exceptions, the knowledge gathered over previous centuries, which created a methodology from empirical practices. They are detailed in treatises of Chinese acupuncture for the controlled delivery of a stimulus akin to, but not necessarily inflicting, pain (in any case, a subjective sensation), for clinical use. The parable of looking for 'the keys' where the illumination is best, is progression to science; *but, also illustrative of this history is a possible loss to fathoming value, while considering specific traditional knowledge or, ignoring the centuries that created its programme for adding to or developing the therapeutic potential of acupuncture.*

Acupuncture Awareness in Europe

The scientific explorations of Acupuncture follow from a previous awareness of its potential. It was not a recent recognition in the West; it was the

Colonial experience of medical aides who provided the evidence of its therapeutic possibility a few centuries ago. A Danish surgeon, de Bondt, serving the Dutch East India Company in Batavia, Java, toward the end of the 16th century, is on record for miraculous cures for a list of illnesses using acupuncture, a technique known to him as a Japanese innovation. Twenty five years later, a few of his enthusiastic accounts were incorporated and criticised by the Dutch surgeon, Wilhelm ten Rhijne, in his more elaborate publication on the subject.

Other Western physicians have featured in publicising acupuncture through service in the East: French, Polish and the notable German, Englebert Kaemfer[ii]. The University at Uppsala offered him a post but instead he chose to serve the Swedish Embassy in Persia for a few years. He also worked as a physician with the Dutch East India Company. Much travelled through India, Ceylon and Japan, his posthumous publications offer interesting insights of the latter. His medical treatise makes extensive reference to Japanese acupuncture and moxibustion and shows details of acupuncture treatment of bowel ailments and the points used.

Colonial academics worked their respective disciplines to discover, interpret and extract value from traditional knowledge systems, and thus brought them to the notice of scholars in Europe. Traditional therapeutics interested some physicians. Gerhard van Swieten, writing of acupuncture and moxa around 1755 said, "—[they] seem to stimulate nerves and thereby to alleviate pains and cramps in quite different parts of the body in a most wonderful way. It would be an extraordinarily useful enterprise if someone would take the trouble to note and investigate the marvellous communion which the nerves have with one another, and at what points certain nerves lie which when stimulated can calm the pain at distant sites. The physicians of Asia, who knew no anatomy, have by long practical experience identified such points"[iii]Gerhard van Swieten shows a perceptive appreciation of the empirical contents of another therapeutic system. He expresses the hope of finding explanations for them within the disciplinary competence of his practice. Medicine was commencing a sojourn in Science. His suggestions may be viewed in the light of undoubted developments today but also with innumerable presumptions about the subject. To find the evidence for acupuncture's therapeutic possibilities may be elusive in the present reductive methods of clinical research. We assume that practices stated in metaphysical epistemology are consequently lacking empirical insights.

Scientists in neural physiology generally regard therapeutic acupuncture as a function of sensory physiology, a modality of Peripheral Sensory Stimulation (PSS). Few groups have, however, investigated the traditional precepts or practices with interesting and useful results. The possibility of such investigations, as mooted by that 18th Century writer specifically of needle stimulation used some distance from the site of pain, has since found confirmation in a series of experimental studies by the Le Bars group[iv]. "—[C]ertain nerves—when stimulated can calm pain at distant sites", is seen to be possible with high intensity stimuli.

Today practitioners have developed the use of short bursts of intense, painful stimuli, needling at locations remote from the site of pathology. Patients with ailments, especially with chronic or acute pain[v], benefit from this form of treatment. The exercises for finding relevance for acupuncture in evidence-based medicine include the practice of acupuncture in forms of traditional usage. As a system of clinical practice for patients world-wide, its traditional usage continues to a greater extent than recent forms of acupuncture innovations.

Fusing a tradition within a prevailing medical culture?

Systems of knowledge from past civilisations, including the Hellenic, have played their part in the evolution of present therapeutic knowledge. Certainly problems that traditional therapeutics pose in our modern context should be understood within the evolving history of medicine and its applications. They follow from particular contextual necessities but the patterns of their origins are also evident in the transmission through translation, borrowing and adaptation. We regard Science and the history of scientific Medicine as commencing in the Renaissance, a demarcation distinct from knowledge as it had evolved over many past civilisations, during centuries of growth and with extensions over an Eurasian land mass. There are, however, continuities from the past to be considered if only to retain objectivity to some of the clinical disciplines of the day. The knowledge that sustains any discipline, whether of the arts or science, must recourse its past for understanding value in the present

This chapter and the next briefly traverse the general importance of the historical interactions that created knowledge, while special systems like therapeutics had varying influences on one another across civilisations. In particular contextual and historical necessities, medicine advanced in the regulations of a research paradigm of science, and relegated to an irrelevance epistemologies which were, for instance, the rationalisation of Traditional Chinese Medicine (TCM) and acupuncture, one of its specialised systems,. Methodological problems repeatedly encountered in clinical trials may well be due to investigating acupuncture without recourse to the empirical practices derived from its epistemology. Metaphysical theories formulated the practices in the first instance and, undoubtedly, those theories gradually became more complex in time through developing extreme academic formalism. If acupuncture is to be transacted in science its practices cannot be dismissed, but must be attempted *in*, at least their pronounced empiricism. The content of TCM finds rationality within the logic of its epistemology and thus supports that practice, while the versions that the scientific investigator assumes to be acupuncture is another form of practice, finding explanations in neurophysiology and microbiology.

The paradigm of science cannot find in the reductive analysis of clinical trials convincing protocols for the inductive practice of TCM, but that deficiency is not regarded as detracting from the value of acupuncture. The extent of interest in acupuncture is considerable and is presently demonstrated in innumerable studies. But, to regard merely an intense sensory input as acupuncture, the essential approach of neuroscience, denies the history that developed this empirical practice with its innumerable facets of treatment that are held together within TCM theory, and possibly seen as of little relevance to science. A reason for not attempting traditional usage is that traditional practice does not accommodate to the present strictures of investigative methodology. Whether acupuncture remains valued as an application for patient pathology, one way or the other, is answered at best in investigations that rarely retain the processes making up the practice of acupuncture.

Transactions of medical science with therapeutic traditions can be considered as a historical continuity. Systems of healing have developed in exchange with other systems even those outside its own civilisation. Today exchange alone is insufficient; any system that can heal or cure, must base that claim not only in a patient's perception but in the evidence that has *biological* and analytical support in a patient's *response*. Should it, for instance be in assuaging pain, there are methodological regulations to objectively test what essentially is a subjective outcome for the patient. Her perception of pain reduction is dependent on many circumstances or variables. In the past the answer to therapeutic utility was an arbitration, the patient's stated response to his physicians' questions and a value judgement followed; that now is considered 'anecdotal' evidence. While traditional therapies retain a validity for society, clinical medicine requires that evidence for them be obtained in a strict method for arriving at their therapeutic value.

Sensation, in the present context of discussing pain, a biological response to stimuli, must be expressed in patient perception. Therapies seeking to assuage pain have to be assessed for their effectiveness. In analysing effectiveness to therapies in general, resolving the holistic and inductive element of its content counterpoised against the causal. Reductive analysis by medical research places the utmost stress on the latter for ascertaining therapeutic value, while traditional therapeutics would evaluate the total experience of the procedure on the individual patient. There is no denying the impact of therapy on an individual, variably mediated in social and cultural factors. The physical contact, like therapeutic massage, physiotherapy, acupuncture, defined as hands-on therapies have holistic inputs in special techniques and do not reduce to a single essential ingredient of therapy as would, at least clinical research suggests, a pharmaceutical, in eliciting patient response. Protocols of study that measure the pain response of a patient as the result of ingesting a pill, the dosage biologically determined would not quite fit the bill for hands on therapies. Acupuncture has both, a sensory biological input from a needle insertion into the tissues, treatment that is conveyed in many factors which include skill of hands making that insertion, often apparent to the patient and others interlinked to the therapeutics of acupuncture. The method of investigating pharmaceutical products is fairly standard procedure in evidence based medicine. Even so they have control procedures in their protocols which presumably demarcate the artefacts which confuse patient response to the essential ingredient being investigated. Extending without adaptation that method to holistic therapies defeats the purpose of evidence for the effectiveness of such therapies. Amongst present medical procedures, whether for surgery, rehabilitative medicine, even psychotherapy, patient response is also to the interrelated inputs including those mediated beyond a fundamental one; to mention a few, the therapist with his skills, physicians ability to communicate and patient expectations about procedure, important to the outcome for the patient and not necessarily to be side-lined as artefacts to treatment.

The attitude of clinical research towards acupuncture in Sweden suggests an extended deviation in history. Scientific colleagues find a functional relevance for this tradition in treating patients and its use as a health resource[vi]. Aspects of history touched upon here relate a view of civilisations developing systems of knowledge, highlighted by the particular therapeutic offerings which preceded the Renaissance. Previous therapeutic systems were mutually understandable even within their respective epistemologies: philosophical divergence was not a constraint and concepts and ideas in translation and transmissions allowed systems their separate developments.

Medicine evolved as an art of healing from similar beginnings in most parts of the world. Inputs came from many sources and knowledge from other times: the medieval, for instance, was a period that had an immense influence on the development and codification of systems and the practices of medicine before it involved the sciences. The influences on Medicine in Europe and on Traditional systems of Chinese Medicine and the context for their respective development differed. But, in antiquity and later, each had the opportunity for contact and access to the other[vii]. Physicians collaborated and intensive contact for the times developed between the prevailing specialist cultures of Greece, India and China. (See later, Greece West Asia and India) which each brought perceptible enhancements to the content of others within their identity and development.

Newer resources beyond local traditions gave direction to further development. To Medicine, the Renaissance was, undoubtedly, a separate impulse toward Science. Yet the Medicine we practice has continuity within a more universal history. The clinical scientist may ignore it but in doing so may be denying inherent value from a past which should not be ignored by science. The immediate example is when clinical medicine having established a method of therapeutic validation assumes that Traditional Therapeutics (TT) can divulge its value in that method. But their epistemologies reflect empirical discovery which could with profit be examined in clinical studies. In the history of its transmission westward it is not my contention that bringing acupuncture within the purview of science would answer the larger questions that hang over traditional medicine in today's socio-medical culture, but it may offer pointers. Attempts to understand or use acupuncture now in certain ways are reminiscent of attitudes that go back to the years of Colonial dominance when academics felt their homespun disciplines were adequate for exploring and explaining 'native' knowledge. They were normative disciplines and the methods designed essentially for problems of their own context, whether social or environmental. We tend to pursue acupuncture similarly in many studies.

In contemporary practice there are other issues which relate to TTs for society. In their epistemology they largely impinge on programmes of Primary Health Care. The responsibility for maintaining their adequacy rests with modern medical practice and within the culture of Science. There is a need to know that past therapeutic procedures have scientific relevance. The issue of patient safety and therapeutic evidence are naturally important and both are better served by therapeutic procedure that can, at least, be related to the pathology and diagnostic problems presented in medicine. Angioedema is a hazard, an allergy may occur with any medication, including the herbal, but to recognise the condition is to provide immediate remedy—neither of which is available in therapeutic practice previous to medicine.

Therapeutic Traditions and Paradigms

The method of hypothesis and experimental verification is the benchmark for evidence based medicine (EBM). The models for verification in scientific medicine form a revolutionary paradigm which can contend with empirical precepts. Those are testable, but not the metaphysics which formalise them. The history of medicine, evolving as a science and finding confirmatory evidence for its processes and products by methodology is a comparatively short process. Controversies have arisen regarding the concept of paradigms which can sustain only a line of application or singular methods of verification. The paradigm is understood by the community of scientists that put it in place for their line of study. Some medical research in solving defined problems is trapped in necessary but reductive consequences of the paradigm. Development is determined by the method of the paradigm, and while progress may be phenomenal for the particular field for which the paradigm was constituted, problem solving is constrained beyond the remit for which it was designed. The need for rethinking paradigms is constant as the nature of the problem to be solved changes. An example can be seen in the features of acupuncture with its many variables in empirical usage. These tend to be set aside in the methods for verification to the neglect of the system's value which may be more comprehensive.

Medical science can demonstrate dynamism sufficient to handle diverse epistemologies. Traditional therapeutics offers some, and medicine is obliged to consider them. The present signs are that traditional therapeutics has a value for society and a popular appeal, but that value is mostly unsupported in evidence. We have arrived at a stage of health care where there is no choice other than a common medical culture inclusive of tradition or, as at present, there will be diverse therapeutics and parallel cultures within our social health resource with insufficient statutory control over many of them.

TTs are widely encountered today but the extent of their use varies across the world. For some countries with adequate health care they provide esoteric alternatives, sometimes in self-medication, while for others where substantial or consistent policies toward health care are lacking they are the mainstay of primary health delivery, sustained in the socio-cultural acknowledgement of their validity. Establishment medicine may be sceptical about TTs which is an added reason for their not featuring in policies or health programmes, and this completes a circular problem of statutory recognition and public safety in primary health care delivery. These questions are to an extent confronted although largely confused and hence unresolved.

Reservations relating to clinical trials

Basic acupuncture research is essentially about the organism's response to needle insertion into skin and underlying tissue. Important information has been gained about the responses. The main thrust of clinical research is through studies on patients to establish evidence for its use on diagnostic categories. The protocols of study usually are analytical and reductive exercises, hence, shorn of much of the necessary procedural practice vital to therapeutic acupuncture. The traditional, multiple and variable methods of delivering acupuncture to an individual patient mostly contradicts reductive trial protocols. Randomised clinical trial and blinded or placebo controls are the methodological standby of evidence-based medicine and the method takes precedence over the therapeutic measure being investigated.

TTs like Ayurveda and acupuncture have been in use for millennia, but the implications for their continuance depend on their safety and evidence-based value. That is essential to progress in the medical culture of the day. However, the present reductive methods of investigating the clinical efficacy, of acupuncture, offer a range of disparate evidence, and no convincing conclusions can be reached based on them. The clinical scientist investigating a subject like acupuncture makes assumptions, amongst which that the methods designed for modern therapeutic procedure must transpose to its investigation without modification. Evolving methods for research may advance should collaborations be possible between the practitioners of the respective systems. The holistic aspects to a practice should be researched, at least in pursuit of its empirical content. The call for reviewing clinical research methods does not merely concern therapeutic procedures but also many modern physical and medical therapeutic procedures.

There is a growing awareness of many shortcomings to the process of finding the evidence in 'evidence based medicine'. Clinical trials in psychotherapy[viii] within the usual protocols for conducting them may be cited as an example. The theoretical structure of Psychotherapy, a disciplinary off-shoot of Medicine, is a distant call from TTs and their separate epistemology. If the Randomised Controlled Trial (RCT) for the former is defective in the quality of evidence it has provided, it is hardly surprising that the RCTs for the latter so often convey contrary evidence.

Traditional therapeutics must account for features in its delivery. Accompanying explanations and regulations are of consequence to the patient response and hardly comparable to swallowing a prescribed pill. The physician's supportive explanations, such as of restrictions to diet are a routine contribution to total therapy. The selection of acupuncture points is specific not just to the individual patient but encompasses a choice duly varied in the natural history of a disease. After insertion the needle is manipulated in different degrees of intensity and duration, and the frequencies of treatment depend on the patient and the progression of the ailment. Each practitioner handles the process of insertion and manipulation of the needle based on his own experience—a variable in study protocols that may not be ignored. Surgery and devising adequate controls for investigation often require adaptation to the particular procedure, and hands-on therapies in their complexity present analogous difficulties for research. But clinical trial methodology might attempt them rather in more naturalistic than standardised protocols which would go some way towards such incorporation.

The reliability of the Randomised Controlled Trial (RCT) is a sine qua non for Evidence Based Medicine (EBM). Any modality which claims to provide therapeutic utility must demonstrate it in the RCT. Insurance companies tend to favour products which pass muster in the evidence, and practices need hardly look beyond them at better alternatives for patients. Such promotion has very wide implications for health care, which is a separate issue. Here the stress is on the shortcomings of RCTs when attempting to obtain evidence for the efficacy of acupuncture.

In evaluating evidence, the 'control group' assumed least controvertible is the 'placebo' control, a dummy procedure which mimics the therapeutic ingredient, and in the patient's awareness is indistinguishable from it. 'Bias' is another factor which vitiates the evidence and may be well avoided in a double blind trial where the therapist is unaware of whether his treatment is genuine or placebo, and the investigator assesses the outcome without knowing which control group the patient belongs to. These are investigations designed and feasible for pharmaceutical products. Randomisation at the trial entry point and 'blinding' of patients and therapists is standard clinical trial procedure established for investigating medication and pharmaceutical products having standard potencies and dosage. Protocols at present are hard pressed to go beyond the stipulated regulations of reductive research to investigate the value of therapeutic processes. They apply to surgical and rehabilitative procedures—which may by contrast to a pill be defined as 'hands-on' therapies. Hands-on therapies certainly represent many categories of therapeutic procedures, some of medical science and others through tradition. Many are effective therapeutic measures, but patient response is agent-dependent, reliant upon his particular methods and application skills.

Medical science has the dynamism to consider Traditional Therapeutics in their diverse epistemologies. The present signs are that TTs have popular appeal and a culturally based value for society, this value mostly unsupported in the evidential process of medicine. There is little choice for society but for a common medical culture inclusive of tradition; or else we continue with diverse therapeutics each offering primary health resources within their separate medical culture. An associated problem is of statutory control which is established only for modern medicine; the others are out of its ambit.

TTs are widely encountered today but the extent of their use varies across the world. For some countries with adequate health care they provide esoteric alternatives, sometimes in self-medication, while for others where substantial or consistent policies toward health care are lacking, they are the mainstay to primary health delivery sustained in a socio-cultural acknowledgement of validity. The Medical Establishment is justified in its scepticism about the evidence for their therapeutic use and consequently they are not featured in Health Policies in programs concerned with the issue of their safer use. This becomes a circular problem since without statutory recognition there is no possibility of control over TT practices which may endanger patients while the evidence for utility and safety is required to precede establishment recognition of TT. These problems are confronted to an extent although in some unresolved confusion. The extent of recognition of TTs differs from country to country, unlike the universally acknowledged legitimacy provided for Medicine by its statutory Establishment.

Whatever the shortcomings in the approach of medical science to traditional therapeutics many institutions of the West, in pursuing a subject like acupuncture, have undoubtedly highlighted the need and sustained interest for a far more considered evaluation of a tradition, which could be emulated but has not been followed with other TTs in the lands of their origin. China, on the other hand, has made great strides with acupuncture in both basic medical and clinical research. Countries like India, where traditional medicine is a massive support system to primary health care, are yet to come to terms with the need for re-evaluating their medical traditions in the methods generally accepted for modern Medicine. The criticisms offered about the methods pursued by science should in no way detract from the value of studies and contributions from Western interest in Eastern therapeutic traditions. The process is emulated to a great extent as a scientific pursuit in China and the Far East.

Taking account of the historical transactions of many other systems before science was established may stimulate the investigation of therapeutics in other traditions, and in particular of realising acupuncture as a therapeutic modality within the science and practice of medicine. It is essential for Traditional Medicine to attempt its function within a scientific paradigm. In no development other than in research is it possible to realise safe treatment for the public and reasoning for its potential for practice by physicians who function in an evolving medical culture.

Biological Tracks from Tribal healing

Assuaging pain, healing injury and curing aberrant behaviour was a need recognised of societal function amongst tribes in prehistory. If nature wrought havoc and disaster she was also responsible for the tribes' food supply, the sufficiency of the hunt or, as early settlements came about, for the agricultural produce. Illness and abnormal behaviour were also attributed to the forces of Nature and, if suitably addressed, her more benign powers could be directed for tribal benefit or in assuaging individual ill health and suffering. Belief systems originated through the knowledge that the tribe's means of livelihood and well-being were subject to the vagaries of inscrutable nature and beyond human control. Anthropomorphic images, idols or other symbols particularised for the tribe, were installed and supplicated or suitably placated to intercede with Nature on their behalf. One amongst them was chosen, usually from amongst the elders, to propitiate Nature, in trappings which recognised and marked his power to mediate in specific rituals on behalf of the laity.

The shamans, witch doctors, priests or temple-keepers possibly made up the earliest organised agencies to codify and derive therapeutic possibilities from the intense bonding of the individual to his culture. They were the early interventionists who, by ritual and magic, ministered to illness or physical pain, or who cast out malignant spirits that had 'possessed' the victim provoking deviant behaviour. Rituals, imagery and the patterns and forms of supplication conducted in view of the tribe re-focussed the individual's intense attention on the cultural model which could assuage his pain or suffering.

The 'witch' doctor had accessed the biological potential of his subject. By virtue of the position he held in tribal society, he interpreted the reasons for an individual's distress in terms understood in the tribe's culture, and established an effective ministration. Authority and ritual utilised a very powerful biological mechanism that could be mobilised to inhibit pain in an individual, or initiate processes toward ameliorating illness.

The interventional recourses in such imagery were models which evoked neural mechanisms: multisensory stimuli, auditory and visual; or modalities of sensation—ranging from touch through to the more intense, the heat of the ritual fire, or sometimes even more painful and intense as with flogging. Their effect on the subject, including the inflictions initiated endogenous inhibition of pain and reflex, restorative processes towards healing injury and other afflictions. The empirical observations of such healing possibilities were, of course, recast in metaphysical terms, primeval theories of illness and methods for their control. The shamans had noted the effects on pain or illness when the intensely held beliefs of the tribe focussed individual attention on the powerful stimulus of the ritual. These neural reflexes related closely to culture and environment.

The Placebo and Nocebo responses

The neurobiological responses continue down the millennial ages to the present, but the cultural models evoking these endogenous mechanism changes down human history. Today, however, in the circumstance of fathoming evidence of the true value of therapeutic modalities, the response is considered an artefact, and in clinical studies protocols are designed to attempt its isolation. In-built responses like pain inhibition and the inflammatory response to injury are developed in the evolutionary history of the organism and aid survival and healing: they gain more environmental and individual variables as they arrive at the greater biological complexity of the cognate human organism.

The witch doctor, shaman and, later, priests were acknowledged healers. Their power could on occasion be used to the detriment of an individual, even to his destruction, as when taboos were violated, social customs disregarded, or authority rebelled against. We are aware that human pain may be inhibited or accentuated by intense attention, or in anxiety, fear or guilt. Amongst many rural populations worldwide a person who feels or senses a sting, if he sees a snake moving away from his vicinity, assumes that he has been bitten and promptly manifests symptoms of poisoning. The snake in reality or the image of the serpent in the culture of many such societies has dire and powerful significance.

Medical science recognises in the 'placebo' a conditioned response. The availability of the response, within the comparatively brief period of human cultural history as against human evolution, constitutes a behavioural trait, although the evidence is that it may be elicited by appropriate models amongst many vertebrate species. The response is initiated by a sensory stimulus and may, for instance, reduce symptoms such as pain. The 'Nocebo' response, its counter reflex, is again initiated in conditioning. In the above example conditioning is in culture and strong belief systems.

There were forms of therapy in early societies which did not require an interventionist. Empirical therapeutic ingredients from a variety of natural resources were discovered by the group at large, and this common knowledge gradually transformed and developed in its lore. Tribal medicine or other methods of dealing with disease, even today, works through these practices, know-how that is available to members of the group. Folk medicine was for use by society and did not necessarily require the insights of a specialist agent. Knowledge and myth, were handed down the generations with little change and used to social advantage. Nuggets are documented in some developed societies but amongst many, particularly those living in tribal relationships in an underdeveloped world, such can be approached only via tribal memory.

Treatments continue their utility for certain aspects of health care in modern society, exploited and sometimes reinvented by industry, often without the evidence to support therapeutic value or identify possible hazards to patient safety. It may serve both community interests and prior rights to intellectual property if state policies were to provide legal safeguard to protect such rights so that benefit accrues to those who first discovered the medical uses. Presently they are unprotected from the exploitative proclivities of the pharmaceutical and other multinationals. Simultaneously there must be directives, required evaluations of the products in medical science.

The story of the Hoodia cactus and the San tribe of Southern Africa are illustrative. The cactus is used as a hunger suppressant by this Kalahari desert tribe as they go on the hunt for long periods of time during which food is even scarcer. Of course, the potential as a hunger suppressant for the overfed and obese is considerable. The pharmaceutical industry has been quick to exploit that market, yet sidestepping and hedging on the question of intellectual property rights and due compensation for the San, a tribe already subject to depletion in numbers by their Bantu neighbours. Even in the exploitation and unsavoury proclivities of today's practices, an age-old discovery has possibly been enhanced but, again, without acknowledgement of the origins, in a one-sided exchange.

The Enterprise of Knowledge. Beyond a Greek Heritage

Changes to prevailing winds are possible in scientific method and debate. The academic world of medicine is suspicious of the publics' attitudes to therapeutic systems of other cultures, generally tending to be dismissive of them as they were not cast in the scientific mould. The general non-acceptance of therapeutic systems of the past which were considerable intellectual enterprises, of disciplinary study merely support the frank prejudices once in vogue. With variations they are familiar precedents in the historiography of science. Studies were carried out purporting to demonstrate the superiority of brain dimension along racist lines and, even more, there were the notorious anti-Semitic studies of the late 19th and early 20th centuries[ix]. Neo-imperialism and anti-Western reactions are movements that continue in Science, to demonstrate the virulence of ideologies extolling the virtues of identities which by now should be archaic. Academic pursuits cannot be credited with objectivity when these spill over, however diluted, and colour respective studies with degrees of dismissal for the knowledge of other civilisations. Eastern, West Asian and later Islamic contributions have, however, recently begun to feature in publications, after the pronounced hiatus in acknowledging their presence as even possible. The well implanted idea of Greece as the fount of Science, and Europe the inheritor in any case has skewed the contrary evidences of history for a while. *The fact of such historiography losing out on the nature and importance to the enterprise of knowledge in non-European spaces marks an objective loss to investigations, especially of medical tradition.*

Following centuries of writing and investigation in Egyptology, many scholars surmised that ancient Egypt lacked in mathematical astronomy or even mathematics. To credit Greece as the sole fount of genuine science, academics of the last two centuries either discount or misinterpret the significant and prior contributions of the civilisations of Egypt and Mesopotamia to early Greek science which had in the past been accepted and elaborated upon by other intellectuals of ancient Greece right down to those of the European Enlightenment. Even a few decades ago, Morris Kline could summarise the history of mathematics of other civilisations in three out of a seven hundred page volume devoted to the cultural history of mathematics. In comparison to what the Greeks achieved in this field, his statement that, "the mathematics of Egyptians and Babylonians is the scrawling of children just learning to write as opposed to great literature" can only be attributed to this historiographer's self-imposed Greek blinker, though sufficient evidence to the contrary exists and should have allowed him a wider field of vision[x]. Historical documentation and evidence get short shrift in the attempt to make facts fit a premise, but objectivity is the casualty.

Over centuries crests have followed ebbs in acknowledging the sources for Greek achievements. At present we are in a phase of denial, and paucity of Egyptian influence on Greek science is suggested, whereas its primacy was previously taken for granted. The reasons for a lengthy sojourn in Egypt by Eudoxus of Knidos, the great Greek mathematician and Plato's younger contemporary are of interest. Despite evidences to the contrary some academics go to the extent of denying that he ever did spend time there. That he lived in Egypt protected by the Pharaoh, befriended by priests, shaving his head and learning their language has been known and recorded since as long ago as the occasion itself and confirmed somewhat later by Strabo, the Greek geographer of Amasya (b. about 53 BC). He was shown Eudoxus' house in Heliopolis and his observatory in Kerkesoura "where he determined certain celestial motions". Finding material for his investigations, which presumably was not available in Greece or elsewhere, substantiates Eudoxus' period of residence in Egypt. Beyond this simple fact are attestations from the ancient Greeks down to present-day scholars. Eudoxus' 'Dialogue of the Dogs' in all likelihood translated into Greek certain texts from the Egyptian 'The Book of the Dead'. Yet, for philologists of today, it offers nothing of greater value than literature with an exotic if somewhat salacious content, the Dialogue of 'Naked Priests' and their predilection for animals; notwithstanding that Egyptian priests were, as Giorgio de Santillana says, 'decently swathed in linen'. The fact is dismissed that Eudoxus, a considerable mathematician of his time, required access to matters that concerned him in astronomy: the unravelling by Egyptian priests of planetary movement, of the Zodiacal figures that within their myths indicated the cycles of visibility and invisibility of stars, their heliacal rising, the phases of the moon and so forth. Since 3000 BC the Egyptian priesthood were, by observation and their mastery of astronomy and mathematics, able to measure time and space, serialise planetary and astral motions and conjunctions, and further, with that knowledge of the heavens and with the merkhet, their instrument of mensuration, help engineer and supervise the building of the pyramids and their orientation on earth, within 3 inches of error[xi].

It was not only Eudoxus of Cnidus who was intrigued by Egyptian methods. Centuries later Isaac Newton expended considerable effort in trying to fathom the methods behind Egyptian mensuration to support his theory of gravitation. He was convinced that an accurate measure of the cubit would yield the correct geographical latitude necessary to prove his theories. Efforts to decipher what were considered in the 17th century to be mathematical calculations of perfected geometric proportions that preceded the construction of the pyramids were hampered by an inability to approach their defined base because of the accumulated rubble of centuries. At least in his early writings Newton was unequivocally convinced of the priority and primacy of Egyptian astronomy and the vital importance of knowing the exactness of the Egyptian system of linear mensuration. Although he later shifted the attribution of priority to the Old Testament and Israel, it was, nevertheless, not to Greece[xii]

Egyptian priests may have, out of secrecy necessary to maintain their social position, shrouded much of their astronomy in allegory, mythology and religious or metaphysical texts. While the acquisition of knowledge was to guide their superior souls to gnosis or spiritual insight, they were well aware that it also entitled them to immense temporal power. It enabled them to understand the possibilities of famine, flood or plenty; but for the superstitious laity it was the magic of the propitiatory rituals over which the priesthood presided that predicted these events. Within their allegories of Osiris or Isis, or the Lost Eye of Horus stolen by Hathor as a Cat and recovered by Thoth as a dog-headed ape, they had secreted and described planetary conjunctions, celestial motions and the seasons of the year. Newton, in an early edition of his Principia Mathematica, acknowledges that Greek Vestal ceremonies were derived from the Egyptian, designed originally for the laity by their priests, and concealed a profound astronomical knowledge.

In denying Egypt the science of astronomy, our historians and philologists leave us with stories of Gods as animals, wolves, baboons and dog-faced men. If 'Orientalism' finds nothing but earth cults, sun cults, libido and sexual perversions, patricide and incest in Eudoxus' 'Dialogue of the Dogs' which he derived from the original literature of the 'Book of the Dead', then the specialists move Egyptian culture toward their narration of the 'Orient', first imagined, then confirmed, by distorting evidence. Scholars are held fast in the cleft stick of a major premise of the day: Greece as the springboard of Science, when indeed more than a few primary sources of Greek science were from Egypt and Babylon. But in their interpretations they would rather make nonsense of any contrary evidence merely to confirm intellectual stances.

Empirical and methodical priorities.
Science before Renaissance science.

Disciplines and, frequently, societies may lose out on the value of cumulative discoveries of the past if science is narrowed to definitions that exclude such enterprises. The recent flurry of interest in intellectual rights for genetic patents, stimulated in the aftermath of industrial predators and global geopolitics, reveals the extent to which the agricultural and biological sciences have bypassed the potential of age-old human activity and organisation since these have not been systematically explored. Exclusion is the result, a remoteness or often motivated selectivity by disciplines, of the content of cultural history. As yet today's agronomic, pharmaceutical and medical sciences in certain areas of the world have hardly gathered a base data for their immense indigenous vegetable and therapeutic wealth, nor has there been any sustained exploration of their origins, their evolution and use; in short, the history of a human function interrelated with the environment. In some known instances knowledge-based developments took place over centuries. They related to change in social organisation, and the compulsions that followed migration. Societies alter as a result of a variety of external pressures and self-generated impulses; but the activities remain and develop in the changing nature of investigation and the innovative organisation for basic constants, *the need to feed themselves, and to assuage pain, heal illness or mitigate its* effects. The methods were no less *than* science in observation, experiment and application. Whether those endeavours are to be recognised as such has depended on definition or presumptions. Science must be ante-dated and applied to the wider world space; the European Renaissance provided a qualitative shift but its roots should be set, not just in ancient Greece, but far more universally.

In viewing annual religious festivities associated with the harvest one is made aware that one is in the presence of specialised forms of knowledge. Vegetable foods and herbal pharmacopial wealth were created in abundance centuries ago, sustained and improved in quality today. Such efforts were under way in empirical hybridisation processes well before science was defined or the abbot Gregor Mendel experimented and formulated his 'Laws'. For all purposes the manner of conducting those activities—often called low technology—cannot be considered anything other than scientific. Man in his curiosity and astuteness looks beyond what is obvious in his habitat, its flora and his heavens. The ability of that ancient onlooker—investigator or worker, not necessarily exalted in status as an agronomist, physician or astronomer, lay in his understanding, through observation, trial, error and replication with wild seed, to be able to make improvements on what he saw and benefit his group. It was experimental science for an essential universal human activity, if not Mendelian in investigative quality, as much in the proportions of their produce.

Discoveries and technological leaps have taken place within the civilisations of Egypt, Greece, West Asia and the Indian subcontinent, during different or overlapping centuries, with yet another of considerable quality in the contribution by the Chinese from the 5th to 11th centuries CE. Each had contextual compulsions and projected finally into the European Renaissance.

The endeavour of science, throughout history was often halted but never extinguished. Systematising knowledge was part of the fabric of social activities. The Renaissance and, later, industrialising societies, offered tremendous advances, enabling universalisation to the endeavour by using mathematical models for the methods to discovery. It was undoubtedly a qualitative shift in place for the context of an Industrial Europe[xiii]. Technology and applications followed in rapid succession earning society many benefits, but the stimulus was the competitive advantage for Europe's nations in an era of Empire building.

Changing Societies and cumulative knowledge

One instance of a specific activity evolving over centuries of societal change is the gradual improvement of the olive from the original scraggly and thorny Mediterranean wild scrub to its economic importance and gustatory excellence. It was not science as we define it, but it surely has some hall marks of scientific activity. The story of science is complex in that it involves a continuum of specialised activity through history, and its interrelated societal influences change its character, determine its practitioners, the methods they adopt and the rate of its progress.

There was a continuing movement and shift of peoples along the Syrian and Anatolian sea-board before the fourth millennium BC, when nomadic tribes hybridised with indigenous peoples and they evolved into more stable societies with new rituals and needs. They had developed and brought an improved and 'oilier' olive to Crete. There they continued to cultivate and transform themselves and the olive and, having prospered through its virtues, they felled the native timber for other uses and extended that land for the further cultivation of olive trees. Selling the olive and the timber of Crete to their neighbours, the dynastic priest-kings of Egypt became an attractive commercial proposition. Over the centuries man's ingenuity engineered mutant varieties and then, by selectively cultivating them, improved the quality of the produce. But while he initiated improvements of cultivable products, man tended to ignore the wider implications of their cultivation. The olive produced the wealth of Crete and its peoples, but it drained the richness of the soils it grew on. The manner of improvement, controlled certainly by societal needs and implemented by its managers and cultivators, depleted the land and in time attenuated, then destroyed, the society dependent on its fertility[xiv].

It may be that definitions exclude this effort as a discipline of science, but it certainly influences its history; the manner of improving the qualities of the olive over centuries involved understanding nature and employing her vagaries to advantage, long before any principles of agronomic theory were laid down. But even had there been a set of theoretical rules then available, without concomitant societal regulations that activity was destructive in the long run. Such situations are paralleled today by a variety of ecological depredations. As an activity, the worth of Science is never self-evident. It may be invoked for societal betterment, institutional aggrandisement and, of course, to the universally destructive proclivities of nations in varying scale.

Borrowing but excluding source knowledge

The many civilisations of South America, the Aztec, Mayan, and Incan, commenced in bloody territorial invasions and conquest. Even human sacrifice was a feature of certain propitiatory rites. Unlike other hierarchical civilisations, whose early achievements included astronomy and mathematics, language, epics, poetic compilations and a sizable literature, philosophical and systematised explorations in religion; the brief Incan civilisation was without many such attainments It lacked even the elementary technology of the wheel, and yet for its time, the unparalleled culture and knowledge of food production must mark it as a civilisation. Oriented as they were to more worldly, sensory and experiential satisfactions, the Incans had developed a highly sophisticated alternative science close enough in its methodology to an agronomy which enabled that civilisation to extract from nature foods of an astounding variety.

Agricultural produce grown by the peoples of the region in previous millennia were improved upon in Incan programmes. They developed techniques to improve its tubers, vegetables and fruit on a grand scale. For example, the Incans experimented on the potato, by cultivating it in different soil qualities and in the naturally varying temperatures of the mountains, in the shadows or sunlight of their slopes. They evolved prodigious potato varieties, different in textures, size and colour, and suited for cultivation in differing soils and climatic conditions. They also experimented with a host of vegetables, corn and grain, producing newer and hardier varieties, paying close attention to blights and crop disease. Some of the terraces of the legendary Machu Picchu on the high altitudes of the Andes were created for vast programmes of seeding or planting on serial plots of experimental soils. Massive carved stone was used to build these functional terraces, arranged to catch the sunlight in its different daily phases of light, shade and duration, and to conserve water from the natural snow melts, channelling it through the stone for both irrigation and drainage. It was research conducted 500 years ago, unprecedented for quality and in scale; but sparse in historical narrative[xv] and its systematised knowledge only now beginning to find acknowledgement[xvi]. Machu Picchu, though, evokes speculation and interpretation with such suggestions as to its purpose as a resort for the highest of Incan society or finding their peace and spiritual resolution amongst vestal virgins. The orientalist flair for explanation is persistent; the lore of the civilised intruder in foreign climes encountering motley 'savages' and postulating bizarre interpretations of their lives and culture even when other evidence may point to down to earth knowledge.

Without the appellation of science, applications evolving over the centuries have been with far greater awareness of social responsibility and respect for the environment[xvii]. When the Incan potato-cultivating practises were not followed in transplantation to another continent, initial crop success there was followed by substantial losses and then disaster. The reasons for European interest in the potato as a food source were understandable. The Spanish Conqueror, in his arrogance, naturally was unable to credit the Incan with any intellectual resources and remained ignorant of the systematised experimental methods that went into cultivating the many varieties of potato. Incan food products were the result of social skills, organisation and astute methodology. The history of the translocation of the potato to Europe by the Spanish and English shows an unawareness of soil qualities, need for pest protection and other inputs. These were known to the natives, systematically garnered by experimentation with cultivable produce, monitored and reproduced for quality, delicacy and hardiness. In Europe the potato was grown for quick returns, ignoring much of the knowledge that went into the original cultivation. Europe's communities were initially slow to accept the potato as a nourishing replacement for grain but, once the benefit as food was realised, her populations no longer subsisted at levels near starvation. However Europe's ignorance of husbanding the product consequently led to the advantages of potato crops being rapidly lost to blights and pests.

Recent reappraisals establish the evidence of projects for improving farinaceous and horticultural produce in an experimental science by a people who had no writing and little mathematics as we conceive them. They had, though, the means of accounting and conveying information across the great distances of their extensive empire by relays of runners. A feature of Incan organisational skills was their manner of maintaining interrelated and updated information of agricultural produce, weaponry, livestock and population records in all districts, and to speedily transmit such information amongst themselves and to the administrative units of the capitol within 24 hours via runners placed at distances for optimal performance and physical efficiency. The runners carried the quipu, knotted cords further supplemented with colour codes, providing the computational system of their data based in numerology[xviii]. The decoding of their system may not yet be completed. Without doubt the Incans were able to provide their society with a good measure of food security. They were able to communicate orders, regulations and requirements to the appropriate hierarchical authority. Their organisation was of a calibre that only a civilisation is capable of, yet accomplished without the facility of the written word, the wheel or beasts of burden, the stipulated hallmarks of civilisation. The Spaniards ultimately destroyed them in the 16th century, but the potato came to the Old World, with the Spaniards from Florida and the English via Virginia.

It was soon obvious that the potato was a staple food of remarkable nutritional quality and easily cultivable on a large scale. Its high vitamin content offset many of the deficiency diseases that the peoples of Europe were subject to. After two centuries of religious wars Europe had been ravaged, the countryside impoverished from constant famine, and populations depleted by depressed fertility and disease. By the 17th century comparative peace endured. The extensive cultivation of the potato in Europe and its introduction as a diet staple improved nutritional status to an extent that the population soon began to multiply. In Ireland, for example, the ease with which the potato could be cultivated and its widespread acceptance and integration led to a doubling of the population within a hundred years. While the potato was easy enough to grow in its newer location, to know how best to increase its yield and at the same time to control susceptibility to pests was another matter. But in Europe that was not discovered until well after crops had been destroyed by blight and ensuing famine had once again decimated populations.

It was only when the science of agronomy came into its own in the 19th century that methods of improving crop quality and yields began in earnest. Centuries earlier the Incans had demonstrated in their remarkable series of soil experiments how it was done. Today agronomy is a burgeoning 'science'. In the earlier period any suggestion that there could have been supporting knowledge to secure the cultivation of the potato was not considered. Valuable knowledge was lost as surely as the crops were during those disastrous famines that followed its successful initiation. The potato had arrived but the benefit from the cumulative wisdom that originally went into its cultivation was left behind[xix]. Whether it was due to unawareness of the optimal environmental conditions that were gradually established during its original cultivation, or by failure to understand that pests could be controlled, there was hardly ever the possibility of considering the knowledge of a conquered people to contain inherent worth. In this instance, Ireland and much of Europe paid a disastrous price in the decline of potato cultivation once it became the staple of their diet.

Incan methods of cultivation can be contrasted with those prevalent on the mountain slopes of South Western India today, where agricultural universities and well developed governmental departments are available for promoting scientific agronomy. The cultivation of potato, certainly, and to some extent of tea, an agro-economic industry, as well as the introduction of acacia and the incongruous water-guzzling eucalyptus by the British, have all been at the expense of the genetic variety of the hardy native flora. They have changed the landscape of the mountains and depleted their underground springs, causing climate and temperature changes. Far poorer acidic soil derives from the newer foliage; the large scale erosion and seasonal shortages of water occurring within the past few decades are hardly a matter for surprise.

The Colonial Enterprise and Native knowledge

Objectivity and the neutrality of scientific method is to be sought after in research, its attainment is often compromised. The broad area of Oriental Studies during the centuries of colonial contact is a case in point. Innumerable disciplines were brought to bear at the instance of the coloniser, encompassing law, social relations, public health or medicine according to his understanding and for his benefit. In the process, the Orient acquired another character, distorting its myths, social philosophy, art and architecture as its critical appreciation and perspectives were shorn or disconnected from the considerable presence of the local narrative. A disciplinary methodology specifically for studying social relationships within a cultural context was put in place, without access to the peoples who lived their cultures in an experiential immediacy to their environment. The disciplines were formally devised to serve societies as they evolved, understanding the social relationships of industrialising civilisations.

Interpretation and narration of social relationships or knowledge systems of hitherto unknown cultures were included in the disciplines developed onwards from the 17 century in Europe, often an arrogation which distorted inherent value. Viable social relationships, whose essential functions had been fashioned over centuries, were lost in interpretations which suited the requirements of newly installed Colonial institutions. Post-colonial questioning and deconstructions are taking place in the many fields of historical study[xx] including Medicine and Public Health and the 'Oriental' slant subject to correction. There was considerable disruption to the social fabric of the colonised at many levels; but the introduction of the Industrial Age with its technology and knowledge had a considerable influence on those societies and their culture. Political certainties changed rapidly, with a marginal effect on cultural values and social order, but the impact on the world of the Colonist which introduced that Age was far more consequential.

Social Contexts and Knowledge Exchange

Colonial intellectual enterprise contrasts with the manner of earlier exchanges and assimilation of systematised knowledge. They had brought to Europe some of the remarkable achievements of specialised knowledge from West Asia. Contributory sources from Greece, China and India were transformed into the highly sophisticated systems of medical education and therapeutic systems in Persian institutions. The remarkable flowering of medicine made its way both East and West; and, as the evidence unfolds, formed an important contribution to the epochal Renaissance leap of science.

Attitudes to medicine in West Asia were changing. From metaphysical classifications and the *humours* as a cause of disease an important empirical shift toward classification based in a disease aetiology of symptoms and signs came to be recognised by renowned scholar/practitioners of Persian Medicine. Further centuries passed before the philosophies that developed Paracelsian medicine become part of those changes. In Europe, the newer ideas suggested natural configurations like liverwort to reveal disease of that organ and therapeutic answers were to be found in nature's produce. It was a speculative approach and hardly empirical yet, even so an advance on the past. It lacked the experimental quality and the sophistication of West Asian medicine which already had advanced systems based in hospital practice and the sustained observation of patients.

Modern classificatory systems retain the structure of that advance, enhanced by detailed pathology and bacteriology, later disciplines of medical sciences but ones which, it must be emphasised, had material to build its science upon. The sources in that Age were not formally acknowledged nor was it required to do so. But, the likely discourse between West Asia and Europe in the field of medical knowledge is difficult to deny, considering the traffic and wide availability of the medicine and its earliest demonstration as a present science. The advent of traditional therapies into the present culture of medicine is continuity to an established history of medical developments. The relevance of pursuing acupuncture in medicine is a matter of historical objectivity through observing traditional possibilities in its passage to neurobiology. For a dominant medical culture that carries the hubris of science, extracting relevance from knowledge systems belonging to other cultures and their unfamiliar epistemological territory should be possible, designed in paradigms of science.

The Industrial Age, Colonisation; Knowledge Enhancement in Civilisational Conflict and Ideological contention.

The phase of imperial expansion advanced science and the industrial revolution. Nations extended the trade and commerce well developed before imperial acquisitions. Following them, vast plantations provided raw products like cotton, tea, cocoa and sugar. Estates owned by members of the landed gentry of Britain, for example, were worked by the colonial or by local indentured or translocated labour. The latter, isolated and without the moorings of the culture of the lands they were transported to, were generally easier to manage. They added to the native stock, in the Caribbean, for instance, with implications to demography, creating complex cultures and influencing the political development of those countries. Colonisation was dispersed across the Americas, the Caribbean, Africa, countries of the Indian Ocean and the Far East beyond the Pacific. Cocoa, tobacco, tea and cotton were transported back to Britain for processing, and the finished products made for great profit, hardly to be seen as trade being unequal or forced upon the colonies or wherever else power could be asserted. Originally a few families with landed interests dominated in the colonies, but they expanded into large commercial houses and became a physical presence established widely across the many ports of the globe. Plantations and mercantile interests provided massive profits, vast fortunes and stately homes; wealth accumulated, increasing the resources for industry at home. Amongst the newly endowed, the creative artist found a place along with the wastrel and the effete.

'The Word' in Europe, available on paper for a while and soon in print, was the stimulus for propagating new ideas. Theological arguments were easily perverted for political ends, and disaffected populations readily assumed identities followed by civil strife—the usual blood-letting and the destruction of hallowed places of worship. The nations of Europe were constantly in conflict, and as the political landscape changed in Christian dissension between Protestant and Catholic, the countries had readier reasons for war. The printed word, however, was a stimulus to general curiosity, yet led to more disciplined learning; the 16th Century was undoubtedly one of intense intellectual enterprise. A ferment of reformatory ideas preceded revolts, revolution and the Imperial onslaught but the industrialisation of Europe increased National rivalries and hostilities. The peasantry of the mainland obtained some rights to land and a livelihood in agriculture. Critical thinking was more widely dispersed, and a wider spread to reading, if not to education, gradually initiated marginal changes to political power and class structures. The functional divisions to society now provided a very substantial class of merchant traders who gained influence as the holders of Capital and assumed a new importance for the economy of these nations. The power equations were changing, and with them the nature of social contention. Larger sections of the population were becoming participants in the changing scene, with immense implications for society and the sociology of knowledge.

A slew of new technologies laid the basis for rapid industrialisation. In Britain whole communities were drawn in from miserable rural conditions to work for wages. A livelihood was more secure although the conditions of new urban townships were even more benighted. 'Among those dark satanic mills' was a new wage economy for miners within the accompanying squalor of the mining towns. A new labouring class raised Britain as a leading industrial power and laid the foundation for Imperial enterprise. Expanding industries, promoted by higher and improved technology and steel, provided rapid transport, a system of steam powered railways and sea-faring vessels. Naval power was established with superior gunnery, firearms and navigational systems. The cotton industry was mechanised enabling the looms to run off merchandise in quantity. Coal from the collieries of Wales and Lancashire, from the deep and damp seams of the earth and under the sea-beds, was excavated to run the machinery. The miners brought unparalleled wealth to the new industrial barons at the cost of their lungs and lives; labour was cheap for the wages paid, and the conditions they worked and lived in was abysmal. The manufacture of mass-produced cloth out of the raw cotton shipped from distant lands to the cotton mills of Lancashire, and its sale back to Egypt and India at lower prices, led in turn to the devastation of native populations whose occupation were weaving the cloth and its dyeing, from the fields of cotton and indigo. The entrepreneurs provided capital for an enterprise: the last great Imperium. And the world moved on, also in the gain for Science and its disciplines.

Colonisation had followed from a foothold gained in early trading enterprises established in foreign ports, often bringing the nations of Europe into conflict with each other or with local rulers. However, for those in the areas of contact it marked the experience of new and more efficient technology, and the ideas that were becoming a powerful influence in Europe. There industrialisation had created a new labouring class, workers who gradually needed to be trained, and hence required education for at least a minimum of competence in handling machinery and familiarising to technology. A demand for empowerment arose in the ranks of organised collectives of workers; a new class and culture was emerging in industrial society with a considerable impact on the sociology of knowledge. Elementary education veering to universalisation was a feature in late industrial societies as working class power was established. The impulses of the times stimulated a demand for the disciplines of the natural and social sciences and the creation of diverse educational facilities to meet the needs of industrial society.

The accumulation of wealth changed social relationships and instilled a new order of intellectual curiosity which was reflected in the rigorous disciplinary method of the sciences. The physical sciences fuelled a technological revolution, vital for industry. A notable feature of modern Science was its universal function and applicability, unlike previous sciences or related knowledge which had marked cultural orientations. Universality characterises the method of science which had been transformed into a global enterprise.

Finally, for the reshaping into organised nationhood of countries that were colonised or who had succumbed to Imperial might, it was necessary to get beyond territorial fiefdoms and feudal enervation. Violent imperial incursion and social devastation preceded the recognition that to repulse Imperialism there was the need to shed or break the shackles of tradition. This was possible only by retracing the ancient genius of dormant civilisations in the fresh acquisitions to knowledge, to assimilate and often to adapt the new intellectual ferments that commenced beyond their own time-worn world[xxi]. For example, Confucianism as a philosophy for political discourse was hardly viable for the times. The old order had to be dismantled to overcome China's disunity and disarray. The leaders in uprisings were often an erudite elite, educated in the West but in contention with it, who influenced or installed a sequence of minor authoritarian regimes. The regimes changed in the activism of increasing numbers of China's people across the countryside and the students in her cities until finally Revolution consolidated the Chinese nation in a Central Authority. This, in its turn, brooked no dissent or political debate, a policy which later led to the worst famine of the century, man-made starvation and mass death in authoritarian intransigence.

The Indian experience of repulsing Imperial power was in many ways in a contrasting ethos. Indian philosophy and her classics were in Sanskrit and Pali. The contents and the language of the former interested Western scholars for its Indo Aryan origins, and were the first to be translated by them into German and English. Otherwise, the knowledge of Sanskrit texts was essentially the domain of Brahmin hierarchies, who ritualised religious literature for the use of society at large. Aurobindo Ghose was one amongst many noted scholars and philosophers in a newly emerging Indian bourgeoisie with an English education who used their heritage to great effect for newer aspirations. Mohandas Gandhi, later the leading light in the movement for Indian independence, was initially called to the Bar in London, then set up a practise on another continent where he experienced racial injustices at first hand. Much else, such as life in a community that he organised, and extensive study which included readings of Tolstoy, shaped the political philosophy of Indian passive resistance. Non-violence as a political movement on that scale was, nonetheless, a revolt which involved the masses as enthusiastic participants towards the accomplishment[xxii] of Independence.

The mainstay of Colonial might was an army extensively manned by the Nepali, the Sikh—Indian sepoys, whom Britain repeatedly used not only upon recalcitrant Indian subjects but in subjugating other colonies if her writ was ever challenged. These soldiers had sworn loyalty to the British monarch, and the reasons for such a loyalty have not had sufficient survey. The fact of the Indian rather than others as the mainstay of colonial soldiery recruited to the armies of Britain in her many wars across the globe is a generally glossed-over sociological enigma. Apart from and despite the mutiny of 1857, The British Indian army has received only plaudits for its performance in the interests of the foreigner. However, the Chinese, during repeated revolts against Imperial aggression, suffered the Indian mercenaries' batons and bullets had nothing but contempt for them, and little reason to understand Indian travail in their own country. The passage of opium across to China, a profitable trade for Indian merchants as well, was further reason for ill-will.

However, Indian perceptions began to change. The demonstration of Japanese power during World War II against former Imperial hegemony, and in particular Britain's humiliating defeat by them, had demonstrated the vulnerability of a former Imperialism and its waning power in India,. There was increasing uncertainty about the role of the Indian in the British armed forces. The culminating act prior to the British decision to withdraw from that sub-continent was the revolt of personnel in ships of the Royal Indian Navy and the prospect of further mutiny within the Armed Forces. It loomed large not only to the rulers but its portent to an Indian leadership negotiating independence that was unwelcome. The Labour Government of post War Britain appreciated that revolt as 'The Point of No Return'.

Reflections on disciplinary narrations of 'the other'.

Often it is the nature of earlier European contact with the rest of the world from the 16th century onwards which played a dominant part in the scholarship of the many disciplines interpreting the character of their new found space. Newer disciplines and methodologies derived from this contact had anchored students and votaries firmly but narrowly to them as specialists. Post-colonial and post-World War II, there has been reappraisals of many disciplines. The history of Sciences and lately, the perspectives, textual myths, and methodology of medicine and public health are being reviewed[xxiii]. The scale of the re-accounting of the historiography of the social sciences is quite considerable and concerns fallacies of content. For instance, previous colonial narration related a public's state of health to climatic and even to racial differences.

The nature of clinical practice since its inception as a social function was fairly seamless, through the ages in universal social characteristics. Changes relate to phenomenal new knowledge but its ethos, seen in medical cultures through history and across geography, still fits Hippocratic essentials. The idea of the clinic and the special relationship of physician to patient contained altruistic value in its functioning and belongs to the history of all civilisations. In today's culture of corporatisation values are shifting to the measure of the market. Alarm bells should be sounding far louder from the keepers of medicine but the subject has not exercised the practitioner, and the concern of most medical scientists suffices in finding the funds as methods of research get increasingly expensive. Within the decades following the intense debates of post-World War II, when the disciplines of social sciences established health welfare as a public utility amongst the nations of Europe, the many benefits that had accrued have been steadily pared down, or jettisoned in the belief that competition would improve the functioning of institutions responsible for societal health and public welfare. Those institutions convert to other marketable products which fit the prevailing economic ideology of value-addition through competition.

The immense benefits from the establishment of Welfare as State policy and were seen in the measured indices of Health for their populations. Yet, for some nations Welfare is anathema, while others more mildly regard it as the socialist nanny, debilitating free enterprise muscle. Needless to say a giant structure of corporates has developed, thriving on the exaggerated taxes, private health insurance and pharmaceutical profit; even as citizens are increasingly subject to ill-health in the default commerce of sales without statutory control, or pre-emption to a market in edibles of nutritive content unstructured for health needs. Concepts of primary health care increasingly damaged by free enterprise require new initiatives. There is a ballooning expenditure for the polity of some developed nations: the price for allowing private enterprise its free ride into a nation's health, and in following such models there is even more damage for the undeveloped. Such experience is contradicted in the evidence of the Scandinavian countries, who return the best indices to health in improving regulations of the Welfare State.

The Colonial interlude and its appraisals of local knowledge.

The arrogation of worth to the disciplines that arrived from the civilisations of Europe was for their scientists also an exploration of the knowledge systems in place before and beyond Science. The manner of that performance has pertinence for academia right into the present. The reaction of practitioners of traditional therapeutic systems was very naturally to hold fast to their own ways, a disdain for science disallowing the possibility of development. Vandana Shiva characterised the tendencies in the opening address at the 4S/EASST conference in Goteborg in 1994, where, in a sweeping summary, she said. "Between 1492 and 1992 Europe's meeting with non-European cultures was actually no real meeting. The interaction by the colonised was always experienced as invasion and by the colonisers as discovery. The experience of invasion as discovery has been facilitated there through which European men had constructed a world in which evolution was understood to have created two separate minds—one for themselves and one for all others".

Nowhere was this better exemplified than in the attitudes of the Colonial disciplinary investigators to the knowledge and institutions of organised humanity in a non-European space. Yet today, while attempting an understanding of the medical sciences of a traditional body of knowledge which did arise in that space, we must assume some acquaintance with their history and the widespread practice of traditional medicine in developed or undeveloped societies of the world. With traditional therapeutics the medical scientist is aware of certain implications to their practice but barely has to acquaint himself with their content. Traditional Medicine is often the sole recourse to primary health care for many amongst world populations especially of countries that return abysmal health indices. As Complementary and Alternative medicine it has found a considerable attraction for those in the developed world as well. Credulity and cultural acceptance combine in motivating populations to seek help from traditional therapeutics. Self-medication becomes a problem when entrepreneurs promote un-researched products of traditional medicine for that growing market. These are hazardous to patients, a problem common to both worlds, which could be minimised through better coordination between medical establishments, scientists and traditional practitioners. Public health is jeopardised if Traditional therapeutics is counterpoised merely as an alternative to scientific medicine at any level of health care.

'Discovery' in this way amounts to interpreting the unknown in the terms of what can be explained by, or fit into the disciplinary parameters of science. The traditional functionary will consider such reductive interpretation by the scientist to be ill founded, a presumptuous dilution of complexities that lie beyond the ken of science. While a popular medical tradition like acupuncture is introduced to programmes of clinical investigation for validation or in primary sector health care, one is reminded of a trajectory followed previously in science and the reasons for the term 'invasion' to describe some of these efforts. Assumptions are made about the value of previous knowledge, but hardly in familiarising with the systems of therapeutics evolving over centuries. Scientists are aware of bio-therapeutic possibilities in traditional methods, yet the history of their disciplinary enterprise was governed by attitudes as they came upon these systems. It was to minimalise their content, disregarding epistemology for the little that could be interpreted in science—a position that has been resisted with some justification by the traditional practitioner, since clinical investigation was hardly directed to a scientific explanation of his practice.

The advent of the Colonial into indigenous systems

For a considerable while Colonial academics interpreted cultures, or the specialised knowledge of the alien, in narratives that were directed to the benefit, understanding and power of administrations ruling over foreign space. The study of extraneous cultures, no matter if in the field of the arts, philosophy or the sciences, was limited to the context of a colonial enterprise "—to create other forms of knowledge about the people they were ruling—", says Cohn[xxiv] and to continue with his perception of the imperatives that regulated the disciplines, "Most investigative modalities were constructed in relation to institutions and administrative sites with fixed routines. Some were transformed into 'sciences' such as economics, ethnology, tropical medicine, comparative law or cartography, and their practitioners became professionals."

How, for instance, does a separate medical discipline 'Tropical Medicine' come about? It obviously derives from the diseases experienced by the colonial in his sojourn in climates and conditions new to him. But as epidemic or endemic diseases they were hardly new, and were once faced in all their vigour in his native lands where they had subsequently been controlled in improved urban conditions such as sanitation, potable water and an awareness and education in better social hygiene. When they were encountered again in the tropics the well-known scourges became transferred to the collection of diseases classified and labelled 'Tropical Medicine' as another discipline. Undoubtedly, to add to that previously experienced collection, endemic diseases such as Leishmaniasis and sickle cell anaemia were also seen the Tropics, and then medical scientists like the Norwegian, Hansen, G H (1841-1912), bacteriologist and physician, and Ronald Ross (1857-1932) to mention just two names of those who pioneered further investigation and discovery in the East, added leprosy and malaria to its medical lore. Leprosy and Plague convert to 'Tropical' disease despite both having ravaged Temperate Europe, while Malaria had had its considerable Mediterranean presence.

The biological sciences developed in the West during the four centuries preceding the present and gradually assumed world dominance. But, either in ignorance or misinterpretation, much of the learning of the lands administered by the early colonist was considered by scholars, at best, as interesting but hardly worthy of pursuit, and certainly not in their 'debilitated' epistemology. Endemic diseases, known as such to the colonial doctor, were known within the respective epistemologies of medical traditions but were not effectively dealt with by them. While bacteriological discoveries in science helped to consign a few diseases to history, other ills were controlled or eliminated through better nutrition, sanitation and social hygiene. For instance Plague had largely been eliminated by public drainage systems and the control of its vector, as well as new cases of leprosy (they have been identified in the US where they no longer present the social hazard they still may do in India). Control of malaria and water-borne diseases owes much to adequate public health infrastructure, sanitation, resource systems for piped water and closed drainage, measures which inhibit vectors of disease from breeding. These measures are abysmally inadequate in many countries of the tropics. The demarcation as a 'Tropical' Disease is arguable for those that are still endemic for the want of sanitary amenities and a basic hygiene infrastructure. Tuberculosis, despite the earlier promise to its control by antibiotics has assumed alarming resistance to them amongst undernourished populations of the world.

Clinical research in medicine could be constructed with a view to maximise the health impact on society in general, an endemic group within that society, or on a diagnostic category of patients. It bears the stamp, in so far as methodology is determined, of the regulations of the scientific culture for problems specific to that society; those same disciplinary regulations when used remote from the one within which it was fashioned, will generally require adaptation based in an acquaintance of the new context.

The supremacy of Colonial Power, its universal impact on individual and social life influenced every branch of scholarship. Notwithstanding the enormous contribution that the disciplines have made to human well-being on a global scale, the methods of study of many social sciences were meant for another space and their constitution for another context. Those regulations and methods were used to study other cultures, subcultures and social conditions, and resistance to unimaginative applications in the new context was not surprising. There were obvious clashes of perception between the ruled and their rulers. The distortion extended to scholars' view of the discipline of the other. 'Invasion' thus was not an unusual perception for the native scholar, but in medicine 'discovery' had occurred but rarely; usually a possibility might be conceded and then a tentative reinterpretation of tradition was made within the existing principles of the new discipline. Another post-colonial term, 'subaltern', placed recognition of the socially unprivileged as its importance, especially in the heyday of Marxist studies; but they never gained impact as they lost their way in Marxist didactics. Dialectics and contradictions were outstanding paradigms for academics to master before formulating the problem for scientific study.

As with Sanskrit and, later, from the wide Indian fund of ancient languages, exceptionally fruitful excursions were made to language, linguistics and related fields of study by respective votaries collaborating in mutual interest toward that achievement. Although, in general foreign interference was rejected in the usual assumption of civilisational superiority, a presumption and hindrance to developing knowledge. Hence numerous applications, and the pursuit and teaching of indigenous systems of knowledge, continue in their preferred isolation rather than in dialogue; and the stasis is supported in Health policies irrespective of their results.

An essential prerequisite to the avoidance of extreme attitudes would have been to acknowledge respective systems of knowledge and to gain familiarity with their contextual importance. Language in translation requires close attention to many aspects, the grammar, linguistic complexity and structure for local comprehension. The quality of a translation thus depends on objective and subjective variables. Interested scholars understand philology, local institutions and their interpretations of data, commentaries on the subject and the later collations. With therapeutic and medical disciplines, development and progress is also possible with insight into ancient systems and this is more likely to happen in collaborative effort. The structures of traditional medical systems do not as a rule concern the modern medical investigator whose primary interest has been to convey treatment results by resorting to the protocols of modern therapy. Constant replications and repetitions calibrate outcomes and clinical assessment of the value of former medical systems; but one suspects that the structure and practices of those therapies do not, per se, fit a modern paradigm for study or the designs of protocols. The enterprise may benefit from the precepts which have furthered valuable exchange within the linguistic disciplines, rather than the assumptions and immutability of modern medical science for obtaining evidence of efficacy.

Outstanding examples of the failure of purely utilitarian approaches are to be found in many anthropological studies, of tribal communities who lived their centuries in cultures isolated and unchanging, and who then were defined as the 'primitive'. The general trend of the studies, however, served the purposes of administrative utility. The specialist functioning in the field may not have had a life-line experience of the subject of his study but that was not an obstacle to his interpretation of the way of life of innumerable small communities none of whom may ever have known an outsider. Strict academic norms have been formulated but their definition was extraneous and not developed for a particular context. An illuminable possibility could exist in methods of the discipline, provided they defined the study for the subject, which most often needs special access across a range of attributes to such communities. Some notable exceptions and remarkable studies have demonstrated the possibility through lived-in contacts so vital for the validity of anthropological studies[xxv],[xxvi].

Social accord and discord, for instance, as defined in Civil and Criminal Law, hinges on property and ownership, a concept as foreign to the subject as the societies for whom those Legal Codes were written. Ownership and the right to property were non-existent in ancient social organisation and custom, and the Law of the alien naturally categorised certain tribes as criminal when they continued helping themselves to whatever happened to be useful to their existence or merely provoked their curiosity. The habitat within which they lived and functioned did not 'belong' to them or any other, but was an essential expression of their humanity. The vitality of communities whose survival depended on a complex relationship with an environment was, for the administrative powers regarded as 'property', and its proprietorship was vested in the State. 'Law and order' follow from the idea of property and the rights pertaining to it, a concept unknown to any tribe. An extreme example but one sufficient to explain that the manner of the introduction of legal science, a discipline conceptualised for another society and in another context, condemned those ignorant of that value as transgressors and criminals. The Imperium has now ceased but long after, that same law without re-examination continues to be the benchmark in the Legal Codes of the present Indian Republic. Ownership of forest land now features in innumerable economic exigencies; the State asserts social and democratic rights, even to the subterranean mineral wealth, in that grand project designated 'development', with a nod to helping our ancient inhabitants to relocate from their forests, or even providing a secular safeguard to a few square feet of land enclosing their deities.

Health Care and the dichotomy between
traditional and modern medicine

The tendency in the definition of science is to contain other discourses resulting from specialised forms of knowledge such as traditional medicine within their time-bound epistemology. Such an approach may find historical significance and some clinical value, but diminishes the possibility of an inclusive medical system of primary health care for nations that are presently more dependent on traditional medicine. Systematic inclusion into a singular medical culture is socially desirable and vital to Public Health. Evidence-based therapeutics provides objectively safer practice when used for clinical indications—disease pathology as described in medicine. That requirement is considered in a later chapter. The process may also be revelatory if the therapeutic facets of a tradition can be explored within its own practice. History, as considered here, suggests the possibility.

From the standpoint of Modern Medicine, Traditional Medicine is given a categorical position attributed to medical applications of the past. It is Complementary at best: or a meagre 'Alternative' to the repast of scientific medicine. Therapeutic traditions are consigned to the nominal category of CAM, an over-arching term. Traditional Medicine by definition is non-scientific. Its acceptance by the scientific community of medicine is equivocal, though occasionally with notable and exceptional scientist interest. Its survival is viewed as an anachronism and the fact of its continuing practice creates little investigative interest for medical policy makers. They are content to allow for it an inevitable presence in its civilisational identity. Traditional systems as a continuing utility in the developed world are related to a mounting public discomfiture with the aspects of general medical practice that people have come to lack confidence in, and its constitution increasingly regarded as a non-social enterprise where Corporates profit from public health needs. In the critical anxiety about trends in medicine, the revealed inadequacies of drugs, their marketing and their inordinate use; and iatrogenic illness, the de-personalisation of hospital systems and even of clinical practices, are all factors of public concern which contribute to interest in 'alternative' therapies. They are regarded as time-tested and less hazardous—a public perception that has little substantiation in medical evidence, though in general their therapists offer attention that is more personalised compared to the institutions and even General Practice in modern health care.

The resulting response of Health Administrations in the West towards a variety of practices which include traditional medicine is to see themselves as representative of the medicine of the 'scientific' community. Within Europe, the differing national responses generally display an insularity, a disinterest towards the socio-historical validity of traditional medicine or the need to come to terms with and evaluate the separate therapeutic methods on offer. Recommendations follow from uncertainty: having to evaluate its worth, Health Administrations delegate that responsibility to bodies whose remoteness from scientific method is an issue, while suggesting they design standards and training programmes for traditional practice. The Netherlands and Sweden safeguard their public largely by involving traditional medicine or acupuncture within research and health care and achieve more towards its safety and utility on a wider scale than the United Kingdom. (See report, Alternative Medicine, BMA 1988. & Socialstyrensen papers). Making necessary distinctions between the plethora of traditional practices bracketed into CAM (Complementary and Alternative Medicine) High powered Committees appointed to look into health practices beyond modern medicine from an assumed monoculture of Scientific Western medicine offer a singular lack of appreciation of the plurality of systems of healing. The assessment fails to address real problems for the public when committees are unable to engage with and differentiate between Ayurveda, Chinese Acupuncture and Bach Flower Healing, Reflexology or osteopathy. Waving them into one of two categories, either Complementary or Alternative Medicine, is an approach that is little help to physicians or patients in making informed choices.

In short, systems of knowledge related to health care which developed over centuries within certain societies are tarred with the same brush as those which can spin a pretty penny for the itinerant mendicant/ physician, his barrel organ and his 'potions'. From the familiar perch of the development and institutionalised practice of Western medicine in less than two hundred years, its Establishment squints at the issues through spectacles with distinct lenses; one for science and the other for non-science. It is scarcely surprising then that committees set up by representative organisations for medical practice go to some lengths to demonstrate the virtues of scientific medicine, recommend it for systems that have come from vastly different epistemic traditions, and end up by suggesting that all those 'Complementary and Alternative' systems should set about putting their respective houses in 'scientific' order. That science itself should motivate Complementary or Alternative Medicine barely engages with the existing social and academic confusions about them.

"If, looking in the street where the light is better for the keys lost within the home, something maybe found other than the keys themselves"

CHAPTER II

THERAPEUTIC SYSTEMS, KNOWLEDGE EXCHANGE AND ENHANCEMENT

Migration, war and demographic change. Biological endowment and advancing civilisation.

There are knowledge-related activities, prime functions of pre-historic collectives which advance to specialised ones as society organises to the demands of civilisation. Amongst tribes groups form to feed people and others use their empirical insights to assume powers of healing and assuage suffering or illness. Specialist activities are increasingly in demand to systematise knowledge and use it, as societal organisation progresses to civilisations.

Warfare or migrations open up territory to other groups and the reaction is to attempt to insulate their respective identities. Extermination is extreme, but previous residents or new intruders may attempt it against one another to isolate or retain intact respective cultures from contamination by the other—group isolation, or persecution and slaughter, were the usual means towards it. Failure is obvious over time. Society changes character; its performance is enhanced in social interdependence and the slow but inevitable mix of peoples. Skills apparent in either culture, or the improvements brought by the newcomer, provide newer tools for use, or even basic techniques, improving capabilities and production. Functionally organised society and the development of specific forms of knowledge are means to the gains and growth of a civilisation. The facts of history show great migrations in antiquity, following which pristine ethnicities hardly ever exist. Yet, such identities maintain at least a nominal survival. They can hardly be sustained in genetics or in biological attributes.

From a base of elementary knowledge how does later enhancement come about? One early means was in diversity of peoples as a result of additions to previous stock. Interbreeding could also change biological determinants, leaving a mark on development. New skills emerge, with improvisation and technology gathering pace. Societies reorganise despite initial trauma of much of their history: technology, social functions and culture advance to new levels of efficiency. Biologically, the changes were not just to human morphology and physical qualities, but in cognitive mental processes which might register new possibilities, at least in some individuals. A means to utilise muscle power and energy output to greater advantage with a log is elementary mechanisation, but to use it as a lever is undoubted discovery in its context. The benefit accruing to one community is unlikely to be lost to another. Notwithstanding nurture, the process of learning and cultural conditioning from childhood, to see differently what once was unremarked upon questioned, developed and applied within the prevailing culture, may be the result of an added neural facility giving further versatility to cognition.

The manifestations of Nature, originally depicted in oral traditions, were later interpreted in language, overwritten in myth or other art heritage of a civilisation. They generally suggested immutability and permanence, a counter to the uncertainty and inscrutability of the world, and were imbued with significances, characteristically conveyed in metaphysical expression. Cultures and traditions seek an order for society which also imposes limitations and absolves in its many regulations, the need for critical thinking. Life-styles and thought are circumscribed. To gainsay the restrictive feature of tradition is often to transcend cultural boundaries. Identifiable and diverse groups and cultural diversity, despite the catastrophic commencement to their arrival on the scene are often the means to revitalising civilisation.

The 'natural' may convey a difference and, importantly, a cognitive shift initiating an individual experience of it beyond the accepted. A need arises for the natural to be examined for another explanation; sometimes the process to discovery or creativity. Another experiential formulation of what, hitherto, was unremarkable, finds in the new a rationality more appealing to society or its peers through having passed some essential test of validity. Knowledge derived from empirical insights and proved in the testing, carries a conviction quite distinguishable from the acceptance of the assertive revelations resulting from hallucinatory or visionary mental excursions of the prophet and seer. Societies living and thinking within entrenched cultures, when subjugated by other peoples or forced to contend with their culture, may find an energy that hitherto lay dormant, for change and toward renewal. Civilisations gain effective knowledge in the constant reappraisals, changing structures of power and social reorganisation when populations are forced into living together. These factors appear to be of greater importance to developing knowledge than the merits of particular human stock.

Better food sustenance and improved methods of production improve society's viability and exposure to the cultures of diverse peoples enhances social organisation. Separate systems of healing can coexist, or new techniques may, in the borrowing, develop into systematic therapeutic forms. The benefit to societal health and longevity is a test of function, as knowledge enhances in expanding cultures. Despite the often turbulent passage of incursions of peoples and newer systems of thought, in history they have repeatedly demonstrated improved means to exploit nature and to control its vagaries, and to move on as civilisations.

A few illustrative models

Patterns to advancing civilisation have largely depended on the mixing of human stock and diverse ethnicities across the spaces of the earth from antiquity to medieval times, and from there at a quicker pace in the centuries preceding the present. With their sea-faring ability stone age tribes migrated across wide oceanic distances from the African mainland to unpopulated land in an Australasian space. That land was not barren. Tribes cast into an unknown environment, without the knowledge or elementary methods to explore newer methods of life support, were trapped and isolated by geography or their preferred insularity. They lost their original tools unutilised over the following generations; techniques of production never had the chance to improve. Their numbers diminished, and in later colonial history tribes have withered.

The Australoid in Tasmania contrasts with the Maori of New Zealand, the latter as an example of renewing possibilities to survival. Of Polynesian ancestry, the Maori migration struggled through and survived. Their common ancestry allowed intermarriage between different groups and, even in the later incursion of the European, trade and other exchange was welcomed! Later their numbers were considerably reduced by the European in deadly wars and, further, in their lack of immunity to the insurgent's diseases. But despite the violence and unsavoury commencement to the meeting with the European migrant, they have since increased in numbers and progressed to demonstrate New Zealand's interesting cultures within a composite society. The country maintains separate cultures in a recognisable civilisation essentially European, which in the impress of time should be a transformed society of intermingled stock.

Over two millennia BCE the history of Babylon was comprised of Hittite and Sumerian war and conquest. The people of the region endured. In time enlarged empires catered to the interests of diverse communities, furnishing the area with newer attributes of civilisation. There was a conveyance of ideas and aptitudes that came with the migrants into the new territory. One such was a codification of laws for regulating civil society. To set up a system suitable for the context required, knowledge, law-makers and institutions particularly as law and order now became the responsibility and vested in the power of the State. The efforts of a visionary Emperor, Hammurabi, unusual for his time, are particularly notable in the recognition of responsibility to his subjects and its diverse groups and to convey the sense of fairness to all. Even the professional classes were in its purview. If a patient died during the course of a physician's treatment, the punishment, also set down in the Code, was to lop off his arm. The compensation awarded against pharmaceutical companies in present litigation is more benign for mishaps of larger scale, and culpability!

Initially the passage was fraught, the migrant unwelcome and ostracised, the invader resisted or isolated. But society is enriched in the eventual absorption, peoples having brought their special talents and other creative and intellectual activities; knowledge, the arts and architecture finding new expression within the exchange. Astronomy and mathematics obtained fresh perspectives, and mutual transactions of considerable value, have followed as in the Greek incursions during their period of immense Empire building. Builders, artisans and artists brought other methods and new architectural forms to the old, and Greece itself gained in return from foreign contact. There is the evidence of transposed humanity, the women and the artisans who followed Alexander's returning armies from his short-lived Eastern Empire whose mark on Greece should be better traceable in the present.

New institutions and methods of statecraft required to be created in response to the challenges of diversity in society. State enterprises brought efficiencies by better management of trade or agriculture. Of the latter we see an outstanding example from the earliest South American civilisations derived from Palaeolithic, Mongoloid migrants of the Old World, and in further population diversification forming the hardier Mayan, Aztec and Incan.

The impact of the potato on the mediaeval history of Europe is well recognised, hardly for their science in its original cultivation and Incan contribution[i], for which hopefully some correction has been mentioned in the last chapter. We now know far more about South American civilisations of varying qualities, most laid waste in the Imperial deluge of the Portuguese and Spanish conquistadores. Virtually enslaved, local manpower was used for the mining and transporting of silver confiscated from the continent's rich mountain streaks. The current dietary satisfaction of our worlds has its price in the ravages; but today potatoes, tomatoes, pumpkins, peppers, the corns and innumerable beans, fruit and greens are taken so much for granted with barely a nod to the genius of its originators. In deconstructed history, reappraisals of the Imperial narrative show the violence of that contact. The conquistador's unsavoury inquisitorial fervours equalled his appetite for gold and, incidentally, also translocated for the Old World populations an invaluable food source in the potato. Its expansive cultivation ultimately provided a substitute for the cultivation of grain with its uncertain yields. In Europe and across to Ireland, countries plagued by the centuries of war and interminable famine, there was at last a valuable and dependable food source which enabled a reversal of the severe population depletion of those years. The contribution of the ancestors of the South American peoples and their inspired intelligence illustrates the need to appreciate the universality of knowledge, its acquisition and applications, without preconceptions motivating the narration about civilisational attributes or where and how science was conceived and to definitions we owe to its history.

Our rich worlds—and poor, owe much to the Incans of South America, to their planned development and progress in the cultivation of innumerable farinaceous and horticultural produce that presently feed the world. The Incans encouraged a societal enterprise for healthy and

45

tasty eating. Certainly a sophisticated food culture is laid and developed in the biology of the receptors to taste, its sensory quality cultivating the excellence of cuisines of excellence of a few nations who take pride in that advancement today! The circular history of development and depression repeats, as parts of South America now import potato from the Netherlands. Today it is a continual struggle for survival and livelihood for the descendants of those who developed what later became Europe's staple nourishment when the potato not only ensured the survival of those populations which had been depleted by starvation in repeated famines but helped increase their fertility and numbers in its better nutritive qualities within a couple of later mediaeval centuries[ii].

Innumerable accounts of wanton and large scale depredation and human slaughter exist: the Crusades, the Muslim ingress into Europe and India, the establishment of the dynasties of China. We have noted European savagery vented on the natives of the New World. Violent death was an option for the 'savage heathen' unless he acceded to the inflicted Christ of the early Iberian Colonist, but even his survival as a Christian was a heavy cross; enslaved and forced to dig out the silver and gold from his mines, and load them onto the galleons returning to Spain. But, once again, we may be less well served in understanding the imprint and its consequence on the bio-sociology of the New World or the Old. The iniquities and transgressions of history cannot be recompensed. The nourishment, wealth and consequent population increase gained for the Old World was rapidly dissipated in reshaping its nations; borders constantly redrawn to accommodate new found identities while pogroms and evictions were reparation for the valuable diversity of Europe. Religious identity propelled its institutions and feudal families to curb and control populations; their armed groups asserted claims to territory, fiefdoms and minor kingdoms. Nations emerged through incessant wars; kingdoms changed names while borders were redrawn and populations shifted.

Human variety brought about by historical circumstance has never been regarded with popular enthusiasm. Populations, in denying entitlements or evicting others who can be identified as later residents or of another culture, substantial though it be, may gain materially in confiscated property, etc., or a perceived safety in insularity. Forms of exclusion are socially justified and instigated for political purpose or to serve the interests of a dominant religion. There is connivance, active support or passive acquiescence, or else, a claimed legitimacy, to a range of manifest inhumanities in the construction or pursuit of an identity—nationality, ethnicity, religion or even social class. The extremes are deportations, genocide, extermination of populations, the massive and obscene violence within memory and, hardly yet, history. Now, those responsible are regrouped into a new Community of Nations and, they never tire in extolling 'humanitarian' ideals in contrast to others. The decimation of other identities continues, brought on in refurbished zealotry. A future to be hoped for may restrict those recurrent frenzies to the flag-painted faces, the spectator-warriors watching international football and cricket.

Slavery, Caste and Chattels. Identities and civilisations.

Early civilisations required vast manpower for labour. Conquests gained territory and ensured a workforce by enslaving the conquered. It was possibly a means to increase productivity. From the cruel waste and inhumanity of the origins of slavery, from antiquity and well into the 18th century in the West Indies and the Americas, local or translocated slaves provided cheap labour. The system also brought biological enhancements to native populations. Forms of serfdom, if that status was gained from slavery, had not necessarily proved too remote from slavery itself. Slave and serf sustained the economies of the State and the wellbeing and comforts of those who owned them. The significance of slavery changes in medieval and in modern history and in its social dimensions, but the commencement was for unpaid labour which, in any form, eventually proved economically unsound. Some societies requiring slaves had profound fears of miscegenation. Male-oriented societies would mutilate slaves presumably allaying fears of virility more appreciated than their own. However, slaves have also risen to significant positions in early hierarchical societies. Exceptional talent could be projected to the highest echelons amongst communities that thrived by might of arms. Mediaeval societies, both West and East have profited from the talents of slaves, promoting them within the family or the polity to esteemed status and positions of power. Mediaeval merchant and trading communities had slaves who were a valued part of the family and business activity.

Discrimination, treating groups, as lesser humanity is not a feature of slavery alone. Even without institutionalised slavery, societies could transfer primal racial prejudice into legislative rationalisations by grading the inherited 'purity' of populations, although this was a biologically baseless exercise. Miscegenation today has many connotations in the consciousness of hierarchical societies, even in those without an experience of slavery as such. We are witness to extremes of social discrimination, exclusion of groups hereditarily restricted to serfdom or forms of chattel labour, or worse, the 'untouchable' in society. The ancient socio-religious edicts that sustain discrimination are powerful enough to have organised society and provided a labour force but the brutalities and human wastage of those cultures continue well past any economic necessity and continue still despite later legal and constitutional mandates for the empowerment and protection of those groups.

The consequences of slavery, 'race, caste and communal identities are persistent and pernicious. A prevailing consciousness amongst members of society who once lived by those divisions, well after legislation directed against its most glaring iniquities, continues to be a social problem, However, taboos toward preserving ethnicity, race and caste or other insularities are unsustainable. The culture persists but social mobility and constitutional safeguards make it more difficult to enforce endogamy as its mainstay. The change is slow and resisted by communities and their elders, but the erosion marks a steady leavening to cultures that are discriminatory. It is notable that in regions making rapid economic progress the communal regulations are less restrictive and freer association is possible. It is also the struggles of the underprivileged and their efforts that wring the change to these time-worn customs, whose purpose is long defunct.

The larger perspective is of changing demographic patterns and variety of cultures adding worth to civilisations. Though we live under increasing pressures of population and require its control, the presence of population variety has a profound social evolutionary significance. In the past burgeoning populations have increased wealth and well-being, their labour increasing production, but the socio-political power structure was inadequate for sustaining it and increased wealth was mostly dissipated in war, the reinventing of nations, and redefining structures of power.

The effects of population influx and cross breeding on original peoples expanded the knowledge base of societies and mark civilisations well beyond the grossest cruelties inflicted in attempts at seclusion. New social groups come about, but the assets to culture are often lost in the broad tendency to historical deconstruction. Byzantine civilisation straddled West Asia and Europe, and in early mediaeval times was a massive influence with immense implications to both. A land mass caught in the fluxes of suzerainty and changing shades of populations also provided an immense fertility to ideas and a variety to cultures but with common recognizable features across those civilisations. Most often in conflict, these unhappy exchanges gave the regions their artists and artisans, memorable art forms and architecture, which leave a recognisable imprint in a dispersed geography from Persia to an Arab North across the Caspian as well as into Mediterranean Europe. There were contributions to knowledge and medicine from a fertile West Asian civilisation, but their later enhancement of the therapeutic sciences as a continuity to that contribution is hardly acknowledged.

In sum, migration shakes up a genetic content of ethnic groups, contributing other shades to constituent peoples, culture and forms of knowledge. Occasionally we note peculiarities that relate well beyond neighbouring cultures, as the language of Finland demonstrates. Causes for its divergence from the three other Scandinavian languages might be immense migrations in antiquity, and linguistically distinct contributions from Asia. Uniqueness to older civilisations is apparent, existing within the reorganised boundaries of nation states, though notable cultural differences are maintained amongst populations marked off as communities. Languages, and within them modes of speech and dialects, mythologies, and the manner of family relationships; differing forms of law relating to property and civil rights; the methods of building—places of worship, palaces or even hovels; musical composition while the themes of the songs of diverse people retain common myths, the art forms to the singing and dancing diverge, as further do the regulations for health, dealing with disease, or the disposal of the dead[iii]—all as a cultural richness apparent in the inherited diversity of any civilisation.

Civilisations. Restricting the sources to historical achievement.

Academic benchmarks define, in specific achievement, the advent of civilisation. One such is the wheel, although its absence has not diminished the quality of the achievements of early civilisations: evidence of notable civilisations established without the wheel is found across the Western seaboard of South America.

Identities, religious or ethnic, Hindu or Muslim, Aryan or Arab, are even more restrictive and do not illuminate as definitions for civilisation, excluding, as they do, the sheer multiplicity of the origins and cultures that make for the quality of a civilisation. Endogamous dilutions by out-breeding, or even loss to a previous identity are considered enervating. But they are undeniable attributes for any civilisation whose richness derives from diversity of her peoples, the historical strands of their struggles and the intermingling.

Pursuing an identity for a civilisation is special pleading, which occasionally, in supportive evidence, verges on the farcical. Harappa, once the site of a notable and researched lost civilisation in the Indus valley dated to between 3-2000 BCE, was possibly a matrilineal agricultural society. This form of societal organisation today has only a limited residue in the very South West of the sub-continent. Arguments have recently been made to 'prove' continuity from that original population for Vedic (Hindu) civilisation in India, up to now regarded as commencing only following Aryan incursions and settlement. The contention is that a Vedic civilisation was untainted by the Aryan foreigner, but derived from, 'wholesome' indigenous peoples who originally inhabited Harappa and Mohenjo-daro. Amongst many evidences for this, the absence of the horse has so far been vital to the distinction between the two societies that inhabited the Indus valley, and its presence on seals and other artefacts have so far favoured evidence for the later Aryan and, together with many other evidences, lent credulity for a sophisticated civilisation. The horse was the logistic mode to the repetitive incursions of Aryan tribes into Northern India. Ingeniously, it appeared as evidence on earlier Harappan artefacts[iv], a distinctive horse with a reduced rib cage—shades of another creation story—. Certainly, to have a horse motif amongst the seals of Harappa's earliest inhabitants disestablished a migrant role for the horses in ancient India. The tracing of horse and peoples way back to the banks of the Indus valley was meant to establish Vedic civilisation in a hoarier past, as a Hindu lineage unsullied by the vagrant 'Aryan'. Such propositions about past civilisations have an appeal for the committed in today's increased identity orientation, showing their need for ethnic 'purity' to sustain the untenable as peoples in diversity live and breed as human species without much consideration for bygone totems.

India

The only stock that can claim a habitation in India previous to migrants and invaders are the peoples presently most deprived and repeatedly damaged socially, the 'adivasis' (first inhabitants). The tribes are scattered around the subcontinent with a presence in the North Eastern and Southern States and the islands around and possibly derived from primary human stock before later land separation into other continents. Social intolerance and mythology deny them, to an extent, the dignity of a culture while civil laws, supporting predatory mining lobbies, rob them of a right to their livelihood. The immense value of the peoples in pre-historic genesis and culture is hardly recognised. Apart from their rightful claim to a civil status, in their steady decline we are losing a fund of irreplaceable linguistic, anthropological and genetic information and such material as offered in their culture—a wealth that the State's short sightedness would forfeit for the exploitation of minerals, and the land and forests which have prior claimants. The traditional abode of an adivasi as property is an unknown concept to him. Language and lore are lost as tribes are forced to disperse, change their life modes or disappear into extinction. A scientific accounting has barely commenced of these invaluable people in the retentive context of their origins, their oral traditions and herbal remedies, still viable and in our midst.

The idea of an Indian is hardly influenced by a pre-history or rooted in antiquity, despite the claims. Rather, he retains cultural uniqueness despite his composite nature following accommodations to incessant invasions and comparatively peaceful migrations of an evolving civilisation. Even after the external impositions following conquest and local resistance, the initial ravages, destruction and turmoil, society moved on into a social compact of living in proximate cultures. Populations of differing descent lived largely in peace without the need to assert their differences. The hordes of outsiders and changing dynasties did not produce revolutionary movements, but political exigencies brought changes which rippled across a civilisational space while settling across a social core. The subcontinent began a realisation of nationality as the narration of a singular civilisation comparatively late within geographical boundaries but, diluted in the older identities of castes, language and corresponding cultures.

Hinduism had its profound impact in shaping the growth and achievement of this civilisation, but its philosophical principles, epics and literary past, a founding source of theosophical ideas, rather than a Hindu theology, inspired, and afforded impulses for her subsequent religions, Buddhism and Jainism. It is useful to remember, pantheism and agnosticism, spiritualism, systematised materialism, and idealism, including the religions mentioned, all find philosophical expression varying in degree of contention, within the intellectual resources of Hinduism. They are repeated in regional languages, in local cultures and their wealth of literature, offering stupendous variety to interpretations of the epics and mythology[v]. The latter over the centuries, in many oral traditions, in poetry, theatrical sources and classical dance, rephrased the struggles and problems of evolving societies; offerings from separate cultures, yet providing the unique richness to an Indian civilisation.

Thus, the 'Idea of India' can hardly derive solely from the culture of Vedic peoples, or any other singular source or identity. A variety of kingdoms within a comparatively compact sub-continental geography, and peoples in different periods of its medieval history, presented a multi-cultural composition to the kingdoms, continuing today in the many regional languages and, within them, groups using dialects of the same source having difficulty in communication with those of another dialect.

The comparatively short lived Maurya Empire (BCE) 304-232 of Ashoka and, Akbar's post-mediaeval Empire were extensively sub-continental. Both have left a profound imprint on posterity. A series of South Indian Kingdoms, previous cultures invigorated by later transformations, made Imperial extensions beyond the peninsula, leaving a distinct cultural imprint on the nationalities of South East Asia. They retain varying emphasis in the cultures, Hindu, Chinese or Muslim peoples lending recognisable art and customs to each prior culture. Now they are become the post-colonial nation States of Burma, Malaysia, Indonesia, Cambodia, Indochina and Thailand. As for the Indian subcontinent, from North to South and East to West, regional cultures have barely consolidated in the political idea of 'India'. But even without the later civic importance as a nation, well prior a rich and composite Indian civilisation existed.

Salient to the Indian sub-continent, undoubtedly, is the repeated ingress of diverse peoples in the waves of invasion, a few outward migrations, and trade. Peoples from the West and possibly the East also, came across the passes of the North West mountain ranges and the valleys of the great rivers; down the Indus and further into the Indo-Gangetic plains. From the earliest times of the Christian era into the mediaeval, a considerable population traded on the sea routes from West Asia, from Egypt, Syria and Persia to ports on the coastline of South Western India; some migrating peoples finding profit in settlement, some groups seeking refuge, and others spread an earlier Christian message. Sparse settlements of Jews and

Christians, beginning at least as far back as the 4th CE, were known in Kerala. Later, along the South Western sea-board, settling in what is now Bombay or Gujarat came the Zoroastrian community of Parsis fleeing Arab suzerainty and the later Baha'i, an interfaith religion emigrated from Persia to retain their identity. Generally, incoming ethnicities have merged with the existing inhabitants; although, some like the above demonstrate a rich culture very open to cosmopolitanism and others, like the small very insular Jewish presence remains in Cochin, S. India. The larger Christian influx from Syria is no longer distinguishable from local populations, but retains in its own considerable theology, or rather theologies, that incorporate further sectarian Churches sourced from an original heretic Syrian Christianity. However, under attack, its religious adherents were totally united, strong enough to withstand the barbaric intensity of the Catholicism of the later Portuguese Colonist which was unleashed against the Syrian Church of Kerala. Commencing in the colonial ambitions of Peninsular Europe, her Catholicism enforced a ferocious interlude, as bloody as two later local Muslim chieftains, onto that novel enterprise of history.

Populations shifted South and East of Peninsular India, with former inhabitants consolidated into communities identified with language or religion, Muslim, Hindu, Buddhist and Jain, conveying recognisable source impulses; or, in the case of Buddhism, in divergences of spiritual content which carried a broad message across Asia, South and East, founding a substantial presence in China. Back home there also was a vibrant materialist philosophy and literature which drew upon the misfortunes of the lowest within a social hierarchy; poets of the movement expressed the content of religion with disdain, and its precepts as responsible for a class held in miserable tutelage within society. Mythology and literary forms find a civilisational identity, but the many Indian languages carry their message for a host of different communities as narrations of the social context.

Nevertheless, the strengths of hierarchical societies and stratified castes are a particularisation that holds. Diverse peoples of differing ethnicities have subscribed for centuries to divine patterns of order and disorder, the universal reflected in their social life and the trajectory of birth, death and rebirth in a timeless continuum encouraging changelessness. At one level corporeal finiteness and the limitation of this worldliness is to stress a consciousness of the divine; but that did not deter the exegetes and Institutions promoting its theology, to material acquisitiveness and wealth common to all societies and religion, land, lucre and gold finding favour with India's oldest Divinities and immense wealth of her better known Temples and places of pilgrimage. However argumentative the philosophies, her ancient religion and its tenets stress an ordained hierarchy to society and its endogamous regulations. There is milk and honey in the rules for social organisation at the pinnacles; rephrased in the idiom of the present, they sustain the many time-worn regulations as a model for modern living. Simultaneously, there is evidence of rapid change in a functioning democracy, which despite many shortcomings, has whittled down the older hierarchies, though they manage to hang on even in democratic institutions.

The Indian consciousness of nationhood as a democratic polity emerged late, achieved in the unified opposition to the previous Imperium. Religious denominations, chauvinism of linguistic regions and civil states, are now further demarcations of identity and loyalties; and there are politicised reconstructions to previous castes. The old social structure has not dismantled in later democratic institutions. Hierarchies are ingrained throughout the system, although electoral and constitutional rights gradually replace those that previously held the disaffected in thrall. The evident reality is a civic society, with large sections still educationally backward, their life at subsistence levels and hence without the possibility of asserting their individual rights. Politically empowered, they are aware of that power only as vested in a communal or regional identity, often antagonistic to secular and national interests. These are worked out through democratic institutions, but restricted to such interests; its members are pawns to the demagogue. Populations are left without the means to reason as individuals, and in democratic consensus find common ground in realising self-serving regional or communal options. It is the will of self-appointed leaders that prevails seeking power through the rabble and conveying identity interests; restrained now but the old identities and previous inter-communal strife are easily revived.

The nation is now portrayed as an economic powerhouse; it draws a veil over widespread hardship, mounting dissatisfactions and the enervation of society, as members are rarely in a position to individually process the available information. The result of limiting access to knowledge is an impoverishment which is reflected in the tenor of its frequent mass agitations. This makes a fertile context for authoritarian edicts, thought-control and censorship, ostensibly to assuage the sensitivities of one community or another. Censorship is the ultimate denial of a heritage of a civilisation noted for its rich diversity. As long as the basic right to institutional education is unrealised, a secular society is not attained, and a much lauded democracy has the brakes on in the spheres of activities that a democratic constitution could provide.

Therapeutic Diversity

The Indian sub-continent features a variety of therapeutic traditions, commencing in tribal remedies, utilising herbal sources and improving them as medicaments, potions and decoctions. The systems then founded developed the more advanced epistemologies of therapeutics, the theoretical structure of Siddha and Ayurveda. Another therapeutic system is Unani-tibb of Arab-Persian descent, acknowledged to have derived from Greek medicine. The system dispersed throughout the Indian subcontinent in mediaeval Moghul incursions and developed further sophistications locally. Unani has an equally popular base in the country as the other systems and has developed a few surgical procedures within it as well. Knowledge in one culture may in borrowing or transmission of resonances from others become transformed or restated.

Other traditional acquisitions in the culture of health and rehabilitation were the physical metabolic control systems of popular Yogic Practices, the movement and postures allowing meditative relaxation with some evidence that the techniques could control metabolism. Anecdotal evidence is the only support for the claims to many of the methods. Mental and physical 'rejuvenation' are, in any case, difficult physiological responses to assess. Yet another related empirical exploration of bodily function was the precise localisation of 'vital spots', an Indian tabulation of less sophistication than Chinese acupuncture points. Controlled pressure on them is reputed to alter circulatory or respiratory function and ancient groups of specialist warriors were trained to study and use them to incapacitate the enemy. These resemblances were formed from independent discovery or developed from possible common sources in India, China and Japan[vi]. Their use in the culture of Asia and the Far East developed for self-defence and presently is a form of sport. Hindu, Jain and Buddhist philosophies underscored their epistemic premise and were systematised further in the prevailing cultures of medicine.

Along with these systems, which have considerable content of theory, are found other local deviant and fringe practices explained in similar terminology: massages and meditation offering entire physical and 'spiritual' recuperative packets, cures for bone and joint lesions following trauma or degeneration, sexual malfunction and so on. The practitioners have a vast clientele, both native and Western tourist who vouch for their claims, but its treatments are not without side effects and can leave patients with intractable complications especially in their use following trauma. There is still confusion as to statutory control over the conflated therapeutic offerings, confounded, of course, by the lack of systematic research before their scientific validity might possibly establish those offerings to the present medical culture.

North America

The civilisation of that continent offers easier access to its majoritarian history since it was condensed into a few recent centuries. Race and other identity was an extensive feature in its development with interbreeding between European ethnic divides, and extended fairly rapidly between European and other stock. Southern Africa possibly offers mixed populations within a short span of historical time but in a contextual space that was quite different. Both are outstanding for the gains to civilisations in multicultural transactions despite difficult social relationships. Unequal opportunities for self-improvement amongst diverse ethnicities from which another cultural model makes progress are viewed from differing geopolitical experience. A cursory survey of the United States in North America conveys the idea of a process of ethnic identities losing rapid definition within an emerging American culture.

Ideas seeped in from the Old World when settlers to North America arrived from England and Scotland, then Ireland and Mediterranean Europe; peoples intensely sectarian Protestant and Catholic, but religion found other than the divisive purposes of the Old World. The vastness of land was a new experience, and toil and enterprise transformed the good earth to achieve the predictions of their shared Mosaic injunctions. The violence of European sectarianism gave way to building and worshipping in different churches, and peace held for common social purposes in the early townships. The initial lack of manpower was also a significant initiative to improvisation, technological improvements and vital communication systems over an expanding world the immigrant could begin to control.

The land was seen as God's gift to the settler, and Old Testament fervour directed his right to it. When that ownership inevitably was denied by its indigenous people it was most brutally resolved. Toil and sweat extracted from that earth its plenty—itself sufficient proof for the settler that God's will prevailed and subsequent accumulation of capital led to further unprecedented possibilities. It gave him independence as a farmer, a new and profound experience. He and his family had arrived in the New World as serf or peasant from the feudal lands of his origins where a living was eked out in conditions of despair between strife, war and famine. It was the context which produced, despite previous sectarian antipathies, the newer sense of community; the creation of early townships in turn unleashing a spate of technologies and skills. Learning, through the following centuries advanced rapidly in the newer sciences and spawned unprecedented industry and discovery. America was founded in enterprise and still maintains that old-time fervour. The socio-political revolutions and crumbling feudalism of 18th century Europe which led in turn to a measure of social egalitarianism is rejected. The American pioneer impulse prevails and though inequality is a feature of society social entitlement is not accepted as the remedy.

The introduction of slavery contributed to the wealth of the nation. For a while, despite the cruelties that the African was subject to, the system was productive, although the culture of the states that practiced slavery stagnated in comparison with other States with free labour and freer enterprise. After the constitutional abolition of slavery there was a slow pace to progress often hesitant due to the resistance of white communities. For the African, his beginnings in America entailed the immense degradation of his humanity, in the merciless and iniquitous institutional trade and ownership of slaves. By now the established Puritanism of England considered slavery and the English slave runner an abomination to God and man. The problems America had encountered as a result found meagre resolution in slavery's abolition and held little succour for the released slave. The aftermath of discrimination, the violence, rioting and mutual hatred, has continued well into the recent past. A recent phase of rebellion led the Afro-American to assuming a separate religious identity as Muslims. It could be seen as directed against the original conversion to Christianity and exposure to a social order which was cruelly discriminatory. The movement was more in protest and gained them little from the culture of Islam, for either themselves or the country. But, in the emerging America there is some resolution; today the American identity is less marked by the colour of the skin. In the passage of the short history of this civilisation, from the terrors of the past to the black American's growing and substantive role, there is a tacit change to attitudes. But beyond it persists the divisive classes and inequality to social entitlements, more visible amongst black communities.

To America, Asiatic and Far Eastern nations offered peoples, usually from amongst more provident groups; and from the nations from the South of America there is a constant influx of their impoverished as immigration policies changed over the decades. Jews found welcome refuge in America especially during the century of ideologically motivated race hatred and European genocides. With intellects generally fashioned in interactions with others over the thousands of years of the diaspora, their numbers now added to America's flurry of population diversity and major intellectual achievement.

It is in the immediacy of her past, and the constant population flux of the present, that a civilisation rapidly emerged. A culture of small town communities, which themselves have only been aware of the world's turmoil in the last century and the present in comparative isolation, but also losing her sons and daughters in her commitment to its solution. Her peoples in their shades of colour, religion and original cultures have found work and occupations, and common social gaols. Cities weaving into megalopolis may leave populations with separate identities, discriminated upon and dissolute, and yet for the most part melding into an American culture. An US-centric geopolitics sees threats to its way of life from without, unless the world falls in line with its vision of world order. There is an egotistical imperviousness, even brashness, to her perceptions of the culture and values of older worlds and their slow maturity.

The jubilant and hopeful Christianity exulting through Luther King's speech is traceable to the age of the early pioneers. The Negro's pain and suffering over the years is transformed and heard in the sung harmonies and the rhythms of an African ancestry; a distinctive music culture developed through the church, and led and conducted as by the pastor through his sermon—a communal experience felt unlike those of any church elsewhere. Luther's speech reverberates the spirit of 'that old time religion' joined to the early rhythms, and leading as it were from his pulpit, to exalt, to carry black and white together into America's 'dream' of a common utopia. For the nation as a whole such values are barely concealed expressions of a settler age, nowadays motivating newer and changed realities. The early puritanism is conveyed in many forms. In America's mid-20th century there was the lurch towards a fundamentalist witch-hunt within its borders related to the intense suspicions and the insecurities of a bipolar post war world.

Assumptions motivate political behaviour and a few can be traced through the Calvinist and related European Protestant fervour to American origins. The life of her own citizenry is valued higher than that of humanity elsewhere, and in overwhelming other peoples in the supremacy of armed might with the added clout of American economic power, those 'awesome' demonstrations carry the injunctions of the Old Testament. The political democracy is, in fact, a plutocracy; the United States has no hesitation in promoting democracy as a superior transplant which yet fails because of its utter disregard of the evolving social history of other nations and their relationship to more recent colonial history. A leadership extolls humanitarian values, while her society is unable to perceive the disproportionate sufferings caused to many millions outside her territory in the unleashing of American might of arms. Not surprisingly, the US is widely resented in those worlds which have only recently shaken off the impositions of older colonialists.

Running counter to the harm and cost of her geo-politics, much of the scholarship of America forms a contrasting culture encompassing a phenomenal range and a capacity to approach universally dispersed and cumulated knowledge in scientific disciplines. Undeniably, wealth and a vibrant mix of peoples have produced many inimitable Institutions of learning. Universities of the U.S. have generally attained stature not only in wealth of intellect but by promoting a democracy to disciplinary functions. They provide a salutary, often a leading role to furthering the arts and the natural and social Sciences. Scientific progress in certain disciplines has been influential, and dominant on an universal scale. Epistemological renderings from the world's fund of previous knowledge, the world's religions, ethnographic, linguistic and philological studies, are a few of universal value in this range, and the departments involved have carried us beyond the methods of study in a previous Imperium[vii]. That they attract a calibre of intellect from many nations is an added fillip. Either independently or in collaboration with local scholarship, their energies are promoted. The result has been a remarkable pace to achievements in deciphering and understanding a few fields of knowledge as they came upon the world through history.

REGIONAL CROSS FERTILISATIONS AND INTERACTIONS.

Europe

Changed political and economic power advanced Europe into a civilisational identity. It suits political ideology to regard it particularly as a transatlantic 'Western' civilisation, but the area is comprised of peoples of both West and East. An important and identifiable aspect to the concept has been the history of ideas and knowledge previous to science and related disciplines. Often unrecognised transactions occurred between scholastic institutions and scholars of many systems of thought across a region, from the Spanish Peninsula, south and east of the countries around the Mediterranean and brought together a few further east from India. Later, a methodical comprehension of systems explaining natural phenomena emerged from secular impulses and an evolving humanism, which came to be recognised as the sciences. These were sustained influences of the Enlightenment, the revolutionary and intellectual movements of the 15th-19th century with pronounced shifts to political power changing an older social order. Among a few nations, feudalism, monarchical rule and the political power of institutionalised religion became subject to a measure of populist control.

Europe's knowledge base was undoubtedly influenced by the worlds beyond; Chinese astronomy, Indian mathematics the considerable developments across West Asia, transforming in the Renaissance passage to science. Prior to it, concepts about the cosmos, questioning of the ideas of Aristotelian physics and the possibility of a sun-centred Universe, had commenced. From the 17th century change was in the air, with newer philosophies proclaiming social egalitarianism. However, in the centuries that followed, previous strife in national or imperial rivalry intensified and, though the old mould of Europe was shattered, the new had not arrived.

Certainly during the period of the founding of a nominal Europe, peoples were in flux over an area well beyond the present demarcated boundaries. This is evident from language and its derivations. In the development of Western thought, Greek, Roman, Byzantine, Egyptian and Judaic ideas are recognisable in the advance of philosophy, the knowledge of nature, and artistic forms, which suggests the exchange and movement of peoples across the continent's broad geography. Despite the turmoil, there is a fairly consistent history of communication, discovery and constant additions to knowledge as it was dispersed into local centres of learning. In antiquity a remarkable, extensive and an undervalued exchange existed between Egypt and Greece[viii]. Before and into the middle ages we see the development of knowledge and enhancement of art by communities with special interests and skills, the translation of manuscripts and collaborative enterprise with local specialists. Sometimes whole communities brought new knowledge and, in contact with those of a similar bent, founded other cultural forms of lasting value, even while moving away from the violence of war or local turbulence. The sources and context for exchange and the cross fertilisation of knowledge were innumerable and varied in Europe's history: to early Greece, for instance, from Sumer, Assyria and Mesopotamia and then, very considerably and significantly from Egypt[ix]. The wars for territory between the Hellenic, Carthaginian, Roman and Byzantine Powers (c 500 BC-750 AD) were the essential background to these advances.

The crusades brought a Latinised Europe to the eastern Mediterranean in conflict but the contact provided Europe with the comparative sophistication of Byzantine culture and access to the systematised knowledge of Arab and Persian civilisation. Still later, invasions by the Berbers from N Africa, followed by Arab speaking Moors, resulted in the conquest and dominion of the Iberian peninsula (800 AD-1200 AD). Those centuries enhanced the cultural attributes of the region, while their learning later penetrated a few centres of Europe. The final phases of religious and political conflict between Islam and Spain were also of considerable cultural exchange. Islamic culture had spread beyond Spain into middle Europe and left its mark on the following Enlightenment and the prelude to the Italian Renaissance.

The territorial expanse of the Mongol empire reached from Europe to the Pacific and lasted for about 150 years from its commencement in the 13th century. It initiated an intellectual advance of a different order and value to both East and West. The violence and battles were constant but also promoted exploration and institutional contacts and the early appreciation of forms of knowledge between West and East. Astronomy and medicine gained from the contacts of the vast Empire. Other achievements came in the form of the explorations of the great scholar-travellers of that age, like Ibn Batuta, reputed for making his way across many countries was one of many other achievements, and in Marco Polo's journey to the East, worlds came a little closer.

The flight of scholars and their sources of knowledge from war, violence and civil strife.

The content and output of Mediaeval West Asian knowledge systems has undoubtedly had considerable influence on Europe. West Asia achieved a remarkable quality to its intellectual life at an earlier time than Europe. Alexandria had been transformed into a coastal capital City and archives of Hellenic knowledge were long preserved there, housed between the Royal Libraries of the Ptolemies and the Serapeum. Commencing with the Roman invasion and loss of Egyptian control, Alexandria was intermittently ravaged and faced general misfortune over centuries. Of that there is not much doubt, but the debate as to who were the perpetrators of the destruction of her ancient and esteemed libraries continues till today (see James Hannam, 2003). A fire started at the time of Julius Caesar's occupation of the city, in Roman revenge for the destruction of his fleet is as likely as not. The Library's existence was not recorded after Plutarch's visit to Alexandria, but in his Life of Caesar he holds its destruction to have been earlier, with an Arab onslaught on the city as the cause.

The Serapeum was burnt by Christian mobs incited by Theophilus, the Patriarch of the Orthodox Church at Alexandria in AD 391. Fortunately, there appears to have been sequestration and transfer of its scholastic content. Scrolls made their way to the ancient civilisations of the Mediterranean within the Byzantine Empire, and to the Arabs in the Caliphate of Damascus. From Alexandria, Constantinople, Baghdad and Damascus Arab scholars were prominent in extending that knowledge to the West. The story of a community of Nestorians, schismatic Christians hence condemned by the orthodox, with a remarkable dedication to intellectual pursuits proved invaluable for the history of medicine. They had preserved Greek knowledge in Latin translation, and in flight and consequent wanderings, carried that material through Byzantine and Arab lands until finally they were offered a haven in the Persia of the Sassanid. This is an outstanding example of the development of medicine in Arab lands, influenced by the earlier sources from Greece and separate from the sources of the further Asian East. (See Garcia D'Orta).

Mediaeval efforts at imposing the fiefdom of Christian Europe on non-Christian lands of West Asia were in battle, but the decimation of non-combatants, peoples regarded as either plundering a Christian heritage or the descendants of those who put Christ to death, was the cruelty of the times. That history slanted Europe as a civilisation with the cultural values of a Christianity wielding the sword. Monarchs owing allegiance to the Pope were encouraged to rally feudal chieftains and armies to restore the birthplace of Christ from the infidel to a Christian Europe. The reasons for this enterprise have begun to be re-examined in a post imperial age. The Crusades, which popular history once made out to be the struggle of Christendom against the Infidel, are better understood now and, as Runciman states were, "the last of barbarian invasions by the chain-mailed knights of Europe against a civilisation of considerable quality"[x]. If Christian zealotry mobilised the means for acquiring territory, which it later lost, there was in the exchange another of permanent value and one which played its considerable part in the later European Renaissance. The channelling and spread of ideas, specialised knowledge and art was facilitated beyond the violence of the contact. The conveyors, though, would hardly be the knights of Christendom, who sought relief from primogeniture and its feudal property restrictions, nor the foot soldiers provided by an impecunious peasantry, readily sublimating their earthly miseries in tutelage to the Church. They pictured themselves as wielding the Sword of Faith in a cause that was blessed, with the promise of a better after-life and, on earth, the prospect of loot. Invariably they were accompanied by camp followers, captives, or the many displaced migrants fleeing the uncertainties of war. Men of learning from either side of the conflict, in time made contact and communicated.

There were possibly results even more significant for Europe from another major confrontation, as Moorish domination gave way to Christian recovery of the Iberian Peninsula from Islam. La Reconquista opened Islamic scholarship of the Moors in Spain to the avid interest of scholars of many markings, Jew, Moor, Arab and Christian. The name of Gerhardo de Cremona of the 12th century exemplifies the spirit of collaboration translations. He translated from the Arabic for Europe[xi]—philosophy, Ptolemy's Almagest and, the known sciences of the time.

The emphasis of history is mostly on the side of the historical coin with the more visible and definite markings—of conquest and retreat, slaughter and destruction. Its obverse is revealed in many evidences in language, architecture and the learning reformulated into local systems. The evidence remains incomplete considering the universal extent of cross-civilisational impact, and remains to be pursued with the disciplinary intensity of that other history. However, that there was a slow acquisition of the systematised knowledge past the confrontation with foreign cultures was an acknowledgement of their worth to the recipient.

The obvious must be emphasised, that the passage of knowledge following collaborations is mutual accomplishment, while in conflict that passage in cultural exchange and borrowing while inevitable loses the merit of study. Exchange and gain to systems of learning was hardly realised in the incessant and catastrophic depredations initiated by the nations of European civilisation in the previous century. It was organised and directed at the intelligentsia, presumably to destroy specific contributions to learning; but most was on a scale of indiscriminate destruction or deportations and population shifts meant to eliminate them. A civilisation consisting of the wealthiest and technologically most advanced nations, unleashed the mass extermination of populations within its borders and well beyond. Even the end of warfare that marked a peace was only achieved by the most destructively fearful technology yet devised. And, within that Peace, the enforced transfers of population to retain ethnicities within redrawn national boundaries continued.

Those who determined the barbarism of previous ages were participants in its execution, unlike the leaders of Nations of today who, in comfortable isolation and remoteness, seem incapable of appreciating the scale of its infliction. This distancing allows them a rectitude to their accounts of the 'crusades' they embark upon, and the Science involved leaves us the dread possibility of a terminal world.

Transactions of value which followed in historical exchange

Byzantium, the Arabian Peninsula, Persia and earlier Bactria (situated in N.W. Afghanistan) lay at the crossroads between Asia and Europe for commerce and exchange. In the civilisations to the East, India in antiquity and in China for a few early centuries of the 2nd millennia CE, science and a vigorous technology had produced many primary achievements.

Indian systems of medicine and mathematics were sought after by West Asia and adapted or enhanced. Notable religious and philosophical interactions had taken place between China and India, and from there into West Asia. Greece was a long-lasting hub for philosophical dialogue and, later, Byzantine art extended her influence. The revealed religions of this area carried within their principles theistic similarities, but dogmas provoked divisions, particularly within Christianity and Islam. Schismatic interpretations considered heretical by the Church of Rome were the cause of power struggles and civil disturbances. Religion was most often the pretext for wars. Islam and Christianity, whether Roman and Catholic, Byzantine, Coptic, Armenian or Russian Orthodox, have been inspirational and influenced architecture and art, and in their execution the singularities and mutuality edify a civilisation. They are to be seen in innumerable enduring masterworks across the countries of a region furiously and constantly disturbed in the battles for ecclesiastical or religious dominance.

Periods of early Greek expansion in India left evidence of mutual influences on language, astronomy and medicine[xxii]. Certainly aspects of astronomy, mathematics and medicine from India were used and developed by the Arabs and Persians, later to reach and transmute in European systems. The early exchanges influence subsequent knowledge, furthering unique systems of thought and applications within these civilisations. Ayurveda became a cumulative compilation with the advent of organised Hinduism and its dominance over Indian civilisation. From the early Christian era a sophisticated system of Indian medicine had flourished. Its knowledge and practice were transposed in studies by West Asian physicians and are to be found in the encyclopaedic compilations of Arab medicine. Refashioned and adapted, they contributed to the development of the sophisticated system of Arab and Persian medical teaching and practice. The medical compilations of medieval Persia are acknowledged for the worth and the universality of their sources. Further study is needed to unreservedly establish in factual detail the extent of their contribution and influence on European medicine and later its science.

Some indication of the complexity of influence on European thought may be seen in the works of individual scholars. One such was Abu'l Waleed Muhammad Ibn Ahmad Ibn Muhammad Ibn Rushd. Better known as Averroes, he stands tall in the passage of some of the systems of historic knowledge, philosophy and religion in European discourse. He was born in 1128 CE. in Cordoba where he received a traditional Islamic education. This was followed by study at one of the greatest Libraries of the period previously established by the Abbasid Caliphate at Cordoba. In his later years he transferred to Morocco and continued to be productive in many disciplinary fields. He must be reckoned amongst influential scholars of Greek wisdom. He made Arabic translations which he then edited, adding major commentaries. His works were later available in Latin, but these were possibly not too accurately translated from the Arabic. He stressed the relationship of religion and philosophy as systems that had mutually nurtured each other, in studies that aroused the natural intolerance of later Iberian State Power and the Inquisition. The secular bent of some of the teachings of mediaeval Islam appeared to the Catholic Church as an even greater danger than to Islamic institutions. Previous to their overthrow in Europe, The Caliphates ruling from West Asia to Spain had demonstrated immense respect for extant knowledge, setting up Libraries in the major cities of their domain and, as with Cordoba, some had a prodigious content of manuscripts. The momentous advantage of paper for transcribing their studies to written manuscripts had by then been put to use, after having learnt of its manufacture and usage in China following the Abbasid conquest of Samarkand in the 8th century.

Averroes had brought Greek philosophy and Aristotelian thought to Europe, awakening a major interest in them at the Universities of Paris and Oxford where the value of his particular interpretations in his translations of Aristotle was recognised. The Universities instituted special courses for Averroes' teachings. By profession a physician, having studied medicine, he left yet another legacy in that discipline.

Latin translations of early Greek works were widely used during the centuries after their salvage from Alexandria[xiii]. Their intellectual wealth nourished the vitality of the regions they were carried to long before it reached Europe. Centuries battling Moslem or Jew undoubtedly colour history, but the long drawn conflict brought their intellectual contribution, a fertility which left its indelible mark on Europe. Yet details of this contact, extending into the Middle Ages, have been largely ignored and require restitution. While the development of Science in recent centuries was unique and in an essentially European context, previous to it were the remarkable exchanges and a diversity of secular intellectual influence promoted by Islamic scholars. There is, however, another narration to Renaissance Science, beginning with the invasion of the Ottoman Turks and the Byzantine retreat. In that tumult scholars fled Constantinople and the 'argosy' the wisdom of the ancient Hellenes returned to Europe which shaped Science from her entombed inheritance[xiv]!

European cultural history from antiquity until the Reformation, Enlightenment and the Renaissance contains the persistent influence of other cultures beyond its geography. Commencing with the long drawn-out achievements of the 2nd millennium BCE from Egypt into Greece they were then shaped in the endowments native to the latter. Contact with Egypt had a profound influence toward the intellectual configuration of early Greece and Rome.

Europe's early philosophies accessed Hermeticism, a school of thought that emerged from the Paganism of Egypt. Intense rivalries existed between different schools but there were also debates with Neo-Platonism and Gnosticism which, in turn, influenced Jewish and Christian theologies. Within each belief system are tracings of another as they developed before consolidating institutional power in dogma. They reappear in the Christianity of Rome. The founding writings of St Augustine to Western Christianity are well known. He was a Berber and a scholar, born in CE 354 in North West Africa. He died as Bishop of Hippo[xv]. Not only mainstream Christianity, but the many deviations, 'the heresies', drew from the theologies of the region, naturally contributing in the development of Islam as well. Confrontation between Egypt and Greece, or in the name of religion, between Rome, the Levant and Byzantium, inevitably produced an exchange if not dialogue. Profound antagonisms were undoubtedly played out; later, they appear as ecumenical influences in sources and myth. The epics of the land area which includes Europe told of, amongst others, Osiris, Christ and Tamuz, each resurrected after death, and then worshipped in their separate religions. Mutually understandable, epistemology and logic, the intellectual attributes, are apparent, woven into social organisation, the arts, the sciences and medicine within a European civilisation of separate cultures.

The Dark Ages

Was it ever a wholly fallow period, a dearth of intellectual activity during the centuries prior to the Renaissance, suggested by the Dark Ages? Historical readings posed that time in Europe as infertile and arid, a virtual hiatus to intellectual endeavour. Ideas, concepts in physics, optics, mathematics, algebra and medicine, and technologies which had been sought after from beyond and developed by Arab and Persian, had reached Europe. Undoubtedly there were centuries of territorial strife, impoverishment and peasant revolts, famines and pestilential sicknesses, while Islamic supremacy was a reminder of the waning power of her nations. Later European historians had naturally found this period most uninspiring, a Europe which lived in the shadow of superior powers into the time of the Ottoman. The 'Dark Ages' was hardly a description of historical reality, more a denial from the vantage of the Renaissance and a later Grand Imperium. European advance was secondary to West Asian achievement before that time.

The road to science led from a knowledge base non-European; from North Africa, Egypt, and through Alexandria where Greek knowledge had been consolidated in Latin and then translated to Arabic and improved in Persian and Arab lands. Arab and Persian medicine in particular had benefited from the previous contribution of Indian systems, major impulses to the earliest science of medicine. Historians in the heyday of Imperialism were naturally disinclined to acknowledge their debt to these later subject nations or that they had contributed to Science.

Were the 'Dark Ages' a lengthy gloom without achievement? Europe was overshadowed by the Islamic peoples, the Persian, the Moor or Arab, with their comparatively immense base of knowledge. Yet that period was not without European intellectual or scientific accomplishment. The scholarship of Europe was favoured in a Moorish presence, and by contributions from West Asia. Centres of learning and healing in Syria, Damascus, Edessa or Baghdad had become Universities, Hospitals and Medical Schools and there was an exchange of scholars with Salerno and Florence, across to Cordoba and Toledo and even as far as the oldest Universities of Britain. They provided vital influences to those thinkers of the Renaissance for whom natural phenomena were no longer sufficiently explicable in the 'given' renderings, but mathematisation provided newer systems for explaining them.

Europe's history has an universality that inheres through the population fluxes and contributions from diverse stocks, a cross fertilisation of minds and thought across a landmass extending to Byzantium and Persia to its East. Its many institutions were the mediaeval contributors, transforming the specific knowledge systems that existed prior to Science. The exchanges which nourished Science are better appreciated as the subject is more intensively explored[xvi].

The history of specialised knowledge acquisition and promotion of more efficient technology for social benefit varies across the world, with its slow commencement over eight millennia ago in elementary applications with many identifiable commonalties. Four thousand years on the pace quickened into a ferment of intellectual activity amongst diverse civilisations resulting in a spate of astronomical and mathematical discovery, philosophical insights and technological promotions, bringing gains, unprecedented in scale, for some societies. In time their importance extended beyond these societies and their boundaries, influencing learning and specialised developments in other civilisations. Paper and printing, magnetism, and gunpowder, discoveries listed by Roger Bacon for their bearing on Science, had their prelude in China. They predated European discovery but their primacy and accessibility to Europe is hardly considered, let alone acknowledged. The facts of earlier discoveries from beyond Europe and their later presence there is difficult to discount, since the evidence of contact alone allows for the possibility.

What was characterised until a few decades ago as "—the background noise of low technology that all civilisations have evolved as part of their daily life"[xvii] is gradually giving way to the recognition of valuable knowledge from other evident sites, those more developed regions, which offered a sustenance beyond life's quotidian necessities, though they only feature as a footnote to the Renaissance in the history of knowledge. We cannot content ourselves with viewing Europe as the birthplace of Science and a few names of its high mark, a Galileo, Kepler, Newton, or a William Harvey for medicine, when unsung, tongue-twister names in languages beyond Europe, have left indelible marks on the history of Science.

"The bulk of scientific knowledge is a product of the Europe of the last four centuries", is not a statement to be disputed, but to preface it today with "—only the civilisations that descend from Hellenic Greece have possessed more than the most rudimentary science"[xviii] can only perpetuate ignorance. It is poor historiography to lock Science into European space unrelated to prior knowledge when the evidence of that knowledge was as far-flung as it was. We require exploration as to how and why the progression to a method called Science happened in Europe, but the explanation cannot be found in facile dismissals of the contribution of other civilisations. Social compulsions within civilisations have a bearing on development but often there are interactions from without. The 'Dark Ages' may consist of comparatively dormant cycles lacking notable discovery, as well as periods of fertile acquisitions of knowledge and technology. Those acquisitions surely must feature as the essential forerunners to the method that defines Science, or even as Science itself. One cannot reduce discovery of the decimal system to 'rudimentary science', unless the scientist is innocent of the history of mathematics.

Scientific discoveries may have immediate functions in application, but a few have an extensive importance through time. To discover that a lodestone had the constant property of pointing, wherever suspended, in singular direction led gradually to technological innovations that accorded to the particular needs of that society. But the principle of magnetism was a momentous discovery for science as is demonstrated in its innumerable uses into the present time. Magnetism was a primary Chinese discovery, and was used by its emerging civilisation in sophisticated applications. Later it featured in many increasingly complex ones over the world. Exceptional development of disciplinary systems relate to the contextual compulsions of a society. There were periods in antiquity when the institutionalised religious hierarchies in India and Egypt provided the growth of mathematics and astronomy; or in China in medieval times, a centralised bureaucracy had in place trained and qualified manpower for her specific needs. Chinese agriculture at the time was far more productive than Europe's; her sciences advanced enough to install technologies based in sound physical principles. The system of grand canals was laid with pound locks and dams, extending the use of her great rivers for irrigation and fast transportation. Only when the great geographical space of China was thus controlled through waterways, and agricultural output increased, could mercantile and commercial interests negotiate the distances and expand trade.

The immense breadth of the survey of Chinese Science, available in the volumes of Joseph Needham and collaborators[7], breaks new ground in innumerable ways, in particular illuminating the immense contributions China made in the centuries prior to European Science. A disciplinary interest has been sharpened toward more thoughtful reappraisals of other epistemologies in various fields. The primary importance of these recent outstanding collections of the Cambridge school of historiographers is revealed in the systematic collection of the evidence from one civilisation which sustains the Needhamian view that science must be regarded as

---

[7]   Science and Civilisation in China, (Cambridge University Press: Vols. 1954)

an enterprise through history[xix]. The group's attestations and references from an array of original Chinese linguistic sources relate the sequence of science, discovery and technological innovations of that civilisation as it unfolded in changing social and political power structures over the centuries. In the context of the periods between the 6th-15th centuries, for instance, from the Chinese land mass emerged a trove of discovery and technology as vital as any to the evolution of world science and its later universality. The volumes are a seminal work in the recounting of the past scientific civilisation of China, the scale of that enterprise equal to the phenomenal extent of a Chinese contribution to world science. Hopefully, it will be an influence that will promote the systematic trace of knowledge across the history of other continents and civilisations[xx].

Non-European contributions to Science and Medicine

The Science of Medicine suggests evolution from previous epistemologies of knowledge, particularly as that developed in West Asia while its history is of further substantial contribution from the neighbouring Eastern civilisations of China and India. It not only reached Europe before the Enlightenment but was the mode of institutionalised practice and teaching before the gradual makeover of medicine into its considerable science post Renaissance.

From surrounding conflicts Alexandria became home to a Greek heritage of learning, having found refuge in the sanctum of its famed Libraries. It was not to be for long. The libraries were destroyed, and the extent of the loss of material and the identities of those responsible are uncertain. Due to its vulnerable position on the coast, Alexandria appears to have been subject to repeated invasions, and damages occurred up to the early 1st century of the Christian era. There was the destruction by an earlier Arab power and possibly a loss to parts of the libraries original scrolls. In the on-going conflicts between Greece and Rome a part of the Library at Alexandria burned. The Royal and The Seraphim, however, were later terminally destroyed. Amidst those sanguinary conflicts, in sectarian riots and the mob violence of communities being directed to set upon one another, Christians of the Nestorian faith, a proclaimed heresy, fled to Constantinople. Their scholars, who had studied Greek teachings in the Latin and nurtured the libraries, managed to salvage some of the material. One of the first scholars, Sergius of Resh-'Aina, a 6th CE physician, in

71

translating into Syriac brought Galen to the notice of the Arab world. He was not a Nestorian, but one of the Monophysite (Jacobite) Christians.

Thus the Arabs, who appear to have initially gained from Alexandria's reputation as a centre of learning, furthered that learning in considerable assimilation and development. Much of this development had reached Europe well before Constantinople fell to the Turks in 1456 CE. Arabic translations of ancient Greek texts were known and used by scholars as far off as Paris and Scotland, while the Hellenic heritage was already developing in the Arab Caliphates and Persia. It came to Western Europe under the hegemony of the Moors and through the conflicts spearheaded by the Papacy to restore Arab and Jewish lands to Christendom and still later while the Moors were in retreat. The intellectual hibernation of Europe, if it happened at all, was never for the want of a Hellenic heritage since its restoration was being mediated in the culture of Asia Minor and the lands of the Arab and the Persian. There the original Greek sources were handsomely acknowledged and the learning transformed.

The routes by which this knowledge traversed were devious, and its traffic interrupted in the religious antagonisms. Greek thought was preserved by the Nestorians at Alexandria. These versatile scholars were the keepers and conveyors of Hellenic sources of medicine and related knowledge. The material survived in Neo-Aramaic translations, and Aramaic provided an easy facility for transfer and use. But the Nestorians were condemned again for heresy following the edicts of Ephesus in 431 CE, and were expelled from their Byzantine interlude. When in need of theological supremacy, orthodoxy of any hue—Christianity was never an exception through history—obtained it with a heavy hand, its pontiffs instigating sects to riot against the apostates, and pillaging, massacring and burning their books. These were the earliest manifestations of a millennium of struggle for political power by the interpreters of the Scriptures which carried into the Crusades and culminated when the Ottoman destroyed Byzantine power. It took a further century of power struggles for the Reformation and a secular Revolution before Renaissance Science transformed Europe.

What remained of the Nestorians settled in Edessa, initiating a centre of scholarship there, but a decade later their travails resumed under Zeno, later Christian emperor of Byzantium. Again they were forced out and moved on to Nisibis in Mesopotamia. They created more institutions of learning but it was at Jundishapur in the Sassanid lands of Persia, and later under the Caliphs of Arabia, where they found welcome, and finally they and their institutions and learning thrived. The Greek heritage was revitalised by translation and commentaries at the zenith of medieval Arab power; yet, it is to the reverence of knowledge and the scholastic achievements of the Nestorian Christian community that we owe a considerable debt for its valuable original sustenance. The applications of that knowledge continued to further Arabian scholarship between the 7th century CE and the second millennium. Arabic, a rich language, facilitated translation and through Arabic and Latin it made its way to Europe in later centuries.

The medicine of Hippocrates and Galen had passed through many lands but the conveyance recreated use and improved it. Its value was initially evident mainly to a composite Islamic culture with a profound respect and appreciation of Greek medicine. There is no dearth of evidence of the achievements of that later period, great teachers and practitioners in Arabic and Persian lands who enhanced its content. The proof is in a variety of medical treatises left by them of institutionalised practice and research which put in place therapeutic and surgical improvement. It was the innovative genius of those physician/scholars, theories from astute observation of illness patterns that are still recognisable within classified pathology, a viable medicine, for its developing science in later centuries.

History so often is the narration about adversarial civilisations: mutual gain of any order discounted in the priority of conflict. Labels as with 'Hindu' 'Islamic' or 'Christian' used as confronting civilisations by some historians tend to ignore a cultural significance in the traces of borrowing and exchange between them, so vital to humanity's comprehensive progress. In the writings of a Samuel Huntington or a Bernard Lewis, a preferred eponym for the 'Christian' may transform to a 'Western' civilisation, conferring on it further value as a democracy, a political ideology, originating once again in ancient Greece, recast from the Enlightenment humanism and developed in the later intellectual impulses of 19th century Europe. Replacing the Christian ethos to loftier secular and humanitarian values, did not reduce strife in that civilisation, on the contrary internecine strife reached scales of depredation in the 20th century, hopefully, never to be repeated. Sustaining European economic well-being for centuries was the practiced imposition of political power masquerading as a crusade of one form or another, the latest, for transferring democracy to foreign shores and 'lesser' peoples ignorant of its virtues. Even so it is not without affecting knowledge as a world heritage within that exchange.

Whether through confrontation or otherwise West Asia enjoyed a cultural fertilisation from Greece, India and China one that existed from earlier centuries between the latter three. During the middle ages we have evidence of it extending to Europe. West Asian intellectual traffic and exchange with Europe was maintained. Sufficient evidence is available for us to reconsider the historical beginnings of the Renaissance. It has popularly been associated with the Turkish onslaught on Constantinople and with the demise of the Byzantine Empire, the sequestered heritage of Greece being salvaged for Europe as its keepers fled there. That must in large measure be discounted. Greek Byzantium had, through the years, often unwillingly acceded to or resisted the pressures of the Latin Church and the Papacy. The relationship of the Greek Church with Rome was always acrimonious, though the inclination for independence from the mother Church was not pressed within the larger context of on-going Imperial power struggles. However, as Byzantine power waned and the old Empire reached accommodation with the Turks and the Greek Church whose theological independence was fiercely asserted but never achieved, was finally relieved of vassalage to the Church in Rome. This is salient evidence[xxi], rather than the climactic convulsion hitherto known through history as 'The Fall of Constantinople' postulating the timing of the treasures of Hellenic knowledge being available once again for Europe.

Medical tracks in History leading to Medical Science:.

Priorities overshadow the uncertainties of history, although the value of Greek knowledge in antiquity for the pivotal role in the development of Science is undisputed. Arab/Persian achievements in the sciences and in medicine are the link between the pre-mediaeval and the mediaeval. In the history of medical progress, there is little doubt that those peoples were the initial beneficiaries of the medicine practised by the Greeks, transposed to their own medical system of Unani. Yūnānī in the languages, Arabic, Hindi-Urdu or Persian means 'Greek Medicine'[xxii]. The name thus acknowledges the source, and continues with Suqrat or Socrates as the philosopher of Unani, along with Buqrat (Hippocrates) and the Hakim Jalinoos (Galen, AD 131-210) acknowledged as founders of this medical system with its wider ramifications both to the East and West. Unani was not merely in the borrowing from the Byzantine Greeks, but developed in composite sources to advance, for instance, beyond therapeutics into public health and disciplines of surgery. In the centuries that followed, their Schools of Medicine were establishments tied into hospitals for practical experience. The widely functioning traditional practice of West Asia has extended to many countries with Muslim populations and their systems prevail in India.

The Firdausal-Hikmat (Paradise of Wisdom) of Ali Bin Rabban, AD 850 summarised the wisdom of Greek and Indian medical thought; and the latter included important Indian works of medical knowledge from the works of Caraka, Susruta, found in the treatises of Nidana and Astragahrdaya. Ali Bin Rabban's most notable student was Rhazes Abu Bakr Mohammed bin Zachariyya Ar-Razi, a Persian Muslim better known as Rhazes (850-925). He was was a renowned practitioner who added to the fund of Unanni[xxiii] and engaged in the study of many other systems of medicine. His studies reached Europe in Latin translations through the Sicilian Jewish Physician, Faraj ibn Sālim (Farragut), who by 1279 completed the enormous task of rendering Rhazes' al-Hāwi as the Liber Continens. This great work by Farragut was sponsored by Charles I of Anjou. Three centuries later we see the works of Rhazes and other Arab medical scholars referred to by Garcia da Orta (c 1490-1570). da Orta studied Medicine in schools of the distant Iberian Peninsula at the universities of Salamanca and Alacalá de Henares. The medical teachings of other Jewish scholars like Isaac Judaeus, an Egyptian Jew of Arab origin, Ibn al-Jazzār, Haly Abbas and and the best known amongst them, Abu 'Ali al Husayn ibn Sinā (Avicenna 980-1037), had reached these Universities during the Moorish dominion of Europe.

Rhazes, who while he translated and studied Jalinoos (Galen) was also critical of him (respect for received wisdom did not deter its questioning amongst the physicians in Arab and Persian lands), developed an empiricism to the practice and observations of his discipline in the hospital of Baghdad where his conviction grew that Galen's was not the last word in Medicine. The Greeks of Galen's time would not have had the advantage that Rhazes and other Arab physicians had—of understanding disease in the observation of greater patient numbers and at close hand within the institution of the hospital. Observation of signs and symptoms and the natural history of the disease and the maintenance of records and data was the rote which commenced the improvements to the methods of empirical disease classification. We know this from his description of measles and small pox as separate diseases, a difference previously unrecognised in the Greek descriptions of epidemics.

His work, the al-Hāwi, is a monumental compilation of disease classification and description which Meyerhoff[xxiv] calls the most extensive Medical treatise ever written by a single man. Its format, when classifying disease, cited Greek, Syrian, Arabic, Persian and Indian authors for each condition, and he then added to each his own observations, experience and opinion. The al-Hāwi is unique in medical history, and must figure for all time, for its encyclopaedic content and the ecumenism of its attributions and acknowledgements. The ecumenism of Science is not novel. South East Asian medicine, Graeco-Arabic medicine and Traditional medicine in the Far East show the considerable imprint of exchange. But Rhazes' works are unique for their scholarship, a veritable tribute to the catholicity of specialised medical knowledge. In completion by later scholars, the original al-Hawi numbered twenty volumes but fifty years later only two volumes were extant in complete copy.

Rhazes was but a forerunner of the many contributors to the fertile climate enabling medical and natural sciences which reached its zenith in medieval centuries. Alchemy was also a science of the time, since ridden by the mystical philosophy of neo-Platonism and Gnosticism. We glimpse on the other hand in Rhazes works an empiricism veering to the experimental. Rhazes in classifying cures recognised animal, mineral and vegetable constituents, unlike the father of Arab alchemy, Jabir, whose mysticism was more pronounced than empiricism or experimentation, although their sources were the same.

Let us note further contributions of consequence from the rest of the world rather than their mere 'background noise'. Numeracy, mathematics, computational tables and algebra, without which Science is inconceivable, featured in China and India and in considerable advance reached Europe. Al Biruni, born toward the end of the 1st millennium CE, was a physicist of eminence and a notable traveller. His 'History of India' is a sizeable record of Indian systems of numeration. It was transformed to the discipline of geometry in the genius of the mathematician and astronomer, Omar Khayyam (about 1000-1009 CE). He demonstrated the unity between algebra and geometry as he resolved the general cubic equation of the third degree 500 years before the Italian Tartaglia advanced it further. Omar Khayyam's fame as the author of the well-known Rubaiyat is less merited;

its translation in Victorian fantasy is over-perfumed, an effete Oriental romance rather than the musings of a philosophical poet.

Another product of Arab science was an amalgamation of Taoist and Pythagorean alchemy. It included a depiction of natural or compounded products used in Egypt in processes like embalming. Alchemy features in early chemistry although it has since been downgraded for its lack of science; but the system retains a historical interest in the development of science. As one of Newton's initial interests, it must be remembered for more than its lack of science. The previous grand leaps of the Chinese in astronomy and the sophistication of their knowledge and application of magnetic phenomena and their technological advances in printing and gunpowder were not discoveries in Science as we define it, but they cannot be denied within any overview of Science.

The science of magnetism had to plod slowly into later European discovery, and stumbled for a while over declination before the nature of the magnetic needle could be mastered in the technology of the compass and applied to navigation. The Chinese had not required to fudge magnetic declination as Europe had to with their early compasses. Chinese philosophy actively searched for inductive effects. It could conceive of effective positions, though spatially separate, influence changes to them, at a single point in time. Inductivity as a principle manifests repeatedly in Traditional Chinese Medical theory. In fact, inductivity is nowadays a feature of the physical Sciences, although in biology causality is of great scientific consequence. Causality is change to an effective position in space, but separated in time.

The stores of literature and knowledge attributable to Arab natural sciences are housed in the many libraries[8] of Istanbul, the Spanish Escorial, in Cairo, Mosul, Baghdad and Persia, and have reached wide destinations in

---

[8]   There is a well-appointed Library of Arabic Science and Literature at Suraj Kund near Delhi, India where amongst others is housed Medical Literature pertaining to Unanni. I was recently informed of a surgical procedure that followed when the routine excisional surgery for an anal fistula, on a medical colleague failed and the fistula recurred. Subsequently the procedure was to run a ligature of non-absorbable material through respective openings of the fistula and leave it in situ. The thread is gradually tightened over the weeks. As the thread cuts through the fistula, the procedure causing a controlled inflammatory reaction, it heals by cicatrisation. This practice continues to this day in the surgical procedures of Unanni, a medical culture older than surgical science. But the origins of the method seem not to have been known to my colleague, a research worker himself at Karolinska Hospital,

Europe. The Iberian Peninsula shows monumental evidence of multicultural diversity within its geography and a consequent enhancement of European civilisation even when balances of political power changed. Sources of attested information are available to scholars presently involved in seeking it. Popular history ignores even what is available as considerable inputs to medical science, claiming the uniqueness of medical discovery as an attribute of the European scientist in those lightning strikes of the intellect and ignoring the contributions of others beyond Europe. The violence of confrontation had often aided the passage of such documentation, but not necessarily an historical appreciation toward the development of science.

The progression of science to an ecumenism and universality has, over the past three centuries, been established undoubtedly in its European transformation. A prior history establishes institutions for furthering the acquisition of knowledge, an interaction between scholars of Cordoba and distant Baghdad, crossing continents and, between their centres of learning, transactions that could only be promoted in translation. Arabic held in the felicity of its language a proficient vein for translation of works from India to Greece; from them into Latin by European scholars, it extended and enhanced the learning of European Universities in the Enlightenment. Eleventh century records show the presence of an African Christian monk, Constantine, from Carthage who, with his medical books, entered the Italian monastery at Monte Cassino[xxv]. The quality of his scholarship may be questionable[xxvi](see Legacy of Islam) but the later establishment of the medical school at nearby Salerno was influenced through his translated works. Amongst them were Hippocratic treatises, Haly Abbas' Arab medical encyclopaedia, the works of the Jewish physician Isaac Israeli and Galen's Art of Medicine: translations of the secular knowledge of medicine, from from Greek, Arab and Jewish sources. Spread through a theological institution in Italy, it serves to illustrate, if not celebrate, an ecumenism to mediaeval medicine, well before that of Science.

The Heritage of Science

Today we take for granted words like zenith, nadir, alcohol, alkali; arithmetic cypher, and algorithms. They are transliterations derived from the content of classical astronomy, chemistry or mathematics from the Arab world or

---

Stockholm and hence, presumably neither to the department of surgery where it was performed. It is amongst the unacknowledged antecedents of medical science.

from India via West Asia. Here again, the Nestorian community played a notable role. There was a latency to mathematical development in the West for the conceptual lack of 'zero' and an inability to progress beyond the abacus and the Roman Numeral. In 498 CE, Indian mathematician and astronomer Aryabhata[9] stated the decimal-based place value notation. The shift from Roman numerals to the decimal system was opposed in the West despite the evidence of its far greater sophistication in calculation. The recalcitrance was partly due to the Greek Byzantine conviction that other methods could offer little improvement to their own methods of computation[xxvii]. Again, when it finally found the value of the system proffered via the Arabs, Western mathematical science strode phenomenally forward in Europe in the further compulsions of the Enlightenment. Very simply, the take-off to Newton's gravitational principles that govern the universe, of mass and squared interplanetary distance, is conceptually impossible without 'the zero'. His was an intellect placed in Europe within the context of great social change, aggressive expansion and to an extent made possible in the general fervour of intellectual endeavour.

From Aryabhata's mathematical treatise, his trigonometry in Sanskrit, completed in 499 AD, and 'Sine' via transliteration of sinus, reached the discipline in Arab lands from his jya-ardha' (chord half). Shortened to 'jya' the word along with much of the mathematics which contained it, found its way to West Asia. Jya meant nothing to the Arabs but 'jiab' did, which means a cove or bay. It is amongst the massive translations from the Arabic of Gherardo of Cremona in Spain (1114-87). His labour brought to the West Euclid's 'Elements', Ptolemy's 'Almageist', treatises on medicine by Hippocrates, Galen, the encyclopaedic medical work of Avicenna and the surgical treatise of abu-al-Quasim-al-Zahrawi (Abulcasis). Amongst

---

[9]   Georges Ifrah concludes in his *Universal History of Numbers*:
       Thus it would seem highly probable under the circumstances that the discovery of zero and the place-value system were inventions unique to the Indian civilization. As the Brahmi notation of the first nine whole numbers (incontestably the graphical origin of our present-day numerals and of all the decimal numeral systems in use in India, Southeast and Central Asia and the Near East) was autochthonous and free of any outside influence, there can be no doubt that our decimal place-value system was born in India and was the product of Indian civilization alone.
       Aryabhata stated *"sthānam sthānam daśa guṇam"* meaning "From place to place, ten times in value". His system lacked zero. The zero was added by Brahmagupta. Indian mathematicians and astronomers also developed Sanskrit positional number words to describe astronomical facts or algorithms using poetic aphorisms (sutras).

Gherado's translations dealing with mathematics are to be found the word 'sinus' (cove). Today, its continued use as 'sine' in trigonometry has come a long way from its Indian origins.

The Passage. Seats of Learning, Universities

The concept of universities, where students live to study a variety of disciplines under eminent teachers, extends far back in history. Medieval Arab universities are likely to have played a role in the constitution of the earliest European universities at Salerno, Naples, Bologna and Montpellier. They were founded in cities with easy access to similar institutions of learning in the world of Islam. So the later autonomic corporations of Europe for the promotion of teaching and, somewhat controversially, research (see Fuller), could well have been inspired by those institutions, like the al-Azhar in Cairo, in Constantinople under Byzantine suzerainty, and in other Arab and Persian cities. While the exchanges of knowledge were, through individual interests, often centred in the innumerable mosque libraries and religious institutions, the content of manuscripts went far beyond into the secular fields of mathematics, astronomy, philosophy and logic, and to those more down to earth disciplines relating to medicine and public health.

These patterns of exchange were followed well before the mediaeval age. Monastic institutions of Buddhist origin at famed cities of learning like Nalanda in Bihar, India, have been described by the Chinese traveller and scholar Hsüan Tsang[xxviii] as early as the 7th century. Between the 5th and 8th CE two famous Chinese travellers to India, Faxian and Yi Jing recorded their interest in Indian health management and medical systems, although Yi Jing was not convinced of any great virtue to Indian therapeutic systems in comparison to Chinese diagnostics, which governed the therapeutic use of acupuncture and moxibustion[10]. (See, Amartya Sen in *The Argumentative Indian*).

The Muslim invader from Afghanistan laid waste, in 1193, the earliest institutionalised centre of learning in the world, burning its manuscripts and destroying the Library. There is considerable evidence that travellers

---

[10] Moxibustion is the gentle application of heat by smoking the herb Artemisia in various ways, usually over known acupuncture points. It is far gentler and more sophisticated an application than cautery in its methods as developed in Japan and the Far East.

had carried with them to China Buddhist teachings from these centres of intellectual activity. Most certainly the ideas generated in such institutions, had crossed civilisations in transmitted knowledge[xxix] well before the ecumenism of the Sciences.

A view of the world that sustained and continues an essential Eurocentricity in many respects commenced in an Imperial age which depicted their Grand project. Scholars in the centuries of Imperialism rarely found systematic knowledge transmitted and exchanged from sources beyond Europe which had fed into their own, of course, with eminent exceptions. There were a few specialists working beyond the general trend who, in pursuing their disciplinary methodology, made novel contributions and enhanced certain areas of Eastern knowledge. The exceptions were notable ones, who often laid the foundation for the lack of such studies in the Institutions of Europe and America. Academic interest has since revived about the stock and diversity of the influence, consistently adding information to selective disciplines.

Classical antecedents to Discovery. Developments to the Physiology of Blood Circulation.

William Harvey is the name invariably associated with the discovery and function of blood circulation[11]. But could it have progressed without the awareness of the pulmonary circulation that had been enunciated earlier? The primary function of the circulation was to oxygenate the venous return of blood arriving in the right ventricle, by a circulation from there to the lungs and then a return to the left ventricle. That was discovered by a West Asian physician/experimenter Ibn al-Nafiz (1210-1288)[xxx]. It is not surprising that experiment as method continued in the works of this considerable pioneer in experimental medicine of the 13th century, following in the footsteps of Rhazes. He hardly featured until recently in the medical history of the discovery of blood in circulation. His demonstration of a pulmonary circulation relates its anatomy to the physiology of aerating blood and predates by centuries William Harvey's model. Harvey did, indeed, progress to demonstrating and describing the human blood circulation and its functions in its most complete form. The implications from earlier discovery of the anatomy of the heart and

---

[11]   in 1628 Harvey published in Frankfurt, "Exercitatio Anatomica de Motu Cordis and Sanguinis in animalibus"

the demonstration of a separate pulmonary circulation were, however, a quite considerable and necessary prelude, and Harvey's access to the works on the subject including that of Ibn al-Nafiz is beyond speculation considering the available information base during the centuries preceding De Motu Cordis. Harvey, it should be remembered trained in Padua under Fabricius[12]. Previous influence and cumulative effects on the notable 16th century transformations of medicine to the methodology of an experimental discipline are not mere conjecture.

Medical history would logically suggest that discovery to establish a functional blood circulation was achieved in stages. That there was experimentation in the medicine of medieval Islam is known. Knowledge of an established physiology of a pulmonary circulation would have come to Europe, considering scholastic translations and the many mutual contacts across West Asia and the schools of Italy. While direct attestation for specific discovery is not available, we know that Giordini Bruno proposed a blood circulation influenced by ancient Chinese ideas, and Cesalpino described a pulmonary circulation in 1571. Considering the intellectual traffic and special interests it is likely that an anatomist like Cesalpino was aware of the 13th century work of Ibn Nafiz on pulmonary circulation. The origins in West Asian Medicine in the 13th century to the physiology and circulation of blood require an acknowledgement, a contribution that was available and no less estimable than William Harvey's.

Explanations of blood coursing the body have come from across many continents and taken nearly two millennia to bring it to its present science. Should we start with Erasistratus, the the Greek anatomist and physician to Seleucus I, Nicator of Syria around 275 BCE who had suggested the link of a blood circulation to the lungs? In expounding acupuncture theories as early as that century, Chinese theorists described a circulation of blood which later gained some physiological sophistication but in an impossible anatomy. Energy was said to be conveyed by meridians (tracts), the ching lo, and blood by the ching mo, in their separate vessels. Blood was portrayed as traversing vessels including capillary-like ones. They were part of the theory of Chinese Medicine during the Han dynasty, early CE, and included a calculation of circulatory time. It came far closer to the true physiological fact than that visualised by Harvey in his physiological treatise. Capillary circulation, though, was not a concept for even later

---

[12] Celestial Lancets; see p 35 in footnotes.

Renaissance workers to understand and remained a stumbling block from Galen's times although the elementary idea that vessels contained blood was demonstrated by him on the field from bleeding gladiators.

The centuries of Galenic and Vesalian error, *of pores transposing blood* were experimentally superseded in the discoveries from West Asia. The discovery of the pulmonary circulation and the fact of a capillary conduit between arterial blood and its return to the heart had advanced the entire idea about circulating blood. The workers from Italy have been mentioned. Valves preventing a back flow to venous blood mentioned in Harvey's epochal work, the De Motu Cordis, with other demonstrations completed the anatomy that could establish correctly the physiology of a blood circulation. But degrees of error persisted in Harvey's physiological exposition; for instance, the time taken for one cycle—"But let it be said that this does not take place in half an hour, or in an hour, or even in a day;—" was way out in terms of the half minute it actually takes for completing that cycle in an average human.

Science and imperatives to Medical Discovery.

Discoveries in medicine are often made in the contextual imperatives and changing patterns to social organisation. Epidemic disease, once seen as a visitation beyond human control, and the devastation as possibly a punishment accepted in most religions, slowly became recognised as within the control of the therapeutic systems of a few civilisations. Transfer of ideas spurred the development of therapeutics and their application. The proof of efficacy and correctness was judged by the outcomes of practice. The evaluation of therapy through the results changed the explanations of disease. Established methodologies were renewed in application and improved by access to other sources. Much of the discovery and progress in the earlier classical practice of medicine was made through physician observation, a filtered perception of detail to the description of an illness. Past the usual routines of practice, physicians observed the unusual, which merited their further consideration. They figure amongst those to whom medicine is indebted for its progress. For centuries smallpox and measles were recognised as an epidemic disease but indistinguishable from each other. In the close observations of Ar Rāzï or Rhazes[13], details of signs and

---

[13]   "The outbreak of small-pox is preceded by continuous fever, aching in the back, itching in the nose and shivering during sleep. The main symptoms of its presence

83

symptoms showed them to be separate entities. That distinction was was not available in the legacies of Hippocrates or Galen but appeared later in Arab classification of disease. The process of discovery and improved classification involved two interacting factors. The differentiation between diseases of an epidemic nature was made possible while bringing an assortment within continuous review by the physician and, secondly, because large patient numbers were gathered in the context of a hospital. The hospital context served Rhazes' empirical observations to advantage. The methodology for observation had taken on a new lease because astute physicians provided bedside records which detailed the history of disease in the changes of signs and symptoms. To discern the periodicity and patterns to the natural history of illness was possible through bedside assessments. In the large numbers of patients, differences between diseases and their response to management or treatment provided diagnostic distinction within the classification of epidemic disease.

Patient care in Rhaze's time in Baghdad was as a social function within institutions. Hospitals, or to revert to the original Arabic, the 'bimaristan', were widely established. They were put in place by a medieval administration under despotic Caliphs who offered a visionary approach to social problems. The 'bimaristan' housing patients was an advance on earlier health care from many points of view, including that of a measure of isolation in times of epidemics. Contagion was by now clinically recognised, and the stage set in later centuries for more momentous discoveries in medicine.

Greek thought contributed to the discipline of medicine but the net must be cast wider when considering its development as science. Early impulses toward medical science as we know it are from the considerable attainments of the medicine of medieval Islam. There is evidence of Chinese and Indian intellectual contribution to that civilisation from previous contacts. The main discourse of the time around the learning

---

are: backache with fever, stinging pain in the whole body, congestion of the face, sometimes shrinkage, violent redness of the cheek and eyes, a sense of pressure in the body, creeping of the flesh, pain in the throat and breast accompanied by difficulty of respiration and coughing, dryness of the mouth, thick salivation, hoarseness of the voice, headache and pressure in the head, excitement, anxiety, nausea and unrest. Excitement, nausea and unrest are more pronounced in measles, whilst aching in the back is more severe in small-pox than in measles" (quoted from Meyerhof's chapter in the Legacy of Islam, Science and Medicine: p 324-325).

from West Asia was by scholars looking for the attainment of peace and spiritual harmony. Alchemy had its substantial following. Rhazes has been mentioned, but alchemical interest or the prevailing scholarly mould did not quite fit his special genius. Abu Rayhan Al-Birūnī (973-1048) has considerable standing—a physician polymath whose interest extended to the mathematics and astronomy of India where he had spent time in study. Significant compilations of his work are extant showing the continuity of contributions to medicine and to its universal transformation as natural and apparent. The antecedent medicine of the Greeks was worked through first in West Asian genius having sources from China and India before arriving in the Renaissance.

Experiment and methods of Discovery.

Aspects of West Asian contributions to the evolution of modern medicine and its universal significance have been discussed.

Medicine owes its progress to outstanding minds, but it is a disciplinary rigour that may further observation and find significance beyond given knowledge. Alexander Fleming noted an unusual change in the character of a staphylococcal culture, was intrigued by it, and wondered if a possible contaminant could have reduced the colonies. A petri dish on his window sill still forms part of that story, and possibly over-dramatises the discovery process of the initial antibiotic, Penicillin. For the research scientist the observation was of the unusual, but it offered an idea; the start of patient and painstaking labour in experimental repetition to eliminate variables and to confirm or deny the hypothesis formulated from the observation.

Again the process of discovery may be in historical continuity, and the effort sustained through cumulative additions in time. The initial recognition of smallpox advanced slowly over many centuries, and methods were evolved for its prevention. Later after discovering its aetiology, improvement to vaccines and safe immunisation were developed, leading to the control of epidemics and finally to the achievement of eradicating the disease. That process came in sequences, in related methods which had occurred across civilisations and in separate developments for controlling the same problem.

To commence with, Greek and Galenic records in medical history are of epidemics of plague-like disasters without further definition of illness[xxxi]. China and India had recognition of the disease emerging in epidemics, for which they postulated methods of control. They developed forms of variolation from cow pox pustules insufflated into the nostril or infiltrated under skin. The effort in principle was to ameliorate the extreme consequences of a recognised disease in exposure to milder forms of the same. Rhazes recognised and conclusively established a distinct epidemic disease, named smallpox. It was a notable step towards clarity of distinction from previous epidemic fevers. After Rhazes, further improvements and preventive techniques were developed in Turkey and the Balkans, possibly by assimilation of techniques from the East. Those methods found their way to the New World and the contributions of Jenner and Pasteur with improved vaccines provided populations with safer preventive programmes.

Efforts for world-wide eradication of smallpox were included in the sponsored activities and international coordination, a few decades ago. A milestone in Public Health was attained by the World Health Organisation, a post-World War II legacy. From the experiments in China and India in antiquity, the concept of this disease had suggested possible prevention. From that time on the eradication of small pox was not by singular contribution. Its history is of multiple forbears, incremental discoveries of many civilisations. The WHO and, indeed, the many public health workers mobilised by each nation for immunising its populations, finally achieved the vision projected by Jenner in 1800. The cumulative process to discovery by scholars transmitting knowledge across continents, of the sociological and medical sciences in international collaboration, finally made possible the relegation to the Annals of History of the scourge that had decimated millions from antiquity and onwards into the 20th Century.

Heterodox Inputs and the development of Medical Disciplines

Improvement to medical science by those beyond its community occurred as a response to social or other imperatives. For Europe the role of the barbers: those few in civilian life with sufficient competence and intelligence provided early elementary surgical techniques which were improved and used in the context of battle. The discipline of Surgery as a Western practice commenced largely outside of the medical establishment of the times, but provided few solutions for complex injury or the excessive blood loss of battlefield injury, often dealt with by amputation

Replacement of lost body fluids had to await further discovery. Blood transfusion was crucial for combating physiological shock; its use increased as surgical techniques for injuries improved in the magnitude of war trauma. Karl Landsteiner, an Austrian physician, of consequence, documented in his laboratories the first three human Blood groups, designated A, B and O. Safer methods for blood transfusion were developed during the Spanish Civil War where the injuries were not only from the battlefield but heavily overflowed into civilian casualties as aerial bombardment as a weapon of war was directed for the first time specifically against civilian populations. Techniques of surgery were improved for the treatment of injuries and large scale body burns. Progress was possible once shock was controlled by the replacement of body fluids.

Modern Accident Surgery in the civilian context became a science, in part consequent upon the experience of surgeons, volunteers, both national and international, to the Republican army in the Spanish Civil War[xxxii]. That war was a historic saga in itself; but it also describes continuity to the thesis of how specific forms of knowledge evolve, even in the experience of war. Surgeons like Josep Trueta, a Catalonian, who had served in the Spanish Civil War, made a revolutionary contribution to the treatment and management of war trauma. After the war he was exiled to Britain and served there before finally returning to his native Catalonia. Norman Bethune, a Canadian, served in Spain and his efforts were spent largely with blood transfusions on the battlefront in that war. He later served in China. Mao Tse Tung's peasant armies had faced many shortages, including lack of anti-malarial drugs during the epic Long March. He records that in their absence, the armies were kept on the move with acupuncture which temporarily reduced the high fevers of malaria. Amongst British medical Institutions, Stoke Mandeville, in Buckinghamshire, England, made its mark in the treatment of spinal injuries under the guidance of the refugee neurologist, Dr. Ludwig Guttmann. Jewish professionals were barred by the Nazi regime from practicing and Guttmann and his family removed to England by 1939.

Trueta's contribution consisted of early surgical interventions performed in mobile field units with fairly comprehensive staff. His methods were the thorough cleansing of all wounds with soap and water, then insufflation with sulfanilamide powder and as much early surgical repair as was feasible. Compound fractures were treated with extensive debridement, followed by immobilisation in plaster casts. These methods made a categorical difference to the outcome of the grosser field injuries. Definitive methods and early surgery in battle situation were previously delayed until the patient was moved to base hospitals. Trueta's regime reduced gangrene and amputations as injuries healed with less infection and disability. An early clinical trial by his team, of over a thousand patients with injury treated by these methods, showed deaths of only 6 patients while the rest progressed to degrees of recovery. Trueta's methods were an immense improvement to the outcome of war injuries compared to the injuries of World War I. The trials were sufficiently robust, without randomisation or controls, in the 'naturalistic' conditions of the battlefield. Those early clinical trials during the Spanish Civil War were sufficiently conclusive as principles for treatment, and were proved in the later development of Accident Surgery as a medical discipline. The benefits accruing to patients in the treatment and management of war injuries were soon enough used for the accidents of civilian life and commenced advanced research for the management of trauma.

Medical professionals and associated carers are called upon to mediate on an increasingly appalling scale to war casualties by devices ever increasing in their potential to cause injury. Developed by scientists and institutions subsidised by, if not on the direct payroll of the arms industry, begs the obvious question. In its neutrality can science, influence a better organised world order emerging from the chaos, or on the contrary does it only continue to serve the time worn political solutions in superior arms as the ultimate arbiter? Wars, following the decades of the most catastrophic ever, continue defunct Imperial interests, and territorial rights are impelled by the ideologies of history.

The industry involved in the manufacture of arms for profit, and those who mobilise and commandeer the use of those products, are culpable of causing the scale of injuries; of those maimed by land mines, villages and inhabitants ablaze in the fire-burns of Napalm, the devastating radioactivity after the bombs on Hiroshima and Nagasaki; or the recent, 'shock and awe' bombing tactics directed against civilian populations. Yet, the Institutions for International Justice and Juries of the World, to date, have practiced their weighty jurisprudence against barely a few—of the lesser offenders. As for those who should be appearing at that Bar, they have not spared us the need for obscene depredations motivated by their hand-on-heart humanitarianism. Their sanctimonious concern over their injured youth and blighted lives goes on, and so do the unceasing ceremonials paying tribute to 'the fallen heroes', now joined by more Nations, on either side of their fences.

Transformations of Health Practices by Populist Perception

Populations may recognise benefits in the healing systems of other cultures and, though the ways of the 'foreigner' may be viewed with suspicion and distaste, his therapeutics may be found acceptable. In the 2nd century BCE, in ancient Mesopotamia, a Sumerian city culture was dominant over a prevailing pastoral one. The edicts of Hammurabi (BCE 1751) included Sumerian medical systems which appeared to be acceptable to the local people. Administrations may also contribute to changes in popular perceptions, and altered medical practice could gain popular acceptance even though commencing with a degree of imposition. The visionary nature of Hammurabi's Edicts and conquest brought a different, possibly more worthwhile, way of life to the conquered.

In Europe the status of the 'red gowned, fur hooded practitioners' was under question from the new ideas of Paracelsian medicine and they had reason to be disturbed by such novelty because it had popular appeal[xxxiii]. Society could assume a value for newer innovations or extraneous cultural mores. Paracelsian medicine (1493-1591) was a materialist philosophy based on chemical elements, which was quite aggressively propagated by a contentious personage against the traditional metaphysical medicine. The older practitioners were unconvinced in their natural antagonism to the introduction of this unorthodox medicine into their fief. Not only his Principles of Practice, but the Purse of the Practitioner was under threat.

Again, we can see medieval Mughal medicine obtaining social acceptance and popularity in India despite the religio-cultural Vedic medical traditions and bonds to the laity. Later still Colonial medicine made inroads although not always in immediate popularity. 'Doctory' as it was called, was certainly against the grain of practice and resisted both by Hindu Vaid and Muslim Hakim. Populations may not have received other medical 'wisdom' without, in the first instance, suspicions and reservations and even resistance.

Colonial medicine in China and India was promoted for the general populace as part of Christian missionary activity. Early missionaries coupled some 'pysik'(cures) with much evangelism, in general both both of doubtful value, offering little succour for the native, body or soul. By the 19th century qualified medical missionaries came upon the scene and, while Christ may not have made the headway his propagators hoped for, amongst the populace there was an awareness of the efficacy of their medical activity. The missionary was not intended for the promotion of Western medicine. That was later taken up by local administrations. The medical missionary and his enterprise was meant in order for native peoples to 'see the light'. But many foreign missions realised a greater fulfilment in establishing institutions of allopathic medicine. It introduced populations to certain values—of public health and the self-effacing dedication in the work of the medical missionary. By then women were included in their ranks[xxxiv]. In time certain of their institutions developed into centres of excellence for teaching and front line medical care. Today they have a much reduced base in evangelism and primarily offer an impressive welfare argument for health delivery: that the best offerings to the health of the community should not be regarded as commodities with a price that is determined by competitive market values.

Missionary effort had, in its evangelical heyday, forced the issue in China. It contained more of the Imperial arrogance which was glaringly evident as the Manchu dynasty went overboard in acceptance of European ways. Traditional medical practices were nearly bludgeoned out of existence by propaganda, and eventually in fiat forcing a public compliance. But traditional practices remained in social confidence and retained its existence. Communist dispensation later revitalised the populist base of Traditional Chinese Medicine, a rather ill-considered revival of policy in the saga of the 'barefoot doctor'. Intense anti-Western and anti-feudal sentiment resulted but was used to promote class ideology. While the barefoot doctor with his acupuncture needles and his potions was meant to extend to the countryside a meagre supply of health personnel, it did not serve for better health care and was gradually recognised for its failures. Later more sustained, collaborative efforts at methodological validation took place within very modern institutions, and traditional medicine returned to a newer acceptability in 20th century China[xxxv].

Popular cultures, Metaphysics and Universal science.

Traditional physicians who presumed that they and none other should have the final say on the merits of an interloping system of medicine were forced to face challenge. The ultimate arbiters of the issue of better medical value were the population who could choose between differing systems. The function of scientific medicine, not necessarily its science, plays a role in that perception. Any medical practice popularly regarded as better value toward health is acceptable. We have, in fact, seen that newer medical practices could be resisted by votaries of an older one when his practice and its raison d'être is under threat.

Modern medicine has found acceptance by any public exposed to science, but science is yet to be understood as an alternative social culture to be accepted when in conflict with tradition. As a result it is community experience that informs the public in determining choice, rather than the individual in his conviction. The efficacy of modern medicine replaces traditional practices, most often in fields of secondary and tertiary health care, but also when traditional practice is perceived to be inadequate. Anecdotal evidence does suffice amongst societies using therapeutics within the epistemologies previous to science that too is essentially experiential. But, for the many life-needs, while the benefits of science are sought, it is not the lived-in culture; hopefully a future prospect in gradual achievement for societies across the world.

Empiricism can provide scientific disciplines with models for the solution of unique issues as they are confronted, even while science contributes over-arching principles and a culture. It is a temper that could pervade sections of society bringing conflicts, especially with tradition. Science attempts verifiable solutions to be confirmed or rejected in application, and its solutions are debatable as much as the methods for arriving at them. The acceptance of Science, its methods of verifying propositions or hypothesis can make no claims beyond the mandate of selected and specific problems. Social sciences contending with societal issues demonstrate that maintaining Health Security for citizens by universal State supported Health Care is a necessity. We commenced with the wasteful economy of States once supported by Slavery. Centuries later the 'Right to Life and Liberty', for the individual, the Citizen, emerged in the Constitution of Nations, informed by political science but made meaningful only if populations have the means to sustain their lives in Health—the specific public policies suggested by the Social Sciences. Following their directive results in healthier populations and is sound economics[xxxvi]. The requisite infrastructure towards maintaining a healthier Nation is an eminent advance of Social and Political Science and the evidence of improved Health indices is reflected amongst nations that have implemented policies for Universal Health and Welfare.

Society has yet to come to terms with and accept the process of science. It may be a means toward resolution of societal issues which reflect on the problems faced by its smaller units. Metaphysical propositions have supported and justified the edicts that maintain hierarchy while open societies move toward questioning and assuming responsibility for themselves and, to an extent, realising the issues pertaining to their welfare. For science, the ideal does not exist, its writ, ephemeral. Open societies debate through democratic institutions, yet may be governed by vested interests and ideologies proffered in the cultures by which their societies live.

In the dynamics of today's social organisation, competition holds the high ground of economic policies whereby Capital and Corporates prevail. In the United States of America a Universal State Welfare system is seen as enervating society; but the government of Canada, and most European ones, have made the Science of Social Health an imperative of policy and find adequate funds toward providing health care on an Universal scale. A developing country like India accepts the need for Health Care as a matter of policy but, in her adherence to the Private Sector, expects Corporates to enter the arena for providing Societal Health. As a consequence, the percentage of funds made available from the public exchequer is paltry. The Private Sector for Health is a forceful player but cannot replace the authority of the State to formulate policies to cater to popular health needs. In business concepts and cost effective policies the Private sector realises a 'product' eminently marketable to a population that can pay. The example of India, in partnership with Private Health Corporates for realising Universal Health Care, is revealing. The Health Indices of India's population have continued to make abysmal reading[xxxvii], even posed against the achievement of neighbour Nations, Sri Lanka, Bangladesh, emerging from their Colonial history, whose gross domestic product does not compare. On the score of GDP India, amongst growing World economies is now reckoned a major player but adulation cannot get past its social well-being which on many scales is comparable to sub-Saharan Africa

Alternative Systems and Health Care

The argument for the inclusion of the many alternative systems within the organisation of Health Care needs to be resolved. They are presently used by the public but no Medical Establishment is seen to be statutorily responsible for overseeing their function. Choices based on metaphysical theories about health issues have drawbacks and hazards and Society needs education and cultural appreciation of a different order for the reasons for ill-health. Therapeutic systems must demonstrate specific value, safety, possible side effects and contra-indications for their products or procedures, within a standardised medical culture, whether the origin is in Traditional or Modern Medicine. Traditional therapeutics and its practice continues within its epistemology but research in science, such as is taking place for acupuncture, is a safeguard and, when explained in the science of medicine, allows newer practices by the medical practitioner. The present research culture, clinical medicine and its *diagnostic pathology* must provide indications for treatment. The development of traditional practice cannot discount pathological indications for treatment in the interest of safer clinical practice. That provides a necessary standardisation and the failure to appreciate that importance can jeopardise public safety. Seeking an uniformity of function based in science does not detract from the value of traditional therapeutics, but there is a good way to go before they are established in the medical culture of the day. The ecumenism which aided exchanges of value amongst previous medical systems and developed them, now demonstrate the need for that continuity in Science.

If science is unique for its revolutionary paradigm that should not be a constraint for therapeutics that are of the past and, if anything, a very functional practice in any population. The insistence that research method can evaluate treatment by ignoring distinct epistemological practices has little merit. Such restraints assume that they are irrelevant to the patient's responses. Medical cultures that came from other traditions are evidently finding more public and practitioner acceptance, despite inadequacies demonstrated in clinical trials: methods, reviews, meta-analyses and so on. Innumerable clinics use acupuncture, for instance, as a possible alternative to other therapy. It is happening without the above validation. Nor have these therapeutics the need for such promotions as are seen for products of the pharmaceutical industry. That a public can give such support without the promotional gambits of a highly competitive pharmaceutical industry is a sociological fact that should merit study.

There is a general acceptance or demand for the many undoubted benefits of science and this extends to modern health care. The legitimate unease toward some of its methods and results is the facet of a problem which may be solved as the debate inherent in issues of Science becomes the warp of society. Until then we continue to depend on the past and its many metaphysical guides in the conduct of our daily lives and even our future. It is not surprising that the votaries of traditional medical systems are able to maintain a popular base and their practice.

Validation of these systems and practices in primary health care should be pursued for evidence, but method was not constituted or even contemplated for complex traditional practices. Traditional therapeutics enjoys popular support, and their use is continually on the increase. There is, for instance, the sheer anecdotal viability of 'herbal' medicine, and where research is removed from that reality it does not cut much ice for clinicians, let alone society at large. 'Anecdotal' evidence suffices[14]. While the Science of medicine has exponentially outpaced others in the quality of offerings, it has not come to terms in a societal context to reconsidering the question of traditional therapeutics, not only as evidence based medicine but in the reasons for their popularity.

Traditional systems of medicine continue a social function, finding favour in a global market with product labels suggestive of scientific validation, just another promotion in the present free enterprise culture. Separating chaff from wheat does not happen by policy declaration, nor even a scientist's determination of what is essential value. In India, for instance, it was proposed that the teaching of medicine to medical undergraduates should be by a curriculum which includes both modern medicine and traditional systems. Proposed by the Indian Health Ministry[xxxviii], it is loose thinking in un-researched policy and un-debated. The basic study of both systems is likely to be diluted turning out ill-equipped graduates in either system of medicine. The sheer fact is that dichotomous epistemologies, of modern and traditional Medicine are mutually inassimilable. While they cannot be reconciled the practice of the past must be examined in the context of the present. Their systems must be investigated, and

---

[14] A hospital with exceptionally dedicated medical personnel, qualified and experienced in clinical disciplines of modern medicine is run for tribal populations at Gudalur, a border town between Kerala and Tamil Nadu in S. India at the foothills of the Niligiri Mountains. Patient needs are special and tribals are trained ancillary workers for sophisticated primary health care delivery, and by highly qualified medical personnel for tertiary care. At the hospital they have no hesitation in continuing with the Herbal Remedies long part of tribal knowledge, in conditions like asthma where they usually make good substitutes for bronchodilators or other pharmaceuticals.

their products and practices sustained in that context before they can be explained, understood and developed. There are inevitable limits to the Traditional in any field of modern life.

A return to Ramanujam serves. "—As often happens, we may not always find the keys we are looking for *and may have to make new ones* (my italics), but we will find all sorts of other things we never knew we had lost, or even ever had". Basic experimental research, molecular biology and neurophysiology have added new dimensions and much new information and enhanced our understanding of treatment based on acupuncture responses. Contemporary relevance must be established in evidence and, where possible, researched explanation in basic medical sciences. A system of thought which past cultures rationalised had a self-sufficiency for the context but is now superseded by Science where their validation is required. To establish a relevance to past knowledge can only be in the critical empiricism based largely in method and experiment[xxxix]. The appreciation of the history of that knowledge offers a few precepts of therapeutic development. We may salvage or improve upon a few therapeutic offerings, perhaps even glean more biological insights from those epistemologies, if ever they are to be discarded.

CHAPTER III

EPISTEMOLOGIES AND THERAPEUTIC ENHANCEMENT

Early Materialism and metaphysics: Ideas and Strengths

Both China and India had considerably materialistic philosophies. In India materialism engaged logic against the grain of the established philosophy that maintained religion, culture and custom. Literature and plays conveyed the social contradiction and, staged or recited, carried a ready appreciation to large sections of society. Popular local sub-cultures, language and literature reflected the aspirations or despair of the deprived. A socially relevant philosophy, in tune with popular discontent diverged from the lofty metaphysics of immutable cosmic dimensions, justifying the earthly divisions of society to perpetuity. The Lokāyata of Chārvāka was a philosophy of 'this worldliness' that proposed an ever changing world, with a profound influence on science and systems of knowledge and widely understood across a popular base[i].

Mathematical and astronomical treatises, those of Aryabhatta and Brahmagupta flourished between 5th to 7th CE in materialistic philosophy. The Susrutha samithi, an on-going medical compilation commencing with the renowned name of Susrutha, a physician of India of uncertain time in late BCE. His medicine and surgery derives from materialist precepts current at the time. Some of the principles he laid down find their way into procedures for plastic surgery after two millennia. Pedicle grafts in re-structuring the shape of the nose is just one example. The principles for the use and survival of local skin flaps and pedicle grafts for repairing defects was an attested ancient surgical procedure in India.

The Susrutha Samitha[15] appears to be a compilation of an essentially Indian Ayurvedic tradition. Procedures for surgery are remarkable not only for the sophisticated techniques described, but also for their availability in translations to Arabic in the 8th CE and then, in the late mediaeval centuries, to Latin, in Italy. These evidences of ancient antecedents to a modern surgical speciality feature rarely, in the history of Science.

From China we note a naturalism in Neo Confucian thought exemplified well in Chu Hsi's work. (CE 1131-1200)[16]. By then the influence of Buddhism was in contention with and, to some extent, for the incorporation of metaphysical ideas. Materialism, as an interpretative outlook, was undoubtedly a part of ancient Greek philosophy[ii]. Its early propositions tended to be looked down upon by the fact of its origins: those engaged in working activities could not merit respect as thinkers! Greek materialism did not measure up to the loftier sentiments expressed in abstract thought, an idealism more expressive of a philosophy by those at the pinnacle of society. However, steep progress in Science was

---

[15]   (The first translation of Susruta Samhita was ordered by the Caliph Mansur (CE. 753-774) who had embassies come from his province of Sind to Baghdad along with Hindu scholars bringing books. The Caliph Harun (CE.786-808) appointed Hindu physicians to Baghdad hospitals and ordered further translations into Arabic of books on medicine, pharmacology, toxicology, astronomy and other subjects. Alberuni who was a member of the court of Mahmud of Ghazni (A.D. 997-1030) mentions the translation of Chārvāka then current although complaining of its incorrectness. The centres of Indian learning in his times were Banaras and Kashmir, both inaccessible to the invading armies of Mahmud. The first European translation of Susruta Samhita was published by Hessler in Latin in the early 19th century. The first complete English translation was made by Kaviraj Kunja Lal Bhishagratna in three volumes at Calcutta in 1907. New sources have been discovered in Tibetan versions, Tamil sources and Mongol versions of Tibetan translations. Indian medicine has played in Asia the same role as Greek medicine in the West, for it spread to Indo-China, Tibet, Central Asia, and as far as Japan. **Chari PS, Susruta and our Heritage** Department of Plastic Surgery, Postgraduate Institute of Medical Education and Research, Chandigarh, India.: 2003 **Vol** 36, **Issue** 1, **Page** 4-13

[16]   Needham (GT, p 38, 39) "—classical language is capable of a magnificently crystalline epigrammatic formulation which is not at all unsuitable for the best kind of philosophical thinking". He goes on to quote in translation from Chu Hsi writing the following as an example from his theory of organic development 'Cognition or apprehension is the essential pattern of mind's existence, but that there is something in the world that can do this is what we may call the spirituality inherent in matter' "To say all this took him only fourteen words" says Needham.

possible, transmitted to and welcomed by other civilisations. Materialistic philosophies provided the premise and possibility for solving social problems in adaptive applications. Functional systems of the ancient sciences and medicine could be understood across India and China, for example, or between early Greece and India, and though originating in separate continents they accommodated well in others within their respective philosophies.

There was a borrowing and interaction of ideas between the Hellenic medicine of Galen and Hippocrates and the Vedic Indian systems of medicine. Chārvāka (1st-2nd CE) contributed by way of exchange to the medicine of the Greeks[iii]. Later as West Asia peaked in its scientific activities there was regular traffic and the concourse of scholars and physicians from Greece, the Arab lands, India and China[iv]. Those exchanges, discourses and translations of material produced mutually comprehensible theories, couched as they were in the metaphysics of those times. For instance, physiological concepts contained in the elements and the humours made sense in Greek, Indian, Arab or Chinese ways of thought, enabling and influencing their respective medical systems.

With changes to social organisation, maintaining the health of a community became the function of individuals or groups and their knowledge was systematised into theories for specialised social function. A gradual reliance on empirical observations and theories related to other significant correlates of culture. Individual health and social stability were attributed to planetary positions and macrocosmic fluctuation had their consequences on daily life, and these had to be considered before individual and social activities, or for actions ensuring agrarian efficiencies. These early beginnings to systematising knowledge about health had recognisable similarities across many worlds. Beyond the change from normality into illness was the influence on the individual of climate and the weather. The cosmos and its planetary signs and configurations were to be interpreted to suit the appropriate time of some daily functions, and for physicians that included the optimal time to treat illness. The readings of natural phenomena were not only accommodated to the expansive comfort of metaphysical principles with a bearing on health and wellbeing, but beyond that, to epidemic disease, floods and famines stalking the land. Metaphysical ideas posed within custom or religion were one form of epistemological specialisation. Those who related cosmic phenomenon to the happenings on earth and social functions were necessarily intellectually gifted, often of a hereditary line within a hierarchy whose capabilities were acknowledged by society. For King and commoner, their interlocution was necessary for many of life's activities, and certainly before embarking on the more substantial ventures, such as warfare.

The regulations of societal functions increasingly stratify in complex metaphysical theory, losing their way from an original relevant relationship to nature which had followed from observation. Early tribal regulations and codes for maintaining laws, familial relationships, health or agricultural efficiencies, as seen in Leviticus of the Old Testament, or in the Vedic Laws of Manu, were based in empirical necessities. But the contextual value of an original regulation changed into an immutability, despite their obsolescence in time, still causes metaphysical proscriptions to hold conservative communities in thrall.

Generally knowledge resulting from early observations was stated in inductive principles. The early thinkers of Greek society in any field, whether of natural philosophy, political or social disciplines, also reflect the instability of the times: the uncertainties due to the violence and the suddenness of change to their worlds are explained in philosophy. Recognising the fluxes in nature, their inevitability and general unpredictability, natural disasters and turbulences and even man-made upheavals were related to cosmic patterns generally unknown, but which could be appropriately supplicated. The known elements, earth, water, air are transformed through fire, the supreme power which realised them (Heraclitus, c 500 BC). Man in his concrete reality was the main Greek concern, though the ultimate beyond him could not be ignored; and Plato informs us that the general idea is the greater reality since it is that which determines the nature of the individual[v].

Evolving methodologies and heterodox approaches.

Across most civilisations philosophy and religion have comprehensible correspondence, being conceived in metaphysics despite immense divergence. The transference of ideas was possible, no matter whether in Greek, Indian or Chinese systems of philosophy, medicine and astronomy. They fertilised one another at times, but their unique ethos stimulated and furthered epistemologies and disparate philosophies. For instance, linear Time was philosophically conceivable for the Greeks. It was not sustainable as such in Taoism, nor does it occupy that position in Hindu philosophy.

Linear Time as opposed to Epochal Time has its profound influence on analytical reasoning, and in the latest development in the Science of Europe that aspect of Greek philosophy is profoundly significant.

The relationship between the experience of a microcosm and the evident existence of a macrocosm beyond it was stated in Laws governed by the disparate yet mutually comprehensible philosophies of the world's civilisations. Timelessness is a theme in Indian philosophy and evident in the mythical stories of the Mahabharata. Conversely, time controls the epochs and should govern social activities. Traditional Chinese Medicine conceived effective treatment and the promotion of healing processes as being dependent on quotidian times of intervention. There are special attributes of Time to be considered in the creation of Indian art forms. In the systematisation of Classical Indian Music the 'ragas', essentially moods, relate performances to the time of the day or night. Classical music performances may commence after midnight and continue till dawn to suit the particular ragas to the context of their time. The ethos and rules for the architecture of temples or the rooms of a dwelling, with their separate activities and functions, may relate to times of day or night which will be propitious when positioned for light and dark.

Metaphysics and Traditional Chinese Medicine

We see that great metaphysical principle Yin-Yang being woven into many aspects of Chinese science and social life. The principle may be seen in separate cultures, allowing it to be understood and lived by, whether in China, India or the countries of South East Asia. In China it is used extensively and effectively for specific functions to living. In medicine it lends itself to adaptation as a qualitative method to assess value both in diagnostics and therapeutics. For its time it carried a sophistication to method, systematised nowhere as widely as in Traditional Chinese Medicine. These 'Basic standards of value'[vi] expressed an appreciation veering to the quantifiable; the further possible gradations of yin or yang within the demarcation of an overall value of Yin or Yang. The increase or decrease of one or the other governs the application of technique for acupuncture stimulation; or the quotidian interpretation of Yang/Yin could control social activity and is used in related contexts. If daylight is Yang and darkness Yin then the period of sunrise to noon is characterised as 'yang in Yang' and the next cycle of noon to sunset would be 'yin in Yang', and so on. These Yin/Yang qualifications offered dynamic distinction and, within its detail, an empirical accord later apparent in pathology and the natural history of some acute and chronic illnesses. Changes to treatment or their schedules were decided by shifts in the yang/yin as a diagnostic configuration. Decisions on treatment thus varied for each patient but were related to the change of symptoms or signs. Their importance was found in statements in the metaphysical theories of Traditional Chinese Medicine, to be interpreted by the physician/acupuncturist.

Metaphysics promoted an universality to understanding and developing systems of previous medical knowledge. In the function and development of all modern medicine the paradigm change discounts metaphysical concepts. But those processes of thought allowed considerable development and comprehensible propositions between the intelligentsia of diverse land spaces well before the universalisation of medicine as science.

The Culture and Epistemology of Acupuncture.

The Chinese discovery of the beginnings of the therapeutic system of acupuncture, the penetration of the skin using sharp objects, goes back more than two millennia. Pointed and sharpened stones were likely instruments used by late Neolithic groups and available to many areas of the world, as was sharpened flint, used to lance boils and abscesses. The origins to the needle were of perishable material, bamboo slivers and thorns which were used for dealing with these problems by many peoples in antiquity.

Acupuncture, though, is unique to the areas of Chinese influence. An archaeological find on an island near Hong Kong comprised sharp needles of quartz, about 3 cms in length, some with broken tips. Its beaches were once the habitation of Neolithic peoples and associated with the find. From initial observations Acupuncture developed into a therapeutic system within the comprehensive knowledge of Traditional Chinese Medicine (TCM), and its evolution from the past in extant treatises to present day publications are available in its unique epistemology (Chapter VII).

The Chinese 'Classic of the Mountains and Rivers' (5th BC) refers to needles as 'stone', used, as many commentators agree, for the easing of painful conditions. Such use is unlikely to have been therapeutic acupuncture. Iron casting developed only later in China, yet a good fifteen centuries before it did in Europe. Technology of an order beyond the elementary was possessed by most East and West Asian civilisations. Further substantial innovation and discovery of social value complemented the special needs of an area of a continentally dispersed Chinese civilisation mostly unified even when overtaken by successive dynastic powers or marauding invaders. A technically proficient bureaucracy with standards for scholastic proficiency ensured a unified administration with some control over the vagaries of weather. In building immense canal and irrigation systems it provided conduits for transport over the land areas and grain for the people. From antiquity onwards discovery and applications undertaken for dispersed societies were inspired by Chinese philosophies, Taoism or Confucianism, and even a version of Buddhism was amalgamated into Chinese thought. It was a culture that accepted influences from without while philosophy marked the structure of theories behind technology and advances to knowledge. The definite spurt to discovery, innovation and a technology with innumerable applications that followed from 8th to the 15th CE was unprecedented in any civilisation before this.

It is not mere conjecture that the immense discovery of magnetism, an observation that is explained as an inductive phenomenon in the logic of its metaphysical thought, happened earliest in China. Philosophy offered a theoretical structure for the phenomenon and certainly the idea that distant bodies in space could influence each other was not a novel realisation. A revolutionary application for oceanic navigation was soon in place; a compass of considerable accuracy followed, through the solutions that overcame a coexisting but appreciated phenomenon, the varying magnetic declination of the needle. The compass was an application by the Chinese while the West still depended on planetary configurations for navigating its high seas. Later even after they discovered magnetism corrections to needle declination eluded the wisdom of Western compass makers.

Not without reason then, Francis Bacon lists three fundamental inventions to changing a world. In 1620, he notes "—these three have changed the whole face and state of things throughout the world; the first in literature, the second in warfare, the third in navigation; whence have followed innumerable changes, in so much that no empire, no sect, no star seems to have exerted greater power and influence in human affairs than these mechanical discoveries". He was referring, of course, to printing, gunpowder and the compass. Each of those have a primacy of discovery in China, but unlikely evidence in Bacon's time for his conviction of their importance.

Metaphysics was no hindrance to discovery in China in a prescientific age. TCM theory is based firmly in the tenets of Taoism. Kho-Hsueh, 'classification knowledge' was the term for traditional science, comprising compilations of observations of nature and natural phenomenon, and of the applications and technologies serving social needs and commerce. Kho hsueh continues as the term for modern science today. The ancient systems were extensively catalogued in, for example, the series of pharmacopoeias, the records of chemical affinities expressed as polarities, alchemical formulae and the many classifications based upon observations of natural phenomena—of astronomical study or the natural histories and varieties of plant life, the diseases of men or of animals.

Numerals and a developing mathematics, termed 'the art of calculation' fit into a civilisational history of more than four millennia, consolidating in the Shang dynasty which commenced around 1500 BCE. A rod system served for numerals, while fractions were expressed in a 'son/mother' relationship for the numerator and denominator respectively and when written by strokes denoted the rod numerals. Addition, subtraction, multiplication of fractions and the solution to complex mathematical problems were, functions in commerce, revenue gathering, taxes and the issues of land surveys and demarcation. The Chiu Chang Suang Shu is a compilation begun possibly in the early Han dynasty and completed at the beginning of the first century AD; the opening chapter, the Fang Thien covers the uses of numeration and mathematics in calculations of field areas, whether rectangular, trapezoid or circular. Similarly eight further chapters of the Chiu Chang form the texts for other social functions. The second chapter, Su mi, 'millets and rice' deals with measurement and percentages or proportions for the trade of cereals. Some of the Chinese contributions to mathematics can be found in Joseph George Gheverghese's [vii] lively, well-documented, recent appraisal for the non-European roots of mathematics.

The Huangti Neijing, the Yellow Emperor's Manual, can be considered a landmark, as an ancient manual of acupuncture. Essentially it is a compilation over centuries commencing from 4th CE, chapters having been added up to the 8th. In two parts, the Su Wen is posed as questions and answers about Living matter, and the Ling Shu (The Vital Axis) contains summaries of the clinical experience of physicians of the Chou and Chin dynasties, some dating further back to the 6th to 1st BCE. The Ling Shu comprises philosophy and theories to acupuncture and moxibustion: the Yin and Yang and the Five Elements, as well as tracts and relationship to syndromes and pulse diagnosis feature in it. (see also in Chapter VII).

The physician and patient problems. The medical culture.

Communication between physician and patient was in a mutually understood terminology steeped in Chinese social culture. The Chinese physician has his information of manifestations and symptoms communicated to him by his patient within the epistemological culture of TCM. While the questioning is in progress the physician observes the general demeanour of the patient, his attitude, behaviour, obvious physical characteristics, pallor, obesity and so on. The major idea that undermined well-being was of 'disharmony', a cultural perspective shared by the patient of physiological dysfunction. Questions and answers were wrapped in the terms of understanding health and disease within the well-knit appreciation of how the environment could affect them. Any communication between patient and his physician whether conducted in pre-scientific cultures or in the medicine of today is within an appreciation of disturbances expressed in respective socio-medical cultures. Even common continuities of symptoms, such as pain expressed down the ages or in geographical cultures, will be communicated within the familiar and with a difference. Along with language and idiom, the expression will reflect that common experience. Clinical Pain Research, for instance, in their standard questionnaires ignore this subjective diversity.

In the metaphysics of TCM health has correspondences to the five elements—wood, fire, metal, earth and water, and is classified in their characterised differences. Another dimension to health was the appropriateness of the Shi and Hsu, general manifestations affecting the body. Roughly Hsu is a weakening, a Yin state, a reduction to energy flows, while Shi is the tendency to plethoric, excess Yang conditions. To commence with, the questioning would be directed towards those perceptions which then were configured more definitively in the conclusions, arriving at patient disharmonies or disease syndromes. Most traditional medical theories, through many lands and in differing periods, subscribe to these ideas with variations within their respective cultures.

A Summary of Examination procedure

More detailed descriptions of diagnostics, method and procedure are carried in translation in the many manuals of TCM. The details below of acupuncture systems stated in traditional theory are entirely from the following reference[viii]. The Physician's assessment of his patient is continued by a physical examination. The condition of the tongue has many descriptive qualities which, along with mal-odour, particularly of mouth and breath, form part of further appraisals. Pulse examination is important, using his three mid fingers of each hand on the patient's wrists, the physician subjectively analyses the sensations detected by his finger tips to decide the quality of the six pulses. In theory they portray the state of organ function. This is a sensitivity that comes only with years of apprenticeship and apparently represents a computational process of many pulse qualities under each of the physician's examining fingers. The physician finally arrives at his diagnosis of his patient's problem, confirmed by the pulse reading. It is not usually stated as a categorised diagnostic entity, but rather as an evaluation of the many factors that require correction, more in the nature of a syndrome of a few individual dysfunctions. These and many other observations in the physician's examination do not, in their obvious subjectivity, offer methods for experimental verification, but the exercises are of interest.

It was not only the frank changes to disease states that interested the Chinese physician. Pre-emption of disease by recognising early imbalances is one of the conceptual possibilities that are important in Traditional Chinese Medicine. TCM stresses the need to recognise disturbances of function manifest in the body's energy systems prior to illness. By his proper reading of imbalance in the patient the practitioner treats and claims to correct states before the onset of frank illness. Pre-empting disease by the practitioner's finding appropriate remedies from his extensive pharmacy of herbal remedies, decoctions and nutritional aids or through acupuncture is apparently possible through the questioning and examination laid down in the propositions of TCM.

Meridians (Channels, Collaterals) and the circulation of Blood and Qi

Acupuncture is one of a few treatments available once patient problems are made in formulations of Traditional Chinese Medicine. There are indications for its use: acupuncture may be combined with medication from the vast TCM pharmacopeia; moxibustion is appropriate in certain indications. Acupuncture is in the distinctive therapeutic form of needling with penetration of skin and deeper tissues once this possibility is envisaged in theory.

Theories in Chinese epistemologies relating to the circulation of blood precede the beginnings of a physiological science enunciated by William Harvey, and were stated in 'The Huangti Neijing', their legendary opus. Chinese sphygmology and pulse diagnosis were essential applications of those theories which again followed empirical observations. Blood was conveyed in a system of Channels a circulatory system, the Ching Mo, visualised as an extensive circuitry of vessels. Chinese phonetics accentuate 'Mo', the differences convey meanings, pulse, channels for blood or substantive Blood. The heart, the 'bellows', pumps blood and nourishment to the tissues and returns with waste products. This describes the appreciation of circulatory function as early as the 2nd BCE. A Quantification to the circulation time had also been made by relating time and heart beat and calculations of the lengths of the great vessels of the heart. It may be calculated to be around *fifty (50) circulations/ day*. These statements, of course, fell within the metaphysics of TCM from observations over 1600 years prior to the experimental initiation of circulatory physiology attributed to Harvey.

Again, we are aware that the historical processes to ideas, stated in systems of knowledge before and including the medical sciences, are often in their correction, and necessarily without finality. In William Harvey's scientific dissertation, De Motu Cordis, we find the time postulated for a complete circulation stated as: "—but let it be said that this does not take place in half an hour, but in an hour *or even a day*; in any case it is still manifest that more blood passes through the heart in consequence of the action than can either be supplied by the whole of the ingesta, or can be contained in the veins at the same moment—".

The circulatory system of TCM finds great relevance for acupuncture in the concept of its conveying an insubstantial system of energy, the Qi. From the Su Wen of the Huangti Neijing: "The heart presides over the circulation of the blood and the juices and the paths over which they travel.—All blood pertains to the heart; all the Qi pertains to the lungs". Hence, this collateral circulation, the Ching Lo, has a less substantive, albeit a vital content—the Qi. It is a theoretical structure laid down for the manipulation of Qi that provides the empirical benefits of acupuncture.

Meridians and Acupuncture Points

Many acupuncture points seem to be originally recorded at consistent locations of surface tenderness and observed with visceral dysfunction. Approximately 160 acupuncture points were early noted. More were defined in time as theories flourished, and their locations and effects were precisely stated and classified into the categories of meridians. The numbers increased to 365 points, with a derived significance to the celestial circle of Jupiter. Twelve channels correlated them to the months of the year and the points settled in the number of days of the year. These became the the regulations for charting the Ching Lo, a circulation of Qi which followed early Chinese astronomical discoveries. The classification followed from early ideas of body functions and the distribution of points on their circulatory channels, a nomenclature laid out in statements of an understanding of those functions in metaphysical tenets which controlled them, such as Yang and Yin, and so on. The theories explained the empirical selection of points for pathological dysfunction.

The classification expounds a pattern for the 12 regular channels. The nomenclature in this presentation takes account of whether the meridians, channels, of the Qi (energy) circulation a) arise in the hand or foot, b) they are Yang or Yin, each graded into further functional subdivisions— Taiyin, Shaoyin and Jueyin or Taiyang, Shaoyang and Yangming, which indicate a quantified content of energy and, c) relates to a Zhang (solid) or Fu (hollow) organ. In TCM an Organ indicates a functional entity roughly approximating to the present anatomical space occupied by that organ. But no further correspondence should be read into an organ of TCM. The pericardium is depicted as an organ and so too, the Sanjiao, which translates to Triple Burner. They are functional concepts with no morphological equivalence to established physical organs of the body.

Their rationale is an accommodation to regularise the 12 channels into 3 groups of 4 channels to each. Each group has its origin in a meridian commencing in an internal organ. It traverses an extended route to reach the hand, whence the next meridian begins—to end in its coupled internal organ and follows its internal course to the next organ and that meridian ends in the foot. Each has either a yang or yin position, i.e. determined by the reach of the light of the sun. The body facing East, *medially positioned on limbs or meridians at the back in comparative shade of the rising sun.* These exercises of Chinese theoreticians were directed at a systematisation of their medical experience. Hence, while five was the number usually encountered in philosophical concepts, classification systems of medical thought turned into multiples of six. The two tables below summarise the circulatory organisation of the 12 main channels in I.

Table-I

Yin	Origin (o) Ending (e)		Zhang Organ		Fu Organ	Origin(o) Ending (e)		Yang
Taiyin	Hand (e)		Lung	→	Large Intestine	Hand (o) ↓		Yangming
	Foot (o)		Spleen	←	Stomach	Foot (e)		
	↓							
Shaoyin	Hand (e)		Heart	→	Small Intestine	Hand (o) ↓		Taiyang
	Foot (o)		Kidney	←	Urinary Bladder	Foot (e)		
	↓							
Jueyin	Hand (e)		Pericardium	→	Sanjiao	Hand (o) ↓		Shaoyang
	Foot (o)		Liver	←	Gall bladder	Foot (o)		

Table-II

NOMENCLATURE	INTERNATIONAL	BLOOD	Qi
The Small Intestine Channel of Hand Taiyang	Intestinalis tenue IT	+++++	+
The Urinary Bladder Channel of Foot Taiyang	Vessica urinaria VU		
The Sanjiao Channel of Hand Shaoyang	San Chiao SC	+	+++++
The Gall Bladder Channel of Foot Shaoyang	Vessica fellea VF		
The Large Intestine Channel of Hand Yangming	Intestinalis grandum IG	+++++	+++++
The Stomach Channel of Foot Yangming	Ventriculus V		
The Lung Channel of Hand Taiyin	Pulmones P	+	+++++
The Spleen Channel of Foot Taiyin	Lien and Pancreas LP		
The Pericardium Channel of Hand Jueyin	Habitatio cordis HC	+++++	+
The Liver Channel of Foot Jueyin	Hepar H		
The Heart Channel of Hand Shaoyin	Cor C	+++++	+
The Kidney Channel of Foot Shaoyin	Renes R		

Table II, is of channels nominally described although with organs translated, the rest in transliteration and the channels labelled by international nomenclature. 12 cycles are fitted into double hours of the day. The time for the complete circulation, according to classical texts, was 50 hours. The contents, blood or Qi in their respective circulatory channels, are dominant or minimal at particular double hours, thus approximating to 24 hours of the day. Such configurations, the dominance by either of blood or Qi in these tracts *or vice versa* and the Shi, Hsu manifest in the syndrome of disease control and determine practical aspects of treatment with acupuncture.

Other channels made a later appearance, possibly to accommodate acupuncture points in further discovery. There are two vertical ones, Du (Yang) channel and Ren (Yin) and their 51 points find consistent clinical use. The landmarks of the former, extend from the midline on the back of the head down the spines of the vertebral column, and the Ren channel follows a mid-sternal line down the midline of the abdomen. Five more channels circle the trunk but their points, in crossing the other 12 vertical bilateral channels, are largely duplicates of those points.

Acupuncture points

Today the named points on the regular channels number about 660, along with the 51 'extra' mentioned above. 'Experience' points keep appearing, as well as 'Ashi' points which are inconstant on the body surface. They are palpably tender on occasion and hence find a therapeutic use. Certain points have special qualities. Five such on the channels are distal to the elbow or knee, and their potency increases or decreases dependent on the direction of the circulation toward or away from the joints. They have an attribution to the *five* elements, on the Yin channels in the order of, wood-fire-earth-metal-water, and on the Yang, metal-water-wood-fire-earth.

Quotidian and seasonal rhythms affecting the patient were elaborated in theory on intricate structural charts which obscured the empiricism of primary observations. Discoidal charts, for instance, were constructed relating environmental energy to a double hour, months and seasons of the year and then to bodily function. To begin with there may have been an empirical significance which Circadian rhythms presently suggest. But classification, in gaining complexity, was impressive theory. It allowed the physician a learned reasoning for the applications of his treatment. As stated to pupils it was more a matter for assent, an acknowledgement of the physician's knowledge rather than discussion or debate. The pupil was, however, aware of the experiential worth of the application and assimilated that experience during lengthy years of apprenticeship to the master. A feature of Therapeutic traditions is that conclusions toward treatment are not debated and failure may yet correct through further weaves of theory and another treatment selection.

If theories were proto-scientific we might not ignore a basic empiricism in the selection of acupuncture points for treatment. These methods as comparative controls, for experiments and clinical trials, without reference to the theories may offer possibility to assess traditional treatment decisions by their results.

Acupuncture Points with Special Effects

The increasing or decreasing scale of potency of points situated below the elbow or the knee is based on the function of the originating organ, the comparative power of the elements to which point attribution is made, and the direction of energy flow in the channel. Considering, for instance, the Lung channel of Hand Taiyin (see fig) the respective potency of two major points below the elbow, Taiyuan, Lung 9, and Chize, Lung 5, is attributed to the element 'earth' having a 'mother' position to its 'son', metal, and these elements control the power of the two points, conferring the authority of mother over son. One set of paired points available on each of the 12 channels, therefore, has special potency if used according to the indications of the syndromes. For reducing excess, Shi syndromes, the 'son' point in conjunction with the 'mother' point but importantly, stimulation to obtain the necessary Qi, which is only achieved in the variations of stimulation techniques. Conversely, syndromes of Hsu may also be corrected by varying the quality of needle stimulation at these two paired points. The literature describes many methodical variants of stimulation and each labeled in evocative language for the quality of their evoked sensation.

Yuan Source Points

Supposedly points at which a Qi of primordial origin collects. These points are significant in TCM for their presence before environmental effects have had an influence on the individual. Each of the 12 channels contribute a Yuan source point.

Luo Connecting Points

These are pairs of points on a related Yang/Yin channel, of use when two such organs are implicated.

Table p325 in E. of Ch, Medicine. The Ren and Du Channel have Ren 15 and Du 1 as the Luo connecting points.

Table-III

Points		Segmental innervation	Organ relating
Back Shu	Front Mu	from Spinal Cord	to Sclerotome
Feishu VU 13	Zhongfu P 1	Cervical 5 to Thoracic 1	LUNG
Jueyinshu VU 14	Shanzhong Ren 17	Cervical 3-5, Thoracic 4,5	PERICARDIUM
Xinshu VU 15	Jujue Ren 14	Cervical 3-5, Thoracic 5	HEART
Ganshu VU 18	Qimen H 14	Thoracic 12, Lumbar 1	LIVER
Danshu VU 19	Riyue VF 24	Thoracic 12, Lumbar 1	GALL BLADDER
Pishu VU 20	Zhangmen H13	Thoracic 12, Lumbar 1	SPLEEN
Weishu VU 21	Zhongwan Ren 12	Thoracic 12, Lumbar 1	STOMACH
Sanjiaoshu VU 22	Shimen Ren 5	Thoracic 12, Lumbar 1,2	SANCHIAO
Shenshu VU 23	Jingmen VF 25	Thoracic 12, Lumbar 1,2	KIDNEY
Dachangshu VU25	Tianshu V25	Th.12, L 4,5 Sacral 1,2	L. INTESTINE
Xiaochangshu VU 27	Guanyuan Ren 4	Lumbar 4,5, Sacral 1,2,3	S. INTESTINE
Panguanshu VU 28	Zhongji Ren 3	Lumbar 4,5, Sacral 1,2,3	U. BLADDER

The Back Shu and Front Mu Points

The Back Shu points are those on the VU channel on the back of the trunk and lie parallel to the spines of the vertebrae. They are located in reference to each spine, two finger breadths (patient's index and mid finger at the level of the terminal phalanx, or 1½ cun, a modular traditional measure) from the midline. They are used, along with Front Mu Points, for deficiencies pertaining to the organs within the thorax and abdomen. The points have evolved from an empirical relationship to those organs of TCM. These VU channel points, for example, penetrate the paravertebral musculature, and at each level the named acupuncture point is located to a nerve supply that relates to its sclerotome. Therefore, the likely effects of their stimulation are on the tissues and organs of that sclerotome by virtue of its developmental innervation. That is often obvious from translations of the traditional name of the point which pertains to an organ; the proviso

111

to be kept in mind is that the organ in traditional Chinese medicine is only partly recognisable as an anatomical entity.

Therapeutic Modes of Acupuncture

The above account ignores much of the theorising of traditional acupuncture. What is considered in that relationship are clinical possibilities which are available from their stimulation. While acupuncture in its Traditional theories and practical usage is very much in vogue, the list of variety to practices suggests no uniform mode to its therapeutic practice. We do not question the term 'acupuncture'—what it refers to and how used in clinical practices or its research. The practice of acupuncture could be **a) traditional.** a number of stipulations need to be satisfied: the pathology of patients requires redefinition in traditional epistemology, and point selection as well as intensities of stimulation are to be determined by the therapist for individual patients. The largest numbers of patients, those in the Far East and many in the Western hemisphere, experience this form of acupuncture. Even within the epistemology of its use there are variations amongst its practitioners and between countries as well. Notably but not invariably, practice within the same epistemology differs between Japan, China and the Los Angeles School in the US, for Traditional Chinese Medicine [ix] **b) at trigger points.** Locations are identified in each patient, and their needling is carried out in brief but painful intensities of stimulation. There is a sensory intensity difference between deQi and trigger point stimulation, the latter mode occasionally used in China and known as needling Ashi points. This is another established practice of acupuncture in recent decades (see Baldry. Travell and Simons). **c) periosteal stimulation.** Felix Mann originated this mode as a therapeutic manoeuvre. It has support in the mechanisms of DNIC (Diffuse Noxious Inhibitory Control) and in the experimental work originally describing the effect by LeBars et al. The mechanism of this type of stimulation is described in the next chapter. As used therapeutically by Mann, the intensity of stimulation is tailored to location of pain and individual response.

There are other innumerable variants of needle insertion developed empirically from an acquaintance with traditional acupuncture, whose exponents have a considerable following in East and West. Some propose biological theories to support their methods while others formulate their own. Superficial insertion of needles has been favoured by MacDonald[x] in Bristol. The Adrian White School in Southampton, practising and teaching Medical Acupuncture, rather strictly adheres to needle effects known to medical science. In Sweden a variant of superficial needling was promoted by Basil Finer. It used a profusion of needles, and the resulting considerable sensory inputs were of particular value in treating musculo-skeletal pains. Vienna has a special school under **Bishko,** which suggests that needles of gold and traditional theories hold the key to its successful use. France has many forms of acupuncture with vigorous nods to tradition, but there **Nogier,** with his needles embedded in the ear, has a considerable following. The ear has properties in tradition also. Needles of special design allow for a penetration of only a millimetre and can be left in place for a length of time. A shape assigned to a foetal configuration controls needle placements and effects on the human body. But a more plausible explanation is in the vagal innervation of the ear, and autonomic sympathetic and parasympathetic responses may underlie treatment benefit. All the above methods provide courses teaching their techniques. The **Jayasurya** school in Sri Lanka has attracted students from many parts of the world for decades, and that school has teaching courses whose participants continue to function back home.

The Swedish model is one amongst the very few countries where most acupuncturists are licensed medical ancillaries with subsequent training in registered courses of hybrid acupuncture. The courses stress the neurophysiology of Peripheral Sensory Stimulation, and acupuncture is reckoned as one such modality in its teaching, while its practice entails an elementary knowledge of traditional precepts, using the channels, collaterals and the acupuncture points given above. The points, though, have been restated in localisations related also to basic medical morphology. Their defined anatomical locations include the tissues encountered in the needle's penetration, the innervation, blood supply and the likely local hazards in ignoring classical descriptions for localisation and penetration.

Many acupuncturists are possibly without knowledge of basic modern medicine, while some may have ancillary medical qualifications. This remains an unresolved problem and is referred to elsewhere in this monogram as a shortcoming to the safer practice of acupuncture. The Swedish method above is a model of teaching to be considered for reducing such risks. The lists of exponents and varying methods of acupuncture are, however, redoubtable in variety and in the practices available to the public.

Evidence Based Medicine (EBM) and Modes of Acupuncture

Neither acupuncture, its variant practices and their methods, nor other therapeutic traditions on the scene have uncritically passed through the needle's eye of EBM. The systems do provide some benefit to patients for a few diseases and many ailments. The critics who cite inadequacy of evidence for those benefits, or who maintain that the conclusions of available research indicate patient perceptions to be no greater than their placebo, have not gained the dismissal of traditional therapeutics. On the contrary, it is ever more widely available for the public, extending acupuncture into Institutional supports for Health Care. Traditional systems and acupuncture continue their utility largely supported by public approbation.

Some EBM practices are of far greater concern than the criticism levelled at traditional therapeutics as a public utility. The intense competition amongst health providers including the powerful Pharmaceutical Corporates and the nexus between them and Private Health Insurance has been repeatedly designed to promote the manufactures of the former as EBM based and 'Best Practice' models. The cynicism involved in promoting Health Care in such Commerce is not lost on an increasingly disillusioned public.

The recent instance of an over-diagnosed Pathology is partly due to the pharmaceuticals supposed to treat it being flogged for a market. Changing social mores begin to have their environmental impact on child behaviour, in unbridled playfulness, tantrums and aggression of a variant child. It finds a diagnostic label as an 'Attention Deficit Hyperactivity Disorder', ADHD, sufficiently important to merit entry in the Diagnostic and Statistical Manual (DSM) categorising Mental Diseases. Specific psycho-stimulant drugs are available to control the syndrome and the expenditure to promote awareness of that diagnosis has 'increased' the numbers affected by ADHD with a subsequent phenomenal increase in the sales of a couple of patent psychotropic drugs. Of course, expensive promotional hand outs to doctors and Institutions in frontline Health Care have helped those sales while presently there may be some reassessments of these specific psycho-stimulants used for children and adults[xi].

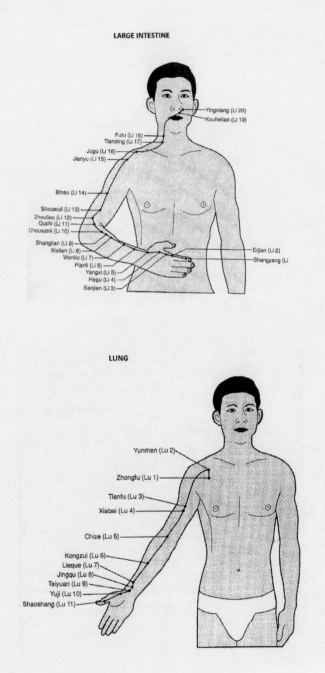

LARGE INTESTINE

Yingxiang (Li 20)
Kouheliao (Li 19)
Futu (Li 18)
Tianding (Li 17)
Jugu (Li 16)
Jianyu (Li 15)
Binao (Li 14)
Shouwuli (Li 13)
Zhouliao (Li 12)
Quchi (Li 11)
Shousanli (Li 10)
Shanglian (Li 9)
Xialian (Li 8)
Wenliu (Li 7)
Pianli (Li 6)
Yangxi (Li 5)
Hegu (Li 4)
Sanjian (Li 3)
Erjian (Li 2)
Shangyang (Li

LUNG

Yunmen (Lu 2)
Zhongfu (Lu 1)
Tianfu (Lu 3)
Xiabai (Lu 4)
Chize (Lu 5)
Kongzui (Lu 6)
Lieque (Lu 7)
Jingqu (Lu 8)
Taiyuan (Lu 9)
Yuji (Lu 10)
Shaoshang (Lu 11)

STOMACH

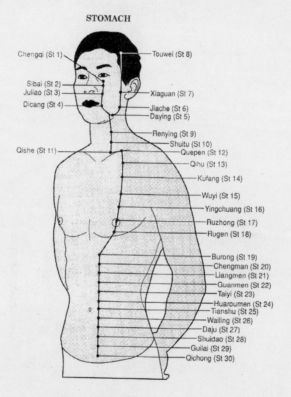

Chengqi (St 1)

Touwei (St 8)

Sibai (St 2)
Juliao (St 3)

Xiaguan (St 7)

Dicang (St 4)

Jiache (St 6)
Daying (St 5)

Renying (St 9)
Shuitu (St 10)

Qishe (St 11)

Quepen (St 12)
Qihu (St 13)
Kufang (St 14)

Wuyi (St 15)

Yingchuang (St 16)

Ruzhong (St 17)

Rugen (St 18)

Burong (St 19)
Chengman (St 20)
Liangmen (St 21)
Guanmen (St 22)
Taiyi (St 23)
Huaroumen (St 24)
Tianshu (St 25)
Wailing (St 26)
Daju (St 27)
Shuidao (St 28)
Guilai (St 29)
Qichong (St 30)

STOMACH continued

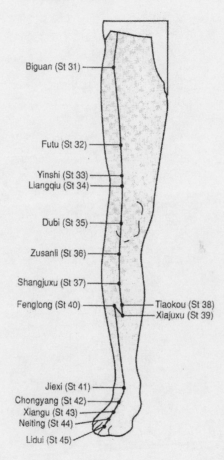

Biguan (St 31)

Futu (St 32)

Yinshi (St 33)
Liangqiu (St 34)

Dubi (St 35)

Zusanli (St 36)

Shangjuxu (St 37)

Fenglong (St 40)

Tiaokou (St 38)
Xiajuxu (St 39)

Jiexi (St 41)
Chongyang (St 42)
Xiangu (St 43)
Neiting (St 44)

Lidui (St 45)

SPLEEN

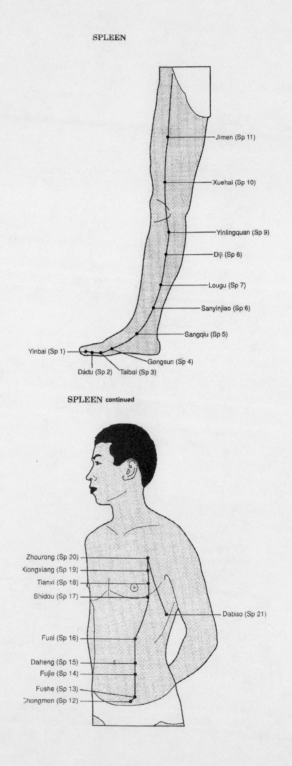

Jimen (Sp 11)

Xuehai (Sp 10)

Yinlingquan (Sp 9)

Diji (Sp 8)

Lougu (Sp 7)

Sanyinjiao (Sp 6)

Sangqiu (Sp 5)

Yinbai (Sp 1)

Gongsun (Sp 4)

Dadu (Sp 2) Taibai (Sp 3)

SPLEEN continued

Zhourong (Sp 20)
Xiongxiang (Sp 19)
Tianxi (Sp 18)
Shidou (Sp 17)

Dabao (Sp 21)

Fuai (Sp 16)

Daheng (Sp 15)
Fujie (Sp 14)
Fushe (Sp 13)
Chongmen (Sp 12)

HEART

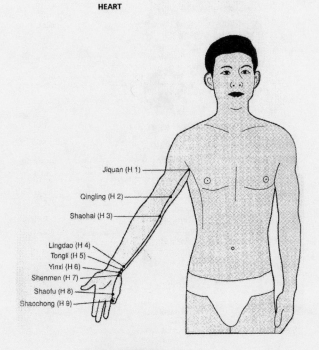

Jiquan (H 1)

Qingling (H 2)

Shaohai (H 3)

Lingdao (H 4)
Tongli (H 5)
Yinxi (H 6)
Shenmen (H 7)
Shaofu (H 8)
Shaochong (H 9)

SMALL INTESTINE

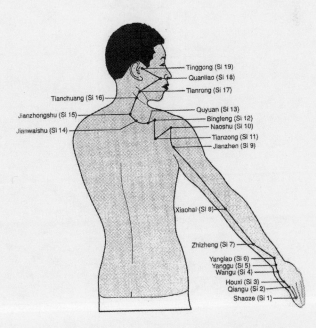

Tinggong (Si 19)
Quanliao (Si 18)
Tianrong (Si 17)

Tianchuang (Si 16)

Jianzhongshu (Si 15)

Jianwaishu (Si 14)

Quyuan (Si 13)
Bingfeng (Si 12)
Naoshu (Si 10)
Tianzong (Si 11)
Jianzhen (Si 9)

Xiaohai (Si 8)

Zhizheng (Si 7)

Yanglao (Si 6)
Yanggu (Si 5)
Wangu (Si 4)
Houxi (Si 3)
Qiangu (Si 2)
Shaoze (Si 1)

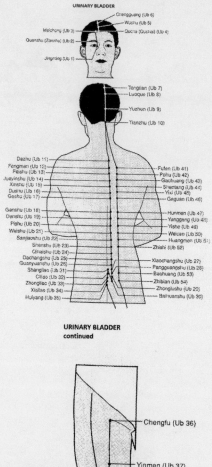

URINARY BLADDER

Chengguang (Ub 6)
Wuchu (Ub 5)
Meichong (Ub 3)
Quchai (Quchai) (Ub 4)
Quanzhu (Zanzhu) (Ub 2)
Jingming (Ub 1)

Tongtian (Ub 7)
Luoque (Ub 8)
Yuzhen (Ub 9)
Tianzhu (Ub 10)

Dazhu (Ub 11)
Fengmen (Ub 12)
Feishu (Ub 13)
Jueyinshu (Ub 14)
Xinshu (Ub 15)
Dushu (Ub 16)
Geshu (Ub 17)

Fufen (Ub 41)
Pohu (Ub 42)
Gaohuang (Ub 43)
Shentang (Ub 44)
Yixi (Ub 45)
Geguan (Ub 46)

Ganshu (Ub 18)
Danshu (Ub 19)
Pishu (Ub 20)
Weishu (Ub 21)
Sanjiaoshu (Ub 22)
Shenshu (Ub 23)
Qihaishu (Ub 24)
Dachangshu (Ub 25)
Guanyuanshu (Ub 26)
Shangliao (Ub 31)
Ciliao (Ub 32)
Zhongliao (Ub 33)
Xialiao (Ub 34)
Huiyang (Ub 35)

Hunmen (Ub 47)
Yanggang (Ub 48)
Yishe (Ub 49)
Weicang (Ub 50)
Huangmen (Ub 51)
Zhishi (Ub 52)

Xiaochangshu (Ub 27)
Pangguangshu (Ub 28)
Baohuang (Ub 53)
Zhibian (Ub 54)
Zhonglushu (Ub 29)
Baihuanshu (Ub 30)

URINARY BLADDER
continued

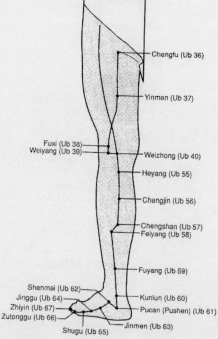

Chengfu (Ub 36)

Yinmen (Ub 37)

Fuxi (Ub 38)
Weiyang (Ub 39)
Weizhong (Ub 40)

Heyang (Ub 55)

Chengjin (Ub 56)

Chengshan (Ub 57)
Feiyang (Ub 58)

Fuyang (Ub 59)

Shenmai (Ub 62)
Jinggu (Ub 64)
Zhiyin (Ub 67)
Zutonggu (Ub 66)
Kunlun (Ub 60)
Pucan (Pushen) (Ub 61)
Jinmen (Ub 63)
Shugu (Ub 65)

KIDNEY

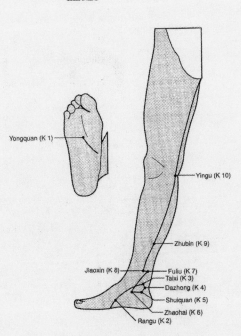

Yongquan (K 1)

Yingu (K 10)

Zhubin (K 9)

Jiaoxin (K 8)

Fuliu (K 7)
Taixi (K 3)
Dazhong (K 4)
Shuiquan (K 5)
Zhaohai (K 6)

Rangu (K 2)

KIDNEY continued

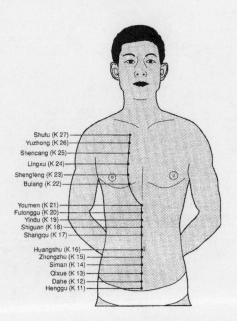

Shufu (K 27)
Yuzhong (K 26)
Shencang (K 25)
Lingxu (K 24)
Shengfeng (K 23)
Bulang (K 22)

Youmen (K 21)
Futonggu (K 20)
Yindu (K 19)
Shiguan (K 18)
Shangqu (K 17)

Huangshu (K 16)
Zhongzhu (K 15)
Siman (K 14)
Qixue (K 13)
Dahe (K 12)
Henggu (K 11)

PERICARDIUM

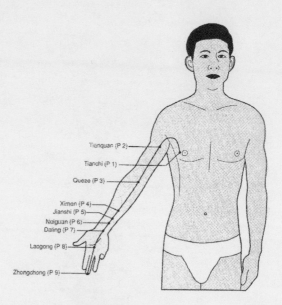

Tianquan (P 2)
Tianchi (P 1)
Queze (P 3)
Ximen (P 4)
Jianshi (P 5)
Neiguan (P 6)
Daling (P 7)
Laogong (P 8)
Zhongchong (P 9)

SANJIAO

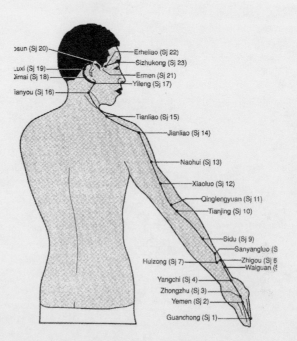

osun (Sj 20)
Luxi (Sj 19)
Qimai (Sj 18)
Tianyou (Sj 16)
Erheliao (Sj 22)
Sizhukong (Sj 23)
Ermen (Sj 21)
Yifeng (Sj 17)
Tianliao (Sj 15)
Jianliao (Sj 14)
Naohui (Sj 13)
Xiaoluo (Sj 12)
Qinglengyuan (Sj 11)
Tianjing (Sj 10)
Sidu (Sj 9)
Sanyangluo (S
Zhigou (Sj 6
Waiguan (S
Huizong (Sj 7)
Yangchi (Sj 4)
Zhongzhu (Sj 3)
Yemen (Sj 2)
Guanchong (Sj 1)

GALL BLADDER

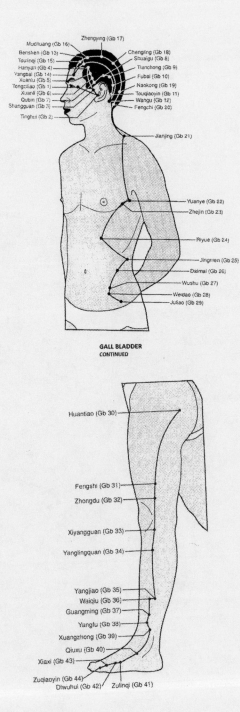

Muchuang (Gb 16)
Zhengying (Gb 17)
Benshen (Gb 13)
Chengling (Gb 18)
Toulinqi (Gb 15)
Shuaigu (Gb 8)
Hanyan (Gb 4)
Tianchong (Gb 9)
Yangbai (Gb 14)
Fubai (Gb 10)
Xuanlu (Gb 5)
Tongziliao (Gb 1)
Naokong (Gb 19)
Xuanli (Gb 6)
Touqiaoyin (Gb 11)
Qubin (Gb 7)
Wangu (Gb 12)
Shangguan (Gb 3)
Fengchi (Gb 20)
Tinghui (Gb 2)

Jianjing (Gb 21)

Yuanye (Gb 22)
Zhejin (Gb 23)

Riyue (Gb 24)

Jingmen (Gb 25)
Daimai (Gb 26)
Wushu (Gb 27)
Weidao (Gb 28)
Juliao (Gb 29)

GALL BLADDER
CONTINUED

Huantiao (Gb 30)

Fengshi (Gb 31)
Zhongdu (Gb 32)

Xiyangguan (Gb 33)

Yanglingquan (Gb 34)

Yangjiao (Gb 35)
Waiqiu (Gb 36)
Guangming (Gb 37)
Yangfu (Gb 38)
Xuangzhong (Gb 39)
Qiuxu (Gb 40)
Xiaxi (Gb 43)
Zuqiaoyin (Gb 44)
Diwuhui (Gb 42)
Zulinqi (Gb 41)

LIVER

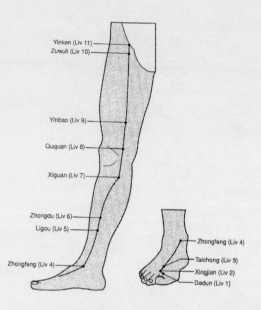

Yinlian (Liv 11)
Zuwuli (Liv 10)

Yinbao (Liv 9)

Ququan (Liv 8)

Xiguan (Liv 7)

Zhongdu (Liv 6)

Ligou (Liv 5)

Zhongfeng (Liv 4)

Zhongfeng (Liv 4)
Taichong (Liv 3)
Xingjian (Liv 2)
Dadun (Liv 1)

LIVER CONTINUED

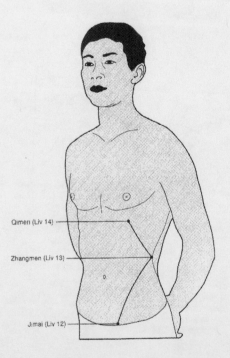

Qimen (Liv 14)

Zhangmen (Liv 13)

Jimai (Liv 12)

DU posterior midline meridian

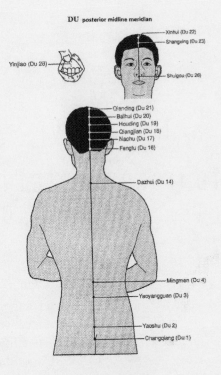

Yinjiao (Du 28)

Xinhui (Du 22)
Shangxing (Du 23)
Shuigou (Du 26)

Qianding (Du 21)
Baihui (Du 20)
Houding (Du 19)
Qiangjian (Du 18)
Naohu (Du 17)
Fengfu (Du 16)

Dazhui (Du 14)

Mingmen (Du 4)

Yaoyangguan (Du 3)

Yaoshu (Du 2)

Changqiang (Du 1)

REN anterior midline meridian

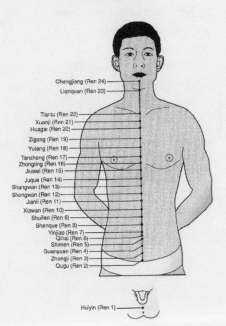

Chengjiang (Ren 24)
Lianquan (Ren 23)

Tiantu (Ren 22)
Xuanji (Ren 21)
Huagai (Ren 20)
Zigong (Ren 19)
Yutang (Ren 18)
Tanzhong (Ren 17)
Zhongting (Ren 16)
Jiuwei (Ren 15)
Juque (Ren 14)
Shangwan (Ren 13)
Shongwan (Ren 12)
Jianli (Ren 11)
Xiawan (Ren 10)
Shuifen (Ren 9)
Shenque (Ren 8)
Yinjiao (Ren 7)
Qihai (Ren 6)
Shimen (Ren 5)
Guanyuan (Ren 4)
Zhongji (Ren 3)
Qugu (Ren 2)

Huiyin (Ren 1)

CHAPTER IV

DICHOTOMISED MEDICINE AND SOCIAL IMPLICATIONS

While systematic theories and rationalisations differed in the practice of any system of medicine, the good clinician augments his practice through experience, intuitively exploited and irrespective of any dominant philosophy. Physicians today have the added reliability of experimental verification for improving therapeutic selection, but intuition plays a part in spite of evidence and 'best practice' recommendation. An awareness of inadequacies of therapies commenced in the present clinical discipline, and the involvement with a more rigorous science promoted newer methods and innovative improvements to medicine. A hypothesis, however, was never a shot in the dark. Scientific method requires a trained intuition to ask the questions out of the routines of practice before new and effective evidence and solutions appear for prevailing problems.

In considering theoretical structures of medicine and its conjunction with practice one is aware of the extent to which a good practitioner depends in his clinic on an acumen that is allowed to stray beyond theory and yet is defined—and limited—by its regulation. This applies to the practice of Chinese or Ayurvedic medicine or the practice of a modern Clinic of the day.

Sound clinical judgement is discernible, whether based in the culture of rarer metaphysical theory, or within the causal, analytical logic of today when the therapist/physician/research worker appreciates the problem on hand and seeks solution within a disciplinary practice[17]. At another level

---

[17]   It would be appropriate to briefly explain what is meant nowadays by metaphysical reasoning. Where the word is not merely used in a dismissive sense when contrasted

it is more than a diagnostic problem, an intuitive appreciation which has much to offer the patient and his individual problem and as such, cultural evaluations play a considerable part to clinical judgement. That relationship with the patient is a considerable aspect of medical practice past or present.

This was brought home to us at our Beijing Clinic for traditional acupuncture where, in the early eighties, we were learning to apply elementary theories of Traditional Chinese Medicine (TCM). A young, unmarried girl with a short history of amenorrhoea came for treatment we were told to understand its cause in the pathophysiology of the five

---

with scientific reasoning, it contains logic that is inductive and synthetic. The traditional modes of reasoning, it must be remembered had generally conceived of time as cyclical and infinite (Indo-Hellenic) rather than the later (Judaeo-Christian), a linear process with its inherent finiteness. The latter was an appreciation apparent in European cultural history and, eventually, the linearity of time offered a most important methodological parameter for scientific discovery. Without appreciating the significance of linear time, considerable discovery and explanations for natural phenomena are noted in China between the 2nd to the 11th centuries AD. Within the Chinese ideas (inductive and synthetic) of the patterns of the cosmos it was possible for an effective positions in space to influence another at the same point in time; whereas, in accepting linearity of time, causality would allow one effective position to change into another within the same space in the dimension of time (see Porkett). Discoveries can follow in either rationality. Magnetic phenomena it might be remembered find explanations much earlier in China within the former inductive systems of thought, where one position is influenced by another over 'unseen' distances. One can appreciate the fact of a discovery such as magnetism and the understanding of the phenomenon amongst the ancient Chinese as it would have offered no difficulties within systems of Chinese thought; its discovery and applications predated them in the West by centuries. Declination, the magnetic phenomenon which distinguishes the polestar from the true North, did not set the Chinese the formidable problem that it appears to have done in the West after its much later discovery of magnetism. (see the GT, Needham, p 21, 23, 46). We need not explore further what is put forward here essentially as two concepts of time, possibly facile in simplification. We understand that science has explanation in the synthetic and inductive, and certainly provided considerable discovery even without the linearity of time. It was that the Chinese who could fall back upon a 'Tao', here the 'Chhang Tao', the 'unvarying way' to explain organic laws of nature. They never needed a Celestial law giver to commission the laws of Nature. The historiography is available in academic detail in Joseph Needham's 'The Grand Titration' in Chapter titled 'Time and Eastern Man', with reference to scientific development in East and West.

Evolutive Phases, the wu hsing (Porkett), and a fairly elaborately derived *Yin deficiency syndrome* was the diagnosis. It was based on a physical examination with stress on pulse and tongue; an examination; quite unlike the physical examination such a patient would be subjected to, at least, by those amongst us who were qualified doctors of medicine. Acupuncture points were then chosen and we were confidently told it was to restore the Yang balance for her Yin deficiency syndrome. We raised the possibility of an early pregnancy but were unhesitatingly informed that it need not be considered as the girl was unmarried!

The context: a young female with amenorrhea in China in the early 1980s; the lady physician had steered her way through the problem, the patient lost no face and the explanation and outcome from treatment was entirely to the young girl's satisfaction. Her normal menstrual cycle was restored in a couple of weeks after the routine schedules of acupuncture treatment. Whether it was in fact effected by an early abortion or, indeed, Yang restored, and if acupuncture played its part in either possibility, what was treated and how it was achieved, were for us still open questions. The physician was confident of restoring her patient to normalcy without asking embarrassing questions. To be unobtrusive and understanding in the circumstances was obviously the importance. The intriguing question requiring a clinical answer remained, while others about a historical therapeutic procedure and the importance of the focus in its culture were to arrive at our doorstep.

THE CLINIC OF TODAY AND TRADITIONAL PRACTICE

A better appreciation of the function of traditional modes of healing requires a minimum understanding of epistemological compulsions. Whether or not they are presently valid they continue in principles to be functional treatment forms into the present. Yet in relegating these systems to 'non-science' compared to the systematised practice of present medicine, whose disciplines seen as scientific, we often ignore a therapeutic social function. Modern medicine and practice fit the paradigm of sciences. Traditional medicine, its empirical observations and theories of inductive and synthetic logic, subscribes to bodily dynamics related to influences beyond them, to a macrocosm, as against analytical and causal reductionism of morphological change in the organisms' limited biological space.

Aspects of the practice of the clinic from the past formed continuity discernible until a few decades ago. It was the manner of deciding the therapeutic procedure or management of disability by a clinician for his patient. A relationship developed, embedded of course in a culture, of society in general as well as the particular intellectual enterprise of medical aid and societal health. The line the therapist follows for his patient, now or in tradition is determined against that backdrop. The therapist, the clinician in any culture, in any age recognises that importance. Altered medical procedure and consequent semantic change in explanation or communication makes some difference to the relationship he develops with his patient and yet, it is a recognisable continuity. Whether it is in the choice of therapy or in management advice the patient is aware of his health partly in the cultural milieu which determines how it is dealt with.

Science in clinical practice

Much of the science is found in the laboratory disciplines allied to medicine. These analyse biometrics or other patient parameters, aids toward diagnosis, localising pathology or causes for patient problems. However, a clinician's acumen, his appreciation of a patient problem is certainly comparable to the older traditions to the extent that it is moulded in the exchange between him and the patient in a particular context, family related or working conditions and so on. The logical position governing that totality is both inductive and analytical in nature. But their respective modes of operation are within different theoretical paradigms, the medical culture of today having a far more dispersed base, some in other specialised and collaborating disciplines. The direction of that collaboration ought to be for the patient's benefit, but today there are deviations from this priority

Innumerable strains accompany the pursuit of medicine as science, influences which are well removed from scientific culture. To the extent that science has penetrated practice, medicine differs from its past, and though societies continue with past traditions, will approach modern medicine for its undoubted benefits. Science is an appreciation of necessity rather than a part of its culture. The popularity of Traditional medicine continues in the level of sophistication relating to the interaction between therapist and patient, but there were hardly any external influences to strain the simpler relationship.

This discussion begins with an outline of the manner in which Clinical disciplines function. Specialities like surgery, internal medicine, paediatrics or dermatology, as examples, either formulate a diagnosis or offer possibilities in differential diagnosis. The method of practice evolved in the history of the clinic, while other supporting disciplines have emerged beyond the history of a clinical past. They have developed from the basic inputs of physics and chemistry specifically to resource biological sciences, and their present role is largely in the supportive investigations for the clinical disciplines. The basic sciences of anatomy, physiology evolve and accommodate greater pathological detail while laboratory sciences like haematology, biochemistry and radiology improve that detail in rapid technological advance. Pathological data is time-bound and must alter through the disease process. Their sets of values or visual readings may be seen as aberrant from normal standards and significant either as pathology or deviant from normal physiology. The newer sciences investigate metabolic or biochemical parameters at cellular levels and microscopic tissue abnormalities for bodily dysfunction. Thus diagnoses progress in far greater precision than in their clinical past which entailed little more than the clinician's physical findings. The general patient context is subject to the above parametric details, none of which can exclude the physician's sensory and communicative faculties; and sometimes a further intuitive facility may decide the choice of management and therapy.

Chemistry and molecular sciences are involved in developing pharmacological agents, the therapeutic restoratives or aids to minimise the effects of disease, but depend on the clinician's assessment, his information base enhanced in communication with the patient, the details of symptoms and relevant signs from the physical examination. If a respiratory problem was apparent, the clinician noted in particular the structure of the thoracic cage, intercostal space (between ribs) configuration, the posture adopted for maximising deficient lung function, and so on. The trained physician intuited the extent of emphysematous change in a diagnosis of asthma, which then decided his management and medication alternatives. For respiratory dysfunction, as for other systems, clinical assessments have been enhanced today but still would only complement clinical judgement.

Data from biochemistry, haematology, or visual ancillary aids and the quantified data of other parametric tests make information on patient and pathology less speculative and more analytical. Therapy or management can be tuned for greater effectiveness. In the example of respiratory dysfunction, the variety of parametric information and tests for respiratory function together with advances in therapeutics determine the alternatives. Changes to medication and management can be further controlled by follow-up tests which monitor progress with the further possibility of juggling medication. The variety of broncho-dilators allows more focussed action at different cellular locations and, in combination with advances to the delivery of steroid therapy, obtains greater amelioration to acute and chronic respiratory ailments. The patient has better management and control for respiratory diseases like asthma, especially if treatment is undertaken when young, by running through gamut of technical improvements and pharmaceuticals. However, basic etiological problems remain to be solved.

There may be justification for the older patient in his feeling deprived of the physician's keen eye and appreciation of his personal history relating to illness. The hands on the patient's chest, fingers spread, one middle finger percussing the other, drumming his chest for tell-tale signs of auditory significance and the attentive auscultation; the clinical senses tuned to discern in their specialised sensitivity, conveyed to the patient confidence in the attentive concentration of his doctor as he decided the problem and its solution. Patient confidence, indeed, provided therapeutic benefit; though for science it is a variable, to be separately assessed in study protocols so that such benefit may not be confused with the 'value' of the pharmacological product or what is conceived to be the true therapeutic agent. Described as 'bias' it is the clinicians' standby, but in relation to evidence of product efficacy it must be disallowed. A more realistic analysis of patient benefit is not necessarily obtained by discounting a response or eliminating a possible one. Evidence of patient benefit to be obtained in 'method' alone for evaluating drug efficacy is a reductive simplification of therapeutic efficacy. The inclusive reality of therapeutics is within the patient/ physician relationship and not an artefact of medication, technique or procedure (see in, Patrick Wall, Text Book of Pain. Chapter 'The Placebo and Placebo Response)[i].

In dialogue and communication, physical examination and the contextual interpretation of test results, the physician instils confidence, most often veering to an expectation of benefit within objective possibility. Whether in the practices of modern medicine or those of a few decades ago, maintaining communication and confidence are an essential therapeutic input. The older pharmacy has been replaced. It once supplied recipes from items prescribed by the physician which he often tailored for the individual patient. Individualising prescriptions is a therapeutic necessity in TCM; in concoctions from its vast pharmacopoeia of herbal and other ingredients, or in combination with acupuncture: 400-500 points precisely localised on the surface of the body, provided choice for effective responses. The therapist, of course, reduced his base options from experience and could combine both treatments in deciding on an optimal selection for the individual patient. The physician of medicine later continued the valuable tradition of communication with hand written recipes for an individual patient; linctus and pills were put together by his pharmacist and delivered with the necessary instructions—therapeutic ingredients modified for each patient, but which was only a part of the procedure sustaining health needs of a community.

Today, the service is replaced by the retail outlet of an industry with global players which siphons for its products the research output of many medical disciplines and academic institutions. Pharmaceuticals are designed for ailments or pathology, and medication tends to standardisation. Drug dosage in experimental studies is in simple multiples, often determined in an animal model and calibrated in relationship to its weight and mass; culminating in a dosage causing a lethal outcome. Potent and safe dose requirement for the human is standardised from the data provided by the experimental work and then further investigated for clinical efficacy for pathology in a group of patients. The individual physiology is ignored in the grouping patients, the cohort. Allowance is barely made for age-related variations to absorption, or other likely individual problems that could change the standard of an effective dose. Drug tolerance based on gender and hormonal periodicity, or in circadian rhythms, genetic or other variability has a nodding recognition but these barely influence the physician's choices to a patient problem. They were considerations in past epistemologies but of course not verified evidentially in the terms of a hypothesis. Human pain in its variable individual aetiology is an example where, beyond the critique of trends and nostalgia for a past, one can visualise a time when designer drugs, made possible by research and attention to variables, will be developed for the individual[ii]. The pharmacy, however, is replaced by an industry, and the discipline is now a part of a leading global business venture. Scandals relating to clinical trials periodically surface, suggesting the extent to which science may be perverted, but responsible voices and influential journals protest to some effect[iii].

Clinical decisions increasingly rely on parametric data or investigative results. Previously when a physical examination unravelled primary information on a patient support came from an X-ray which only generated varying tissue densities in a single plane. Without perspective it therefore had to be interpreted then reconciled to the clinician's findings of the likely pathology in bone or soft tissue. Today, multiple scanning techniques offer better perspective and localisation of pathology. Vastly advanced visual aids increase the clinician's dependence on technology, most often providing improved diagnostic aid, but the process has certainly diminished the visual and tactile senses and instinctual acumen which continue a multifaceted importance to a physician's decision.

Industry also offers tailor-made products for the results of certain investigative procedures. Scanning techniques for coronary artery insufficiency may indicate an atherosclerotic plaque if stenosis of the artery is visualised. The line of treatment recommended is a stent to allow increased blood flow. For a knee eroded by arthritis a particular prosthesis is offered as the answer to pain free function. Therapeutics of this order may reduce the importance of clinical judgement. Further assessments of the patient in context might be required, rather than off-the-shelf solutions. Better visualisation of localised narrowing in a coronary artery does not diminish overall the importance of considering the patient's many circumstances. Age, diet, genetic proclivities and stress levels deriving from life style and habits; these are factors that maintain or increase risk, and must be factored in with signs and symptoms before elective surgery for mechanical correction.

The patient living with a painful knee may not benefit, invariably, by excision and replacement. Pathology deduced from a radiological finding might suggest benefit from a prosthetic correction, but closer attention to other circumstances of the pain may reveal it as an inappropriate choice. The surgeon need no longer delve by clinical examination to localise the origin or reasons for pain—a neglect that visual technologies may not answer for, however great the detail. Pain continues to be looked upon as a symptom of pathology but need not relate to the pathology provided by radiology since pain has its own aetiology[iv]: for example, in neural pathology. An informed surgeon goes beyond a routine dependence on the X-ray or scan, and would consider the possibility of avoiding a surgical solution for a patient's pain. But today the trend is ablation of the joint and its more expensive artificial replacement, based only on visual investigatory information. Bio-mechanics, by their constant technological improvements to prostheses, allow considerable restoration of mobility and relief from pain for particular patients, but a prosthetic replacement is not the invariable answer to all or to early joint problems. Surgical specialities and surgeons need to be aware of developments in pain research. A few patients suffer chronic postoperative pain, which is possible as an iatrogenic consequence of surgery, but surgeons are sometimes unaware of its prevalence and the reasons for it[v].

Corporeal data on function are necessary and increasingly important but can only supplement the vital experiential and cognitive information that is available to the clinician in his direct contact with the patient. Blood pressure, an ECG, a biopsy, all have temporal constraints while visual diagnostic aids, the many scanning procedures, are readings restricted as much in time and the space it investigates. The point is that data do not reflect the dynamism of function or disease change, and data which relate to anatomical spaces require interpretation as they are not reliably conclusive of pathology. Biometric data from the patient and medical investigative technologies, therefore, are values or readings recognised as limited, to that slice of time when the material or data was obtained from the patient. They offer information which can be likened to a 'frozen section' biopsy, a microscopic section of a patient's tissue without a physiological input. Undoubtedly, such aids are invaluable and provide informative advances to decision making and remedy. But they do not record dynamic change, and it is for the physician to consider a natural history of pathological change. Parametric results are generally subject to these limitations.

On a demographic scale there is a developing tendency to the use of similar information. Certain cohorts are known to be at greater risk to particular pathology. The screening of a male population over a certain age for prostatic cancer, for instance, can lead to unwarranted evidence that bypasses a need for clinical assessment of the individual subject. In suggesting an age group, and then eliciting data from that cohort with increased prostaglandin levels, assumes that group is at increased risk from prostatic cancer. Statistics, for instance, suggesting that a group having lived to an age of 75 is more likely to have had an accident than a similar one at age 40 is no solution toward accident control!

There are developing techniques, however, able to record system changes over time: for example, the protein which allows a long term evaluation of a patient's blood sugar, or an ECG halter monitoring coronary function which yields greater dynamic data of change. Somatic alterations and change can be monitored, but when some are intensely influenced in the psyche or the environment of the patient assessment by the clinician is required. The information based on microscopic analyses—a tissue biopsy, quantified readings on blood analysis, or system readings such as in radiology, are relevant but static data. They need processing in the clinician's perceptions of an individual. The patient can be reduced to a diagnostic category, like an 'unstable spine'. This describes no particular pathology, but the diagnosis has a categorical answer in expensive surgery by internal fixation[vi]. A moderately expensive investigation reveals coronary artery plaque (atherosclerosis) in men after a certain age. The CT scan may be of significance if associated with symptoms and signs, but by itself offers no dynamic information as to whether a plaque is eminently unstable. The definitions on high-powered investigation get directed to the use of material or gadgetry designed by the health industry for a surgically expensive procedure and offering correction for what is seen. It need not necessarily answer a patient's problem.

Recompense for Health delivery.

Today, medicine and its practice tend increasingly to become a 'product', and the 'market' commands its value. Its development as science by the medical research worker or the physician in his practice of medicine continues within a changing commercial culture which tends to undermine previous values fostered in a social enterprise and the esteem in which its main actors were held.

One is yet to see changes of quality to social and health indices that can be evidentially related to institutionalised market practices, privatised medicine and Insurance if posed against policies based in Social Health Insurance and an Universal entitlement; or, again, when the ethos was service and devolved on the degree of dedication. The recompense for it could be, in preference, a transaction directly between the physician and the State Health Administration.

I recognise contradictions by referring to earlier times—as a raw medical graduate sitting in with a friend whose practice was in a remote village in Kerala, South India. Indian health needs were, and continued to be, met in modern medical and traditional practice, but the attitudes and values of any practice prevailed in traditions especially of the countryside. My friend, an older graduate from our medical school, commenced a morning's schedule at 7 AM, and until 11 AM was busy with a load of fifteen to twenty consultations. This might include minor surgery, a tooth extraction or a paronychia incised with a digital block, but also a physician's usual rote, patients with respiratory illness, fevers, gastro-intestinal ailments and paediatric problems. Patients comprised an assortment of landlords, traders, a few officials from the local bureaucracy, plantation workers and fisher-folk. Their respective numbers decided our menu when a break for our breakfast followed; the uncertain earnings of the morning usually determined whether we could stretch beyond coffee and a boiled banana to a bit of fried liver, an egg and bread as well!

Despite centuries of separation, one can understand the clinic has an essential ethos and a continuity in therapeutic practice, as divergent as clinical medicine is today from past traditions. The acupuncturist treating a patient in China receives special responses from the patient; a mutual awareness of disease as with 'perceptions' of energy alterations and progress with treatment. The therapist helping him would explain the patient's requirements in terms within its specialised culture. The means for illuminating the patient's problem by the clinician and his method for dealing with it are also within a relationship which is straightforward and not subject to considerations beyond it. The recompense for service, though a nominal factor in the relationship, is dependent on circumstance, and even that may be dispensed with or defrayed at the clinician's initiative. Traditional, though developing, societies in many parts of the world are still closed communities, and they recognise poverty and financial hardship amongst its constituents. Dispensing elementary health welfare was the clinician's duty; the requirement to recompense that service is accepted but often left to the discretion or means of the patient or his family. The relationship prevails with traditional practices. It was emulated by the modern physician for decades but its passing, hopefully into better organised health delivery systems, is not without regret.

The clinician in a Western medical practice (the practice modern medicine rather than its geographical situation) is required to help the patient whose information about the problem of his disease informs the choices available for solution and are to an extent found in many interests extraneous to the relationship. A vast area of health provision is a business venture rather than social welfare. The industry for health products is increasingly influential, promoting their products in advertising, organising seminars attracting to them many groups—research workers and clinicians, in junkets and other aggressive sales pitches. Further, insurance for health cover offer terms that may influence a clinician's decision to choose solutions that differ from an adherence to the physical examinations of signs. A striking example is the resort to prosthetic joint replacement when the natural one may yet be adequately serviceable for the patient's quality of life and the least expensive alternative. Stalking such decisions are legal institutions specialising in the area of health laws and claims for compensation; a fertile and important issue in the USA where health care contends with private enterprise. These factors influence the clinician and his practice and may undermine patient relationships. Wittingly or unwisely it does lead to decisions which should be focussed more directly to the patient's health and well-being.

Choice of treatment and management, while increasingly dominated by data from the ancillary medical sciences and industrial inducements, should not be paramount in clinical decision making, which could yet remain inductive to the circumstance and context of the patient. Closed analytical thinking may answer his problem if the supportive data available are conclusive, but often they are insufficient, requiring to be weighed against the variables. Data may sometimes be ignored or, on occasion, judgements made despite results of biometric tests suggesting another alternative. The armamentarium of medical information should not rule decision making but be used to affirm a clinical choice, or perhaps a pointer to a different one. Unfortunately, there is an increasing tendency to rely on parametric data as finality to choice. Communication between clinician and patient is not merely awareness of of the illness, but of the complexities beyond, and to help a situation which the illness had brought about. These were basic concepts in traditional therapeutics: the inductive principles individualised treatment, with the clinician's ability to see the patient in his milieu and the special nature of his patient's dependence on him brought about in illness. Having arrived at health care for society, the patient while benefiting from all the system has on offer may not equally benefit from the confidence of contact with his clinician. Society loses much if the approach overlooks a vital relationship of the clinician with his patient.

Traditional Medicine (TM)

Continuity in application without development.

Traditional medicine as functional therapeutics cannot be directly compared to the clinical disciplines of today. Any exercise towards understanding it will not be entirely served by a direct extension of methods of medical science. What have to be accommodated are the compulsions on the clinician; there were different influences through its history but similarities to clinical practice of modern medicine are also discernible. A development is feasible for any therapeutic tradition in the paradigms of medical science, and put simply it is a contextual necessity of the present. Acupuncture and other therapeutic traditions in fact continue their practice in TM's previous epistemology. Yet there are socio-medical problems in an epistemology that is static because the present culture of health care operates in a greatly different context. By and large society accepts the value of traditional therapeutic culture without question, while the medical culture of science only accepts value in the evidence of its method. The respective positions can only be clarified and stated in comparison, and by reviewing TM's therapeutics in the newer medical culture. This is not to deny sources of knowledge, the pertinence and therapeutic value for health related problems, but they too must pass muster in methodical evidence. The failure of society and the scientific medical establishment to approach the problem in a systematic way has drawbacks and even hazards.

Traditional medicine had many developmental obstacles as empirical evaluations were later carried to preposterous lengths of theoretical rationalisation. Acupuncture, a therapeutic speciality of its time was an empirical science, but its theory was formulated in metaphysical concepts. The systematisation to the use of acupuncture was within the principles of Traditional Chinese Medicine. Pathology was recognised as qualitatively shifting as the organism was in dynamic interaction with the macrocosm, and was classifiable, changing signs derived from Yin/Yang balances[vii]. Normal physiology to observed pathological change was linked to *gradations* of those balances, and described as yang within yin, yin within yin and so on, thus arriving at qualitative differences to symptoms. But the changes in turn were derived from what were observed cyclical recurrences in nature on a macrocosmic scale, then reduced to calendric cycles, yearly, seasonal, lunar etc. Needless to say the physics was comparatively elementary, and medical observations fell in line with the metaphysics and theories of the time. Empirical observation progressed sporadically rather than methodically in experiment, and ultimately fell short, even as an elementary method.

One must not forget that this was a society that had established considerable feats of social engineering and technological innovation in other spheres of activity. It had a unified government with an efficient and centralised bureaucracy; hydraulic systems and canals, reservoirs and lakes leading off from their great rivers, and many other achievements which have been mentioned previously. Traditional therapeutics while obtaining its structure through the empirical, lost sight of it and turned gradually to flamboyant theorisation. Theoretical reasoning was hardly able to keep pace with empirical decision making; therapeutics were well suited as an academic pursuit and complex explanations impressed a patient. A social culture of being cared for by the learned was, indeed, an aid to cure.

The acupuncturist would explain to his patient the complexities of his condition in pathology relating to bodily humours and the qualities of his energy balance as they were affected by any of the five characteristic elemental configurations. His selection of acupuncture points was on a meridian or meridians which had their nominal relationship to what was perceived as a functional organ rather than one with an anatomical structure. The brain, for example, had a privileged position relative to other bodily functions. The meridians, whereon lay specific acupuncture points, were additionally linked to specific trajectories of blood flow. Thus points were very precisely specified along the ching lo, energy meridians but, when punctured, influenced the ching mo system of blood in circulation[viii] thus enabling correction of organic functions. Selection of points, their precise localisation, was decided by the physician for individual patients at each attendance as the variations in the ailment required. If appropriately punctured and stimulated to elicit an adequate deqi (the specialised sensory response of the patient), blood and energy patterns could be restored to the normal.

Point selection was the empirical key. The good therapist was intuitively sound in his assessment of the problems relating to patient and individual complexities as interpreted in theory. It was, however, in the selection of a line of treatment or of acupuncture points made with confidence and more often than not benefiting the patient that, at least, anecdotally validated his long apprenticeship spent in close observation of a reputed teacher, and later in his own experience. It was the practice that possibly could be contrasted with the theoretical explanations to the patient or in the teaching of students. While not without the rationality of a logical system of thought, it tended to be less empirical and more pedagogical in its convoluted detail. It may, however, have helped the patient participating in a complex explanation to understand the grand metaphysical implications to his problem even if it was dubious as a science. The process has held fast. Possibilities of confirming experiential insights by method may have lost out. Many therapeutic systems in the world sooner than later adopted these venerable mantles of academic respectability as their ways of thinking, but the result was failure to progress for the lack of fresh insights or a method which could initiate development. Attaining social status is history for practitioners of medicine. Jargon stifled innovation and theories lost pliability inside that straitjacket. Today, it may be commerce that retards innovative thinking, but beyond it primary discovery is attainable as clinical hypotheses continue a possibility in the experimental method. Discovery, innovation and development are societal necessities; if institutions are found wanting there will be inquisitive intelligence within or without the system to make them.

Traditional Therapeutics. The Need for Development as a Social Imperative.

In traditional medicine there is no unrecognised pathology for illness within the ambit of their all-embracing metaphysical classification. Therapy unlimited in scope is directed to 'cure', and management of illness is not an operative concept. No condition is beyond therapeutic scope. Neither has there been a systematic appreciation that illness unravelled as science made further discoveries; diagnostics in traditional systems of medicine continue as metaphysical exercises following their own order of classification and recognition. Traditional systems today may acknowledge a modern medical diagnosis but their purview of its therapy can only be decided following its own approach to diagnosis. Institutions which undertake the training of students in traditional medicine (Colleges for Indigenous Medicine) will outline elements of modern medicine and diseases. However, that understanding is not a systematised progression to a method for developing traditional medicine into a newer and comprehensive medical culture.

The idea prevails that therapeutics can function at two 'alternate' delivery levels, the modern and the traditional.

Tuberculosis may be treated with herbal concoctions or acupuncture, as the illness manifests in the patient's 'phthisic' constitution, and then deteriorates by seasonal 'increases in external damp'. This cannot be sustained as an alternative treatment for that condition. Phthisis is a constitutional state described in Traditional Chinese Diagnostics as a 'Shi' condition; 'damp' the exaggeration of an environmental factor aggravates a diagnosis made from these considerations. Such diagnostic forays in most traditional systems of medicine have limitations which are deficient in determining lines of treatment if the bacteriology underlying a disease goes unrecognised. It is not sufficient for the management of a disease today with a known aetiology and evidence based remedy in appropriate antibiotics.

The pathology of tuberculosis is understood as a socially transmittable bacillary disease as well as its relationship to immunological processes. The disease is curable when treated by therapeutic regimes which are constantly upgraded and validated. Recognising tuberculosis has virtually controlled its prevalence in most of the developed world. Traditional medicine does not feature an understanding that its remit has limitations. Basing a primary line of treatment for tuberculosis on remedies other than relevant antibiotics is socially irresponsible. A health administration accepting that would show culpable negligence were it to allow traditional medicine as alternate treatment for a recognised transmittable illness. Those limitations of Traditional systems must be accepted if society has to come to terms with rationalised health delivery systems (see panel discussion in 'The Hindu, Health Folio, Oct 2000). In history, the consequences of regarding the earth as the centre of the universe, or the date of its commencement as Sunday, October 23rd, 4004 BC as stated by the good Bishop Ussher in the 17th century, would not be as much of an impediment for society as maintaining certain untenable positions about the value of traditional medicine: increased mortality and morbidity rates would follow for their populations.

Beyond these limitations, one can accept that traditional modes offer treatment possibilities for acute and chronic disabilities in certain circumstances, but must be under the stringent supervision of validated health care systems. Claims for their efficacy can be consistently investigated, and supervision may offset potential threats to life or limb.

Tradition may also furnish a stock of management methods, adjuvants, even complements to the treatment of a patient[ix]. Amongst them are dietary formulations, splintage methods, massages, and a prodigious pharmacopeia to draw on for recipes that may help alleviate the disturbing symptoms of a chronic disease or aid in its management and recuperation. At the other extreme, in the process of denying traditional therapeutics a role in an unified health system, we ignore the need for adapted research methodology and collaborations that can be set in place to begin the collation of the very remarkable anecdotal evidences for their efficacy. Tradition recognises organic and environmental factors that retard recovery. Such aids to treatment available from the past are well within the scope of methodological investigations for the succour that they claim to offer. Obviously these would need to be designed with detailed attention to the nature of the claims.

It is necessary to come to terms with shortcomings of traditional systems in the context of what we know today. It is not enough to maintain that failure of traditional therapies was invariably due to the faulty application of theory. Therapeutic failure must be assigned where appropriate to inadequacies which become obvious from developments in the fields of social sciences. Despite the revolutionary developments in modern medicine and therapeutics, Tradition has not taken account of its own ignorance of that body of knowledge, nor does it doubt its own efficacy when confronted by the qualitative changes to explaining, understanding, and hence providing improved solutions to disease and social health. It does not accept that the constitution of traditional medicine as presently grounded cannot incorporate essential features of scientific progress. For these reasons, to consider traditional therapies as an 'alternative' medical mode is an allowance, special pleading for those therapies to continue within the mainstream culture. Its practitioners, functioning in a previous mode, are not required to comprehend change if they cannot accept the developmental contributions of modern medicine to societal health. Amongst the polity in certain societies the term 'alternative' is of little consequence if the immense spectrum of medical advance, its reliability for some illnesses and unique necessity as treatment for others, is not a choice available for the public on an universal scale. As of the present, Traditional medicine has its continuing role well beyond its capacity as a dependable health provider. Certainly its individualised therapies have their function, but its claims require eventual validation in method rather than in its cultural niche. To do that requires adaptive and innovative thought that would offer substantive but comprehensively safer modalities to health delivery.

Here then are present contradictions that require constructive solutions. The authoritarian nature of traditional medicine presently relieves it of the need for an appraisal of its conclusions; the statement as hypothesis requiring to be tested, and the testing offering replicability before there can be conviction of the soundness of its claims. At one level the culture of authority should give way to discussion and the initiation of methods for substantiating knowledge as a public utility; the merits of the knowledge stemming from antiquity cannot now be distanced from a method of proof. In the widest sense the brake on all manner of authoritarianisms is to empower the public for possible choice, but in science-oriented conviction rather than in terms of insular culture.

The science of medicine is open to question. Acceptance, whether as a theoretical proposition or for application, comes only after methodologically validated statements are appropriately presented in a journal for that speciality. Publication may or may not follow depending on the critical peer review process. The details of published material, protocol for the study, an experiment or the clinical trial, provide for replicability and hence the possibility for refuting the contention of its hypothesis. Or, it may be possible to alter or restate, or even rediscover in another form, in order to confirm or deny its validity. Acceptance may be slow. It follows criticism, debate, and confirmation by a specific community and, once in place, has the added possibility of opening up further inquiry pertaining to its field. The decades spent in initiating the perception of Pain as an endeavour for Science after the initial study published as the 'Gate Control Theory' is illustrative of the process of medical science.

'Truths' empirically established in traditional practices were irrevocable because they were logical, and preserved because of the authority and fame of their promulgator: they passed into the corpus of theory. Practitioners could now delve for answers into the considerable, ever increasing sources where modalities and schedules of treatment were archived and sometimes updated by reinterpretation by a later physician of renown. The essence of discovery stemmed no further than the empirical; but occasional benefit and more repeated failure by the 'given' treatment (prescribed in literary lore or the physician) should lead to questioning. In the first instance, doubts about the efficacy of a treatment could be a start towards designing methods for more consistent answers. But that is another paradigm. Tradition has certainly known experiment, but not as a sustained method to improve empiricism. Traditional medical modes, whether Siddha therapeutics, Ayurvedic recipes, Unanni, or acupuncture and the concoctions from a TCM pharmacopeia attempt to treat, sometimes disastrously by present universal standards, septicaemia, diabetes, an incipient blindness of glaucoma, and unrecognised fractures, or sometimes even recognised ones, by massage. If empiricism continues to be the guide today, that should be sufficient to recognise failure as well as success at many levels. Modern medicine with its own shortcomings has, in comparison, investigatory possibility for redefinition or correction. Disasters are on record and generally, if tardily, recognised and corrections attempted. Similar occurrences are faced by communities in countries where traditional medicine is promoted, but where recognition safeguard and control are ignored.

Society requires to discriminate between what is offered in terms of benefit. That is a qualitative and not a cultural choice. With early recognition certain health hazards can be better treated or managed if the choices available are reasonably adequate. In their absence we still have prayer, divine intervention or the therapeutics attuned to culture. The resolution of the dilemma falls upon systems of tradition also for not intelligibly recognising blind spots, and that in the world of today knowledge can be attained in science as a part of any culture. In many areas stalemate prevails when not recognising illness as requiring redefinition in the discoveries that later passed traditional medicine by. But can a way forward be found?

Inherent Development of medical disciplines.

Consider the discipline of surgery flourishing today: having a commencement which was well outside the hierarchy of Europe's physicians and origins quite beyond the pale of any science. The school of Susrutha in India won even Colonial advocacy for the methods, developed as an accomplished surgeon around 600 BC. For Europe, surgery as a discipline commenced with the barbers' knife blade; it adapted and changed character, dealing with abscesses, localised infection and injury, and a host of empirical methods and tools evolved from this into multi-disciplinary surgical practices in the late mediaeval period. There was a better pecuniary resource for the barber in the toll of war injuries, and his elementary techniques made progress to a life-saving discipline. The barber was of the ranks, but he was in the field and available, whereas the physician by comparison was far less effectual with his salves, medication and bandages and, above all, his delay in attending the injured, since he was likely to be at some safe distance from the gore and immediate danger of the battle.

From its humble, sometimes disdained past, surgery progressed through innumerable vicissitudes, both of human salvage as well as disastrous outcomes. From progress made to the injuries of the battlefield the techniques were applied to patient problems in civil societies, but past all the heroics of their performance, the physician/surgeons were concerned at the catastrophes from sepsis, both in midwifery and elementary surgery. Again developments in other fields were used to improve surgical technique. Achieving a degree of safety for the patient thus came only later, and in the many surgical aids, such as in the profuse use of carbolic acid solutions, initially to control sepsis, then moving on to concepts of asepsis in surgery. We owe much to the process of wine making and the beginnings of microbiology and bacteriology directed by Louis Pasteur for prime discoveries towards safer surgery.

The armament industry brought more effective technologies and enormously increased the capacity for civil destruction and slaughter in the mass. Air-power targeted against cities and towns brought a toll of casualties on an indiscriminate and unprecedented scale as warfare was now directed at non-combatant populations. Gross and multiple head and body injuries, massive burns and compound fractures with extensively traumatised soft tissue were accompanied by blood loss and shock. Existing civilian hospitals were ill-equipped and inadequate to deal with the numbers needing medical attention on an emergency basis. Accident Hospitals with a staff of specialised personnel were required, and surgeons able to deal with injuries in the widely varied anatomical distributions. Their organisation needed Burns Units and Blood Banks, and means for round-the-clock monitoring of essential biological parameters, ionic and fluid balances and blood loss, to support emergency and extensive surgical repair. Patients required rehabilitation following treatment, the further supervision and the specialised management of disability. These newer institutions came into existence and made the difference to patient survival and to their re-entry into society.

Development of many surgical procedures was possible once blood and fluid loss could be controlled, and safer and far more extensive surgical intervention was enabled. Some of the techniques in the care of trauma have been mentioned earlier. (See Ch. II). Today the essential preludes to blood loss control are routine to surgical procedure, whether of elective or emergency surgery. As a profession prestigious amongst the medical disciplines, one might add that a surgeon's recompense holds no comparison to the barber's original mite.

None of the therapeutics of tradition has been remotely able to sustain development sufficient for the changing social contexts as has medical science. Let us return to Traditional Chinese Acupuncture. Quoting from the best contemporary evaluations as to reasons for the hindrance to its development, Lu Gwei-Djen and Needham say, "The dominance of this proto-science after the Thang period was a turning point in the history of Chinese Medicine, for in it abstraction triumphed over empiricism and practical experience. The loss of much older literature in the Jurchen Chin invasions, and the rise of Neo Confucian philosophy, all helped to make physicians more learned in theory than adept in the clinical arts."[x]. The Thang was the dynasty, AD 618/906, responsible for a part of the period known as the Third Unification of China.

While the practices of today by their universal nature alone are a wholesale change from that past where once 'abstraction triumphed', development must be found in methodology for improvement. Even with medicine, notwithstanding constant progress in its technology, one senses an encrustation as science. Technology is undoubtedly a stimulus, but its commerce may put a leash on the development of better science. Through the ages there have been compulsions beyond medicine detrimental to development. But outstanding discoveries have resulted from intellects whose trained insights were not hampered by prevailing theory and practice. Those who could intuitively find in the empirical refreshing applications did so, but for traditional therapeutics discovery as such was a rarity.

Empiricism in traditional epistemologies sustainable in scientific method

There is scant acknowledgement as to what the Chinese or other traditional therapeutic systems of the world gleaned of the macrocosm and an organism's relationship to it. In tradition, phasic change was incorporated in the theory of disease. The macrocosm, it meant related to the organism, in an inductive/synthetic rather than a causal relationship. In sound health the organism maintained its energetic balances in the face of environmental change, which is reminiscent of the stability of the *milieu interior*—a concept in physiology enunciated by Claude Bernard in the 19th century. TCM, however, continued theories of predictable change to the organism by the hour, from day to night, in lunar cycles and in the seasons of the year.

Evaluations of Circadian Rhythms on the human organism is not a principle for treatment today, but for tradition it was a therapeutic concern. Presently times of conducting animal research are protocol statements in the awareness of sleep and hibernation patterns, and hence the quotidian variations in corticoid levels. Animal experiments require the times at which they are conducted to be known, allowing the reviewer to gauge the implications, since endocrine change may be a variable and affect trial results. Yet, while tradition recognised inductive influence on the organism, today it is viewed as an animal's hormonal function, its responses to alteration to light, rather than to cosmic rhythms. The protocols of investigation usually account for this variable.

However, in the standardisation of present day medication there is a disregard for variation in patient symptoms as a biological influence of these 24 hour cycles. We ignore its relevance even while otherwise extrapolating results of animal experiment to human requirements of medication. In the timing of drug use, attention to Circadian rhythms in trials could be of significance for some individuals even as dosages are carefully standardised for age. The susceptibility of human physiology to variation is evident in quotidian and lunar cycles and relates to the pathological. This is seen, for instance, in lunar cycles amongst younger asthmatics; and amongst elderly patients with rheumatoid arthritis whose signs and symptoms vary in intensity with climatic and weather changes.

IMPLICATIONS FOR SAFETY WITH THE PRACTICE OF TRADITIONAL MEDICINE

Public health needs in Kerala are met by modern and traditional medical disciplines. The state of Kerala in S. India has, by Indian standards, a high rate of literacy and gender equality in many spheres of social activity, extending to education. Socialised health care offers a fair coverage throughout the population. Modern medicine and traditional disciplines function within its institutions, and are also available in the private sector, allowing citizens a wide choice of health care. Traditional therapies, including homeopathy are seen to be adequate for certain problems, while informed choice may decide that modern medicine is the answer for others. Choices are made from the many systems available to an educated and well-informed society, but also from a rich heritage of medical systems which had long been dependable and thus recommend itself[xi] (see summary of paper in footnote of p. 9 of The Introduction).

Kerala State is illustrative for a public that has comparatively good welfare services. However, if Kerala presents a fortunate example their public are yet without the requisite information for the safer therapeutic practice of traditional medicine. As of now anecdotal recommendations for the benefits are common currency, but data in the realm of mishaps are uncharted apart from those that may reach a hospital or where the extent to which a patient's tardiness in seeking advice in modern care can be assessed as having jeopardised her future health by having resorted in the first instance to the traditional. Any evidence not deriving from the method of 'Evidence Based Medicine' (EBM) may demonstrate validity but must be confined in the term 'anecdotal'. Such evidence is not without empirical veracity, but for the context has the limitation of insufficient random sampling and robustness to analyses. Much of the evidence for Traditional Therapeutics is restricted to such shortcomings.

Modern medicine requires validation through research, acceptance of its therapeutic products then follows. In principle it is offered to the public after clinical trials and scrutiny by regulatory bodies. The traditional medical practices are based on societal experience which has its ancestral dimension. They are self-recommending without further validation, which does not mean an absence of evidence of benefit. In Lamarckian terms a cultural experience, healing included, may develop heritability in repeated exposure over successive generations. Evaluation of worth and therapeutic benefit is a learnt experience and likely to embed in biological mechanisms provided by specific cultural cues (ref. Chapter I, Tribal Healing). Cultural cues are also significant variables when seeking methodological evidence for the effectiveness of therapy.

Regulatory authorities suggest that research by the method of clinical trial can be conducted for traditional therapeutics which already are in the public domain. Public health policy should motivate collaborative institutional research in suitable method for traditional practices to provide better information and possibly increase choice for the physician if the evidence commends it to practitioners of modern medicine as well. Presently much of Traditional medicine functions in approbation, being viewed by the public as better 'suited' for certain ailments, as the above paper demonstrates. This is insufficient as scientific information. The immediate need is for collaboration between science and tradition for more information relating to the relative merits of therapies. A physician should be able to evaluate modern pathological conditions as indications to justify the use of any therapy. Traditional practices have indications of disease based on Traditional diagnosis, and that is necessary for their practice. It is essential for the safe use of traditional therapeutics that its complications, hazards or contraindications are understood in pathology if we are to avail of immediate remedy, and on occasion in today's context, since the measures are available, to save life.

Underdevelopment reflects in poor societal health and lack of education and could be redressed or eased as seen in the sociological evidence from Kerala, where even for poorer societies better established institutional welfare has made possible. Failure in these essential areas will not be compensated for by high growth rates unless they are simultaneously and constructively addressed. Without education, particularly of women who play a most important role for a better informed public, especially in the awareness of health management issues, there are fewer alternatives to a dependence on the previous culture of traditional medicine. That dependence, especially in the early stages of issues relating to pregnancies and childbirth, is partly the reason for countries returning poor health indices. Access to basic modern knowledge about health and the institutions that provide information and health care are often beyond the easy reach of populations in an underdeveloped world. It is not only health policies that matter, but access to information through better education.

There is a growing demand for the many esoteric traditional alternatives being marketed but only a few countries actually offer alternative therapies like acupuncture within institutional care and with medical supervision. Patients, in regarding them as the less harmful or intrusive than available modern therapies, may overlook a physician's advice and try them out. Such trends resulting from the publics' uninformed interest require to be addressed. Some confusion is evident, and attitudes rather than information is marked amongst medical establishments of the Western world, which reflects in policy advice. We are in dire need of researched clinical assessments of the known, and discovery of whether yet unknown possibilities are offered by Traditional Chinese Medicine, Unanni, Ayurveda, Siddha or Tibetan medicine. Terms like Alternative and Complementary Medicine (CAM) do not resolve problems for the public but confirm establishment indecision and a disinterest of any potential that might be extracted out of anecdotal information, and which could be to an extent resolved in research. CAM is an establishment concept which abdicates a need for their involvement, better information and safer therapeutic practice.

Presently we have in one world a variety of therapeutic offerings but an inadequate infrastructure for extending the Services for Universal Health. And yet, in some countries when institutional systems have delivered interventions on an universal scale, they have had momentous results. The elimination of small-pox and the definite possibility of eradicating poliomyelitis are substantial achievements, the epidemiological efforts against malaria, tuberculosis and HIV are impressive, yet patchy. It demonstrates that the extent of diseases taking their toll over the centuries was never dented by traditional therapies, and the evident progress was only in policy decisions to implement immunisation mediated through specific institutions—a scientific medical solution for epidemic disease. In Western societies traditional therapies usually play a minor role as a Health Service. Both worlds continue a dichotomised function with the modern and traditional, but the Developing World veers to the Traditional out of necessity and limited choice. Their virtue locally extolled and inconsequentially verified, yet those parts of the world in dependence on them return dismal Health Indices especially for infants and women. There are exceptions, as in Cuba, Kerala in S. India, or Sri Lanka, where those measures are markedly above average. The reasons are to be sought not in the therapeutic merits of the traditional but in the general advance of these societies through policy directives spreading the net wide: health infrastructure, education and gender equality are seen as social imperatives having an impact on nutrition, maternal health and infant mortality.

Traditional Therapies in the United Kingdom

Acupuncture in the United Kingdom has training and accreditation by a few modern physicians who conduct short courses and certify the competence of their students who are usually legitimised physicians. These teachers and their practices are quite separate from the traditional practitioners of acupuncture or other CAM practices, the latter having no qualifications which have been assessed by institutions, but nevertheless are in the public domain. The practices of tradition have their role, though its practitioners are not under any supervisory control.

The General Medical Council has a statutory presence for the supervision of medical practice and maintains control since any qualified practitioner of modern medicine is required to register as a member. A similar body does not exist for CAM. The effect of this dichotomy is essentially an abdication of a need for an universal statutory authority to oversee all medicine and therapeutic practices through the qualifications of practitioners. The traditional and majoritarian modern in their different epistemology present inevitable contradictions, emphasising the need for Traditional medicine to have its functional societal role as a part of organised health care, if possible under a single, supervisory body, one that can at least assess claims within the evidence or, if the claims cannot thus be substantiated, decide whether treatments are safe for the public. But the reports of numerous commissions are yet to recognise such a need for their societies[xii][xiii]

Despite the interest shown by special groups within mainstream medicine in some traditions like acupuncture, their continuance is in exotic isolation with a freedom to exploit an uninformed public. This contrasts with qualified practitioners of modern medicine who use acupuncture, often exclusively when by experience they find it a relevant procedure for patient benefit. They are well aware that a therapeutic tradition like acupuncture has limitations as well as indications for use within the totality of medical possibility. Mostly they are unlikely to use the concepts of Traditional Chinese Medicine per se, and prefer to use the methods derived from acupuncture which they choose as the likely therapy for a diagnostic problem[xiv]. These clinicians see the value of acupuncture for specific pathological indications[xv], while the traditionalist pursues it for his patient's treatment, irrespective of the fact that there are better alternatives. No agenda for an organised discourse between the two has commenced. Despite the occurrence of negligible meeting points between the modern and the traditional the traffic is generally one way and mostly channelled into institutional research. The Swedish approach has to an extent overcome the dichotomy and, although well worthwhile as an enterprise, research has hardly secured a necessary dialogue with the traditional practitioner or sufficient transactions with its precepts.

IMPLICATIONS OF DICHOTOMISED MEDICAL PRACTICE AND SAFER HEALTH WITH THE PRACTICE OF TRADITIONAL MEDICINE

Countries which produced and continue in the resort to a plethora of traditional practice for their society is a context which assumes greater significance when no single overall supervisory body exercises control over their variety of medical practices. There are proportionally more dangers for countries like India, Ethiopia, Rwanda, Tanzania and Uganda where the extent of primary health care or mental health care provided by traditional practices for their populations stands at 60%-70 % or more[xvi],[xvii]. Undoubtedly a social need is served by traditional medicine but if it is the means to providing health care to modern standards, we see less fortunate results in comparison to those served by the medical sciences despite possible benefit. It is an anachronism to depend on tradition for up-to-date provision of health needs, and whatever the virtues of traditional therapies they cannot fulfil them to today's standards. These societies are served reasonably well by many traditional therapists in terms of alleviating illnesses provided those do not run the risk of long term morbidity. To safeguard modern health care is the statutory supervision of the providers and the role of an overall Medical Council would be to control by certification and supervision the practitioners at present flourishing without the necessary qualifications for a medical practice. No such mechanism is presently available for traditional therapies. We are left to take their ethics on trust and depend entirely on the merits of tradition without knowing what exactly is provided, if the polity leaves traditional practices beyond the reach of a supervisory authority.

The need for review by systematic assessment of traditional or 'alternative' applications are long overdue. The critical issues to safe health delivery should be understood and defined by collaborative commissions which include representatives of traditional and modern medicine. That practices haloed in tradition are safe or harmless may be a general assumption, but it must carry conviction in more than cultural perception or the ubiquitous availability of a supposedly harmless herbal product through the many entrepreneurial promotions in the health market.

In today's circumstances information about complications and adverse reactions to treatment should be available in the curricula of all medical study, and the therapist be aware that they can be avoided or controlled.

In some instances definite curbs to certain traditional practices should be imposed. We are in a position to assess modern medicine in those terms and evaluate the complications in hard evidence. Social acceptance has come about not only in the performance of the system but in its accountability to society. Traditional systems are perceived to perform by societies geared to accept health solely as a matter of cures for illness, but patients have no means to demand accountability when they cause harm or complications. Isolation of the systems stems from an unwarranted confidence in the virtues of traditional knowledge, but that is a hedge from the remit of normative requirements of health policy. A system of health delivery should include these traditions in unified, not separate, policies, even when modern and traditional practices diverge.

Amongst other features, health policies for a nation should require that that standards are set for traditional practices in the same way as they are for practitioners of modern Medicine; a qualification and a period of supervised institutional apprenticeship must be served to register with a Medical Council before a modern graduate is allowed practice. These norms and others which define due care for the patient should apply to any therapeutic practice. While criticism for its lack may not apply to the better known traditional practices, a total absence of control makes it impossible to apply the safeguards that have become very relevant for delivering safer therapy. As such, mishaps can rarely be rectified and only later be identified by recourse to criminal or civil law, which can be detrimental to institutions and individuals to an unwarranted degree. There are hardly any standards or mechanisms for protecting the public against illicit practices or negligence if anyone can claim some proficiency to treat patients, whether by modern, traditional or dubious therapeutics; all claim to manage the health needs of the public in unwritten licence. Short of mechanisms which help define dangerous practice we face the problem, most importantly, of recognition and early correction of medical mishap and the cause of disability or a disastrous outcome for the patient; thus tangible medical evidence in Law to distinguish between *malpractice and negligence* is not available. Recourse to criminal law and punishment is least likely to circumvent either the possibility of malpractice, or medical catastrophes following bad procedure and mismanagement. Public well-being in this area *requires the scrutiny of law specifically related to the practice of medicine,* distinguishing between practitioner negligence and malpractice. The issue can be scrutinised in better definition and that only by recourse to Medical Jurisprudence, a well-defined system in Modern Law and in the syllabus of undergraduate medical teaching as well. If in place that system affords legal rights and protection to practitioners who have qualifications to function under the umbrella of a supervisory body such as a Medical Council. Law relating to medical practice recognises that mishaps may occur, but it allows confidence for the practitioner, safer health for the patient, and for the public the knowledge that tried and tested medical practice and products are in vogue. In principle if the outcome for a patient leads occasionally to disability, or even death, the assumption is that criminality is not the central issue *but negligence, errors of judgement, omission or oversight; and only at the extreme, and with evidence, can criminal malpractice be alleged.* It is the extent and quality of negligence in the law relating to medical practices that most often defines liability on the part of the practitioner or institution.

Traditional Medicine at present is an area beyond the reach of this speciality of law. Medical Jurisprudence is geared to the terms and definitions of modern Medicine, for example, a Death certificate. It is not possible to point to the negligence of a rural, 'Dai', or a bone-setter whose qualifications for treatment are generally without standards of study, nor are obstetric or traumatic conditions necessarily diagnosed in these terms, which relate to medicine. If resuscitation methods are available they should be known in such eventuality for use for a diagnostic entity; avoidance or correction of iatrogenic complication is unrecognised for lack of knowledge and there is no mechanism for collecting such data and recording it. Under these circumstances a patient mishap through the above practices will be viewed not as medical negligence but far more likely as a criminal offence.

Permanent disability from traditional therapeutic practices is often palmed off as part of illness or the consequence of trauma. Myositis ossificans, the heterotopic bone formation in muscle following massage by a bone setter for an elbow fracture, is not an unusual complication in parts of rural India. Evaluation is difficult for the hazards posed to a patient in the context of traditional medical prescriptions which are concocted from a host of substances for individual diagnosis. While this method of therapy could be commended, in certain circumstances it has drawbacks for the lack of definition and standardisation. It could transpire that a patient is exposed to and dies of angioedema and shock induced by the presence of just one substance in such cocktail formulas. In the countryside, death by septicaemia due to unhygienic obstetric procedure may never be recognised unless the patient reaches a hospital unit. Rather than a fault in a therapeutic process, or a substance or material causing allergy, plausible attribution to an illness will suffice as a cause of death. Standardised drugs have indications for use, and side effects and contraindications are stated. If a drug recognised to cause allergies is injected without a preliminary test dose, into a patient who had stated in his history that he was prone to allergy, a degree of negligence or culpability is obvious from a definitive set of circumstances.

The lack of definition makes it difficult to bring within the purview of medical jurisprudence both practitioner neglect or medical mishap. In those countries where traditional practice continues to be supported by a poorly informed public and where cultural assumptions of value prevail rather than the definitions based on methods of assessing value upon which modern medicine bases its potential, the hazards resulting from traditional practices have not been sufficiently and methodologically scrutinised. Without that information a structure for corrective measures are not possible, *and without them an otherwise competent practitioner may be culpable of negligence for a momentary lapse, but in extreme circumstances and within common law he may be charged with manslaughter.* Modern medicine attributes an individual's death or mishap in terms of modern pathology which is unknown to the practice of traditional medicine. It extends present confusions about them beyond the field of health into the Legal system.

Traditional practices in these countries have a role catering to health needs of society, but policy assessment and decision of how it fits into a system of health delivery is required. Presently traditional medicine functions as a second tier of health delivery, but for many a rural population where the facilities and institution of modern medicine is lacking it is in the forefront for health delivery. The possibility of it being a part and parcel of modern health care has not been comprehensively considered. There are financial constraints, political obligations and a disinclination to upgrade health and education in the order of expenditure of the State or the Nation toward public Welfare. A disinterest of health administrations to evaluating a modern role for traditional medicine allows health policies to continue in administrative default. Present dispensations fall in with the continuity of traditional medicine as a convenience, without coming to terms with the many uncharted drawbacks. The practice lies largely within its epistemological roots, a proposition to be welcomed and sustained provided the safeguards for such practice can be maintained within an already established system which stipulates how safer practice may be affected.

An early Swedish Model for treating Pain with acupuncture.

Advanced societies have problems despite careful policies of Health delivery, and even as a model, policies fashioned in their social context will not transpose globally. In Sweden acupuncture is part of therapeutic health care, provided it is undertaken by doctors, dentists, physiotherapists and, as its possibilities became more appreciated, by nurses and midwives, all of whom study medicine as a part of their specialised training before being licenced to work in their respective fields. As these professionals wished to study and practice acupuncture within their fields of competence, they had to undergo a certifiable training course for its use. A World Health Organisation recommendation introduced its feasibility for the Treatment of Pain in the eighties, which led the Socialstyrelsen (Central Swedish Board of Health) to debate the issue of acupuncture for treating or minimising patient pain. Their decision was to allow its use by the above categories of personnel, while the Health administrations of Landstinget, (roughly County Councils) were primarily given the responsibility of conducting the necessary courses by recruiting recognised teachers.

Chinese doctors and others who trained in Traditional Acupuncture practice were mobilised to teach students. The content of the courses included a few concepts of Traditional Chinese Acupuncture, laying stress on Chinese Acupuncture Points which specify sites and regulate depths for the placement of needles in the human body. The modern relevance of the acupuncture points were anatomically defined in surface markings, along with the blood vessel and nerve supply of their field of stimulation (i.e. the skin and the tissues penetrated). In short, the morphology of the Points on the Meridians were carefully collated in a Compendium for Study[xviii]. The theoretical basis of its teaching was neurophysiology with some understanding offered to the theories which have traditionally guided acupuncture.

The lectures comprised explanation of effects of stimulating peripheral nerves, for which in Sweden there already were many animal and human experimental studies. The lectures outlined the anatomy of neural pathways involved in the sensation of pain and explained how the excitatory component of sensory pain pathways could be centrally inhibited by controlled manoeuvres like acupuncture, which stimulate other sensory pathways. Basic information of the microbiology involved in the neural transmission of pain was by then current knowledge. Stimulation with acupuncture needles, electrical or vibratory stimulation achieves physiological effects not only on the sensation of pain but on the body's endocrine and immune systems. An account of its basic neurophysiology is elaborated upon in a further Chapter. *The essential biology is an enhancement to the knowledge of acupuncture, a science to the continuance and development of a tradition which simultaneously offers acupuncture a clinical role in modern institutions governing societal health.* An important follow-up for the students on this classroom curriculum was practical training with patients chosen for their problems with pain, conducted by a tutor in hospitals or in clinics for smaller groups of students.

The experience of Sweden certainly does not exhaust other possibilities for this tradition. A serious criticism of the content of teaching an ancient therapeutic practice in this manner is a) its abbreviation and b) that it lays the greatest stress on understanding the biological effects of acupuncture therapy rather than its presentation as an ancient holistic model within another epistemology. The latter is prevalent practice and cannot be ignored. Essentially this curriculum gave an arcane system a modern structure and related it to developments of mainstream medical practice. At the time acupuncture in Sweden had not yet been considered for conditions other than for patients afflicted with pain. Since then there have been extensions of its use for other pathology. Since the sixties, pain as a multidisciplinary subject, its microbiology, its clinical and pharmaceutical research and application in Pain Clinics has been an exponentially developing subject in the health care of the West. When acupuncture latched on to these developments, the biological information, both clinical and experimental, that research made, was considerable and the interest continues to be greatly stimulated. Pain clinics are now to be found in many institutions, mostly under the direction of departments of anaesthesia. Many anaesthetists were eager proponents of acupuncture in Sweden[18].

In addition to the morphology of acupuncture points imparted to students, likely side effects and hazards of therapy related to the penetration of needles into tissues was also covered within the Compendium.

---

[18]   Stefan Arnér, Dept. of Anaesthesia, Karolinska Sjukhus.

Over-enthusiasm is encountered occasionally, which can jeopardise patient safety, even with all the safeguards in place in the introduction of traditional therapies. A major hospital in a Landstinget of central Sweden had already instituted a pain clinic under the aegis of its department of anaesthesiology and was also periodically conducting courses for training interested personnel in the use of acupuncture. The relevance and advantage of adapting traditional practice in the manner shown above is hopefully to cater to patient need, but also to impart safer practice. The following is a relevant portion of a patient history and illustrates the importance of policy direction, the training and the study to be organised within it, rather than the assumption that a competence to practice acupuncture is easy to come by in the simplification of needle insertions into patients. Many other matters touched upon in the chapter can be understood in the experience of this patient history.

Case History

A lady in her mid-fifties was being treated at Pain Clinic of the Hospital for her multiple Joint Pain and was recommended a course of acupuncture for Rheumatoid Arthritis (RA). At that point in time we happened to be conducting a course for acupuncture at the Hospital and I was a tutorial member of that course. The concerned anaesthetist who treated the patient was not a trainee from one of our courses but had acquired his knowledge of acupuncture from another source. As an anaesthetist he had a registered medical qualification, and on that basis had used acupuncture in the pain clinic of the Department of Anaesthesia.

A course of acupuncture treatment was commenced by the anaesthetist and, after a few sessions, the patient asked the anaesthetist whether a specific course of acupuncture might not be directed to treating co-existing chronic asthma. The lady had noticed benefit for her asthma from the insertion of needles for RA. The anaesthetist agreed to the treatment (at that time asthma was not yet within the Socialstyrelsen's remit for therapy with acupuncture) and a few further acupuncture sessions were also directed towards treating asthma. The anaesthetist decided that needles over the posterior chest wall would be helpful, and a few were inserted at locations parallel with vertebral spines. The patient was a comparatively diminutive Swede, small in stature, thin in physique, her emphysema adding to atrophy in respiratory musculature.

Poor tissue cover over the rib cage resulted in a few needles penetrating the pleural cavity and at that session the lady developed an acute dyspnoea (difficulty in breathing from lack of oxygenation). Since we were conducting practicals for students nearby this complication was brought to my notice by the doctor. Emergency treatment was immediately instituted since he recognised pneumothorax and a partially collapsed lung in his competence as an anaesthesiologist, the diagnosis confirmed by X-rays. The negative pressure of the pleural cavity was quickly restored since the damage to it from acupuncture needles was miniscule, and the patient soon made a good recovery.

An inquiry was instituted by the hospital authorities, and amongst the details some facts are essentially relevant to the present discussion. Multiple parallel needles down either side of the spine (spinuous processes) in the region of the thorax were amongst those inserted for the treatment. Normally there is a considerable thickness of muscle tissue (trapezius, erector spinae, rhomboideus etc.) in the region of these needle insertions. In the instance of this particular patient the physician lacked an appreciation of the proximity of the pleural cavity to her chest wall and the loss of lung elasticity with emphysema. Ordinarily the normal elasticity of tissues, including pleura and lung, would seal and withstand the penetration of a fine acupuncture needle, all the same a hazard to be aware of and avoided. Possibly there were multiple penetrations through her defective rib cage past fibrous pleural degenerative tissue into the pleural cavity. A pneumothorax ensued. No blood was present within the pleural cavity. Resuscitative measures for a pneumothorax initiated immediately in the department were effective, and the patient revived soon.

Acupuncture and traditionally discernible caveats.

Needles at these sites must be inserted only to prescribed lengths and the depth is defined by the patient's physique. A 'cun' is a classical Chinese measure modulated to patient proportions, the breadth of his/her thumb across its pulp. The Tutorial Compendium prescribes lengths (by tradition) of 0.2 to 0.4 cun into the particular Urinary Bladder points used (see figs in Ch. III), and in ordinary muscle in this region the needles would not penetrate further than the muscle tissue. This patient's thumb would have been correspondingly small, and by prescription needle insertion should not have been more than a couple of millimetres into her atrophic muscle.

However, the necessity for the use of needles in that location might also be questioned by a more competent acupuncturist. Asthma could be treated using needles at locations distally on the limbs, and not necessarily into the chest wall. That was already evident in the response of this lady's asthma to the previous treatment for her joint pains.

That modern diagnostic definition of the hazard of a pneumothorax and its remedial component is apparent in this instance. Traditionally the above eventuality would be diagnosed as a blockage of qi (energy) in the Meridians of the lung or other. It is unlikely to be recognised as a pneumothorax, a pathological condition, terms unknown in traditional theory. The use of acupuncture points are stipulated for general crises. But the nature of this catastrophe *required a different recognition, a pathological definition and resuscitative measures of a dimension beyond the teachings of traditional acupuncture.* Despite some shortcomings of the anaesthetist-cum-acupuncturist in his acupuncture treatment, only the fairly heroic interventional techniques which he used, and which were available to a department of anaesthesia, restored the patient from a catastrophic and defined emergency of this order.

Training and recognised registration must be considered when assessing a degree of culpability. In this instance there were deficiencies, possibly to his training, and errors of judgement in the anaesthetist's acupuncture treatment, but having encountered a complication he had the knowledge required to forestall a likely disaster. He had overstepped the requirement of not using acupuncture for conditions other than pain in Sweden, but as a doctor the treatment for asthma was also within his purview. Both recognition of the pneumothorax and patient resuscitation were successfully conducted by him. A viable process for the patient's protection was in place and she survived. Without a legal background, I suggest that due note would need to be taken of the entire context; consonant with law and medicine today, even had this patient in a hypothetical instance, not survived. Manslaughter could well be a charge against the doctor, but with the applicability of a system of medical jurisprudence the extent of culpability does not have that connotation, extending a notable and required protection for the practitioner of medicine.

One does not need to go into the action taken by the hospital authorities as a consequence of this mishap. The point to be stressed is that a traditional method of treatment was legitimised for use in the medico-social context. The occurrence of such an emergency is rare but possible.

Because of its definition the measures to be taken are in place: invaluable knowledge today in dealing with a catastrophe possibly recognised in the context of using traditional acupuncture, but effectively dealt with only in hospital and by its personnel.

The Need for Unitary Policies toward Patient Safety

Basic to this discussion is the fact that, before conclusions of liability of an institution or negligence of a practitioner can be reached any system, including the law, must be able to draw upon all the evidence and the circumstances relating to a mishap which must necessarily be scripted in medical sciences. Here the safeguards relating to qualifications of practice, teaching procedures, statutory recognition of medical practices, recognition of pathological complications and rapid availability of technology and the expertise for resuscitation, must be available within definitions of science and are essential to establish patient safety in all practices, including traditional medicine. Only then would there be protection for the public in traditional practice on a par with today's practice of medicine. Any issue of culpability or negligence is within the broad framework of safety regulations defined by a single authority.

The areas of traditional practice stipulating safety for the public lie where its own institutions determine standards of competence. The Swedish model is one. Presently, central or state administrations responsible for the health of other societies are unable to bridge the dichotomy, the epistemological divide. Primarily there is mainstream medicine, scientific in evolvement, whose institutions have been set in place to sustain standards of patient care. Peripheral to the development of modern medicine has been the lack of institutions to monitor the scientific relevance and review standards for much of the practices that still remain the mainstay of medical care in many parts of the world. Due largely to fiscal restraints these older systems function by default but also in the merits of the therapy of tradition, since they do offer many solutions for treating disease. It is a convenience to project them as an 'alternative' system of medicine in no way related to the development of science. This is an unnecessary divide which shelves solutions to basic issues of health delivery.

However, we may note the practice of acupuncture evolved in a country like Sweden is not within the field of its traditional epistemology.

In developing countries its benefits to the public are incomplete, not because its practice is within its traditions, but because to achieve safer practices the hazards, complications and the measures to forestall or treat them ought to be uniformly defined in the medicine which has the most up to date means to deal with them. For this reason traditional practices presently pose some danger to the public. In those countries the more expensive but rapidly evolving system of modern medicine with its associated technologies do not contend with traditional systems, since the former rationally occupies the better funded slot and primary importance for Health Care. At present the 'alternative' is not necessarily ancillary therapy but for many in the society essentially the first resort to Health Care in many developing countries, ubiquitous, generally unregulated, culturally understood and approachable in greater affordability. The role of traditional systems can be enhanced and made safer if we consider all health care inputs, traditional and modern as a unified whole within the evolving system of medicine.

While the move toward understanding traditional practice within the biological sciences is taking place, that in itself need not be a hallmark of safe traditional practice. There is an arena of concern for safer traditional practice in the many countries of their origin which need not necessarily reach the sophistication of such a model as Sweden's. At the same time, and apart from the safety issue, one cannot deny that the negotiation of acupuncture with biology is important. This ancient therapy, itself benefitting in those studies, has added researched information to the neurobiology of acupuncture and pain, and provides many indications for its use. That paradigm has offered an enhancement for biological discovery beyond the clinic as it moves into areas of basic research. In advocating a unified system for health delivery, inclusive adaptation could offer similar development to many other traditional systems. But there are elitist votaries who would consider science as superfluous and an interloper to existing traditional knowledge. The development of forms of knowledge was, indeed, an historical imperative, a contextual necessity. Certainly case histories like the above and innumerable other patient mishaps occur within any therapy, but the fashioning of measures to minimise them is overdue and achievable in the advancing knowledge and technology of medicine with support by policy directives.

HEALTH SYSTEMS AND CHOICES FOR THE PATIENT

Today pathology largely accounts for diagnosis, increasingly supplemented by ancillary medical investigations to confirm and devise treatment. The clinician most often makes his decisions because products and processes available has evidence-based experimental support for their choice. It does, however, change the reasoning behind clinical practice from the holistic to the reductive while its application has made tremendous strides in terms of saving life or maintaining its quality.

Developments in prophylactic medicine and primary health care make for an incremental quality of life and contribute to sustaining healthier societies are part of the major sociological change which gathered momentum in the past five to six decades of acknowledging the State's responsibility towards those goals. The information that sharpens decisions on diagnosis and treatment may not be uniformly posed for therapeutic systems, but if the calibre of resuscitation is jeopardised due to ignorance of the pathology of a medical emergency, it is at a cost to the public or a patient. Recognition of this is a universal imperative where many systems of medicine coexist.

Reliance on the commercial sector is entirely inappropriate for the achievement of universal health care. The evidence shows that nations which assumed responsibility for Health Welfare policies return the better health indices, irrespective of their economic and developmental status. Within most societies today choice of therapy whether through alternative systems, including the traditional as against what modern medicine has to offer, requires to be made after the individual patient is able to process the respective merits of systems for his particular ailment. Decisions should be made from informed choice rather than from within cultural slots which often tend to prejudice choice[19]. Despite cultural predilections it should be possible for an individual to sift the value of information about

---

[19] The following was told to me at Kunnumkullam, Cochin, decades ago by Cherukutty a retired Sanitary Inspector of the Raj as it was then. His jurisdiction, while in service, was over a panchayat of Trichur District. In the State of Cochin. His duties were generally to report on and oversee the health of its population ensuring that any public health hazard was brought to the notice of of the District Public Health Officer. Diseases suggesting the possibility of an epidemic required stipulated measures to be initiated by the sanitary inspector under the supervision of the DPHO. Should the threat of communicable disease be imminent, appropriate

therapeutic possibilities with regard to his health. But lack of choice has many social dimensions and it is unfortunate for a patient who is not

vaccination or immunisation schedules of a local population were immediately undertaken to prevent it reaching epidemic proportions

Small pox was the context of the following episode. It had broken out affecting one family and Cherukutty had mobilised his people and the department to initiate the vaccination programme. This village had a prestigious temple and its Vellichapad (keeper and priest of the temple for the deity, Ayyappan) wielded considerable clout amongst the local population, his hereditary position extended to mediating with the deity to preserve the health and well-being of his community. The gentleman previously had brushes with Cherukutty on community health issues. Quite simply the Vellichapad, realised a threat to his position in Cherukutty whose authority derived from the Colonial administration, a power, in those times, more potent than Ayyappan's in some matters!

When the immunisation programme had commenced, the Vellichapad also sallied forth and while Cherukutty extolled the need for the new vaccination programme the Vellichapad reminded the population of Ayyappan's powers and his ability to protect against disease. There being some scepticism about Ayyappan's ability to deal with diseases of this nature judging from previous experience Cherukutty had the edge in this instance. However, the Vellichapad's rod, mediating Ayyappan's power over disease—and health—was out in his hand and being waved over village gatherings along with the sonorous recitation of appropriate slokas (devotional verse). When Cherukutty appeared on the scene there was a shift of people toward him and he explained the elementary principles and the need to vaccinate and protect themselves against small pox. Soon enough the vaccination programme commenced much to the chagrin of the venerable Vellichapad. He knew other forces were out to diminish him, his deity and, of course his livelihood, and he was not giving up without a fight.

He went upto Cherukutty and suggested that he and his team withdraw and leave matters of health to his own priestly ability to intercede on behalf of the people with Ayappan. Cherukutty on the other hand advised that even the honoured Vellichapad was at risk in the matter of small-pox and that he should also be vaccinated. A wordy battle was joined, egged on by the crowd. A furious Vellichapad sensing defeat, waved his tremulous rod at Cherukutty, cursed him roundly in the name of Ayappan and proclaimed he would be dead of the pox, within the week, that no vaccination was likely to protect him from Ayappans power as all before him would see. Cherukutty was not to be outdone. The little vaccination stillette in hand and pointed at the Vellichapad he pronounced that in two weeks he would contract the disease and a week later it would be the Vellichapad who would be dead. Being vaccinated himself and aware of incubation periods for small-pox Cherukutty had the advantage in that encounter. Sure enough Cherukutty's prediction came to pass; the story as recounted by him with somewhat inconsiderate glee.

educationally empowered. That deprivation is seen at its worst where lack of literacy, cultural prejudices and poverty skew opinions in directions where the outcome for the patient is often increasing morbidity or frankly life-threatening. These debilitating social factors and the limitations to the organisation of public health provision allow an autonomous insularity to the health practitioner of different traditional medical systems. Their attitudes and training are inadequate at present to provide knowledgeable advice on the respective merits of therapies for particular patient problems. The best they can offer is what is available from within their own antique cupboard.

Medical specialities and their advancing technology are a scientific culture in contrast to therapeutic traditions. The theories of the latter persist with the ideas of macrocosmic change or seasonal variations affecting the organism's humours and manifesting as disease with undefined causative agents and pathogenesis related no further than to the environment. Earth, Water, Wood, Fire, Air, as presentations of metaphysical theory, may sustain valuable therapeutics, but are virtually static in that dependence and hardly likely to advance empirical insights. In some respects this outlook accords with the requirement of proper sleep, rest and diminishing stress, fresh air and food for the patient, while heat, cold, damp etc., denote some aspects of his symptomatology. Adequate nutrition today features protein, carbohydrate and fats along with vitamin supplements, fluids, with minerals and salts to be controlled for a patient and his disease; we then have moved by experiment the empiricism of environmental factors to specify nutritional needs.

Even today, where choice of therapy for certain ailments is considered, traditional systems do provide satisfactory answers for the patient for a particular ailment or during stages of its genesis. A comprehensive organisation of national health care should be able to offer patients information on the possibilities of respective benefit as well as the limitations and dangers of certain treatments. An integrated system of health delivery is the reasonable option when multiple therapeutic systems are available to society and their practitioners must acquaint themselves with the options, limitations and drawbacks of their own systems through studies beyond their own. Integration of this order should supplant the two tiered and compartmentalised health delivery of the underdeveloped world, enabling the public a choice with confidence.

It is beyond argument that in the culture of medicine today, physician's advice is based to a great extent on tested information. Evidence based medicine is a methodological research process and no drug is marketable without it. Until it is in place for all systems of medicine, practitioners have to rely on the anecdotal values in lieu of the methodologically verified. The fact of traditional therapies for certain patient problems surviving in plausible evidence and through the ages may not be dismissed, even if it does not measure up to evaluations which promote therapeutics and procedures in modern medicine. That evidence is obtained in a method, a paradigmatic shift from the anecdotal. The commencement toward methodological evidence for therapeutics is important; it offers new perceptions, not only to the traditionalist, but for the scientist an awareness that paradigms too may require to change. If a traditional therapeutic procedure is of importance it should not be discarded as a misfit to a paradigm and method. However, aspects of the traditional, although taken out of its epistemological context, as with acupuncture, have many studies based in neurophysiology or clinical applications and provide evaluations for a physician to offer in the interest of his patient. There are intense reviews and an on-going debate over clinical study methodology and evidence-based medicine initiated by the contact between them.

The limits on choice for a physician of modern medicine are due only in part to the lack of proper evaluation of the traditional therapies. Choosing is occasionally a question of aiding a patient through his illness by following a particular therapy best suited to its evolving pattern. Traditional therapies take this procedure for granted. A mix of the modern and traditional for the natural history of disease should have a place in treating certain categories of illness. Postsurgical rehabilitation and intensely enervating syndromes following treatment for malignancies etc. may well benefit from systems of tradition. Such a possibility would assume that available therapeutics is not constrained by practitioner prejudices. At present there are very definite assumptions by those opposing modern medicine and physicians who will not consider anything other than scientific medicine to be the best on offer. The full array of therapeutic choice should be available to patients in 'better practice' routines. Systems of therapeutics need not be compartmentalised; the separate entities today could evolve into routines of treatment schedules.

Contrasting with the marked divergences and dismissals between proponents of the various systems in the culture of medicine today, there stands the mediaeval, as with Persian and Arab Medicine and even that of the earliest colonial context in India, when far more respect and a mutual awareness of systems which offered benefits for specific illness was apparent. The Persians and Arabs previously worked the wealth of medicine of other worlds to transform their own mediaeval therapeutics to the greatest sophistication for the time. It was amply seen in the incorporation of the wisdom of many other medical systems by studying and translating into ancient Greek therapeutic offerings which they had transformed to their own, thus bringing medicine to another level of diagnostic and therapeutic efficiency. The extent of medical advance has since been superseded only in the recent centuries of its science. States can initiate policies and directives to make those advances to Health Care an Universal entitlement as is well demonstrated by a few.

CHAPTER V

ACUPUNCTURE MECHANISMS

"We are the offspring of history and must establish our own paths in this most diverse and interesting of conceivable universes" Stephen Jay Gould.

"To any one brought up in Western culture, the traditional explanations of acupuncture are so strange and archaic that the facts are often thrown out with their explanations." P W Nathan in TINS July 1978.

CLINICAL ACUPUNCTURE

The consideration here is only as treatment for clinical pain. Even today acupuncture is used therapeutically more extensively to treat diseases rather than for pain associated ailments but research advance in recent decades in the neurophysiology of pain offers interesting possibilities for testing some of its claimed clinical effects. Importantly a field has opened up for further experimental work in pain treatment through peripheral sensory stimuli, of which needle insertions, as in acupuncture, is one form.

The rationalisation of acupuncture is not merely in its metaphysical theory. Acupuncture effects are mediated, as presently understood, in neuro-physiological activity and, as with any therapy, supported in individual biological configurations. This traditional practice has many areas of use, and interesting extensions of effects on immunological systems are emerging and being explored. Experimental evidence on how acupuncture modifies inflammatory responses is available, and aspects of clinical pain relief are mediated in the mechanisms generated through the complex neuronal connectivity of spinal cord with central components and the autonomic nervous systems.

The evidence for its utility in treating pain syndromes with a hormonal association e.g. cyclical migraine headaches or dysmenorrhoea before the onset of pain has prompted further examination. If acupuncture can indeed pre-empt such pain, it suggests the possibility of rectifying premenstrual instability. Hypothesising on causative mechanisms for chronic pain and dysmenorrhea in the hypothalamic-pituitary-adrenal axis which could be explored in experimental acupuncture research. A further intriguing possibility is whether acupuncture may offer greater clarity to the biology of placebo, a phenomenon mostly thought of as an artefact to treatment and critically considered as explaining acupuncture effects. A later chapter deals with placebo and its relevance in clinical acupuncture trials. The extensive range of claims for traditional acupuncture for ameliorating disease or easing clinical pain requires far more clinical research—closer attention to patients with chronic problems within the usual clinical diagnosis; but further consideration of pain pathophysiology as nociceptive, neurogenic or idiopathic found both substantive amelioration or lack of efficacy in that differentiation, and such evidence was also notable when using techniques akin to acupuncture. Certain methodological innovation for hands-on procedures were the small patient numbers—limitations that could be critiqued as amongst shortcomings of these studies[i].

Research into acupuncture has progressed in spite of its formulation in the theories of traditional medicine. Practitioners of traditional medicine consider its precepts to be unassailable and, if doubted, assumed to be due to an insufficiency of study of those theories. Adapting for the likely neural response to acupuncture-like stimuli or in utilising variants to traditional acupuncture, experimental and clinical research demonstrates psycho-physiological evidences of effects and mechanisms for therapeutic utility. The approach has also suggested parameters other than the traditional for the clinical use of acupuncture in diagnostic categories of pain[ii,iii,iv].

If the use of acupuncture in clinical studies shows discordant results these cannot provide a reason for some critics arguing that it is evidence discounting acupuncture as therapy. In medical literature, evidence-based medicine provided therapeutic applications that have since strewn the lists of the discarded because of their unhappy consequences, and later rectification of the evidence. In their time such applications were based on 'conclusive' clinical evidence—and in a few instances they have caused disasters for patients and society. By contrast acupuncture appears to have survived a couple of millennia only too well, and continues to gather apace an extensive clinical and research base despite the detractors. There is merit in an approach to acupuncture studies in the presentation of many lines of evidence, both for neural mechanisms and clinical utility. 'Universal' evidence for its therapeutics may be controversial, but experimental responses in areas of the central nervous system activity suggest that its clinical effects relate to the immense individual variability of neural activity and response, with the added problem of subjective human interpretation for assessing responses which cannot be conclusively ironed out by statistical methods.

Acupuncture becomes the more viable a proposition in accepting negation. Clinical trials, for example, could demarcate a quality of its content as empirical[v], an essential for the science of acupuncture to progress. Therapeutic usage may be found wanting, but it could also be that the methods of study need sharpening if they do not sustain its use for the diagnostic categories as conceived for the trials. Dismissal is unwarranted when the neurophysiological evidence for its effects is available in experimental research. Furthermore, provided medical science does not ignore or dismiss credence for the essentially experiential and anecdotal that sustained therapeutic heritages, the practices may unravel improved evidence for selected clinical pathology.

Therapeutic benefit from acupuncture in tradition was found over a wide range of health problems. It was only around the late seventies of the last century that a World Health Organisation dispensation for acupuncture as a therapeutic possibility was conceded for medical practice in conditions of pain. Pain clinics and departments of anaesthesiology increasingly involved with clinical pain were then able to consider acupuncture as a therapeutic 'alternative'. Its use was limited, but in that environment it caught the attention of 'Pain' scientists. From such meagre beginnings within established science, there continues a necessary interest in acupuncture and other such inherited therapeutic systems on the lowlier scientific slopes of the peaks of medicine. But if *complementary and alternative medicine* (CAM), commences in the considered limitation that it is not Science, the position is untenable as the social science research available has posed problems for a public that uses such practices.

A needle insertion initially is a sensory perception which often elicits further responses in the organism. Traditionally the response was explained in inductive theorising as an energy form, signified in the arrival of Qi, which had effects on the normative pathology formulated in the inductive theories. In today's science empirical responses are perceived in neural impulses, and neural transmitter sequences follow the stimulus, an initial sensory input, with possible therapeutic benefit. What has changed from the time of the ancient Chinese physicians to the present neuro-scientists are the respective terms of explaining that response. The language has changed, but not the nature of the response of the organism to a needle in the tissues, which could hardly have altered in the millennia between. Maybe we can look upon acupuncture not as an 'alternative' but as seen in present scientific paradigms.

A word about criticisms of the lack of incontrovertible evidence from the results of acupuncture studies in clinical pain: the problems of pain itself presents" its wild and variable relation to the stimulus that evokes it", a commonplace statement for the clinician, but of considerable research significance by a founder of modern pain research[vi], who stresses variability.

Is inconsistency in a response to a painful acupuncture stimulus or one that borders on pain through the techniques of an experienced therapist be effectively controlled for therapeutic benefit? Patients are perceived to be individually good or poor responders, and mostly their responses vary within grades in between. Such divergent responses are seen in species, and can be accentuated, for example, by inbred mouse strains. Genotype is an important factor in the strains studied, but responses were also influenced by the environment[vii]. As one moves up the evolutionary ladder genetic variation is obviously more pronounced, and divergence of response to a particular stimulus where the inputs relate marginally to pain is all the greater in the human subject.

There are valid criticisms directed at many clinical studies of acupuncture, but the ones that do so on the grounds that results are diverse or inconsistent for patient groups with similar pathology are often off the mark. The outcome, when testing the effect on pain by countervailing acupuncture stimuli in an experimental subject or in patient groups, will show response differences amongst both individuals and groups which are unlikely to be consistent or uniform. Replicated, or comparable clinical studies on pain and acupuncture which conclude that its results do not support those of an earlier study, and therefore the 'analgesia' or pain relief claimed is either a placebo effect or questionable evidence is often surprising. If the present methodology of clinical studies is directed to obtain incontrovertible evidence as the criteria for the medical utility of acupuncture, that is an unlikely pursuit. Cohorts within a similar diagnostic category of pain, even assuming study replicability, will respond with outcomes not necessarily similar in each study, because neither the individuals constituting the cohorts nor the therapists are 'replicable' in relation to the use of acupuncture. 'Acupuncture' does not offer the consistency that is assumed in replicating a clinical trial. The extent of variability does not offer easy solutions in the methodological regulations of a study, nor in statistical appraisals of the results. However, despite overarching negative evidence for the outcome of some studies which may mark patients as non-responsive, there are others who benefit whether from placebo or from acupuncture. The studies are useful in that particular pathology has been subject to study trial, and a few patients respond to acupuncture; at the very least; for the clinician facing diminishing therapeutic choice, it suggests another possibility. This is the reality of many primary Health clinics in the West.

A meta-analyses may assess study quality within the general application of study protocols but oversteps the claim for reliability in a dependence on statements about the protocol claims. For instance, high value is attributed to a protocol stating a use of placebo control. As quality value for an acupuncture study, a claim that it used a placebo control is questionable from many points of view. A strict placebo is inert in respect of the essential therapeutic ingredient. The essence of a needle insertion relates to sensory inputs, and even the best studies claiming placebo design have tactile cum visual inputs, sufficient reason to question the claim. The grading as a better quality study through the claim to have used placebo therefore requires a foundational assessment for a meta-analyses. A correlation between study quality (based in the regulations of study method) and outcomes of treatment is standard meta-analytical procedure. We are no closer to why and how the utility of acupuncture is to be negotiated in the present methods for evidence-based medicine in the outcomes of a meta-analyses. Such assessment of study quality for pain and acupuncture brings us no closer to improving methods for hands-on therapies.

Good study quality proposed by meta-analyses usually relate to: a) the controls, especially whether or not they were stated to be placebo. Examination of the role or validity of placebo for acupuncture may not be the responsibility of a meta analyses, but surely a placebo controlled group for acupuncture in a study protocol cannot be used to measure the standard of quality if a true placebo does not exist. Placebo controls attempted for acupuncture are contrived in order to satisfy method and are hardly convincing as they do not achieve an inertness relative to peripheral sensory stimulation. *We would not witness the present plethora of 'placebos' for acupuncture if it were in fact achievable.* Placebo claimed as acupuncture controls is another acupuncture mode. Subcutaneous needling, which is used in many studies as placebo, has itself has been demonstrated as having therapeutic effects. Macdonald et al. in an elegant paper established this as long ago as 1983[viii]. Placebo mechanisms are generally unravelling, questioned for what is elucidated even in the plausible methods of pharmaceuticals and more general therapeutic studies. Relating acupuncture outcomes to quality on the merit of placebo is about as reliable as to the blind men, in the Indian folk-tale, relating the feel of one body part to be conclusive evidence of the shape of an elephant!

The information that can best be offered on clinical studies on acupuncture lies perhaps in evaluating its methodological quality, provided that the protocols of study attempt to relate to the context of this therapeutic mode. The process of acupuncture intervention requires, first of all, the therapist and his hands-on therapy. Study protocols that attempt to satisfy only hallmarks for quality may not offer the quality of evidence one strives for if they ignore the basic nature of the therapy that is being studied. Hence **b)** In the circumstances of acupuncture therapy we must question the possibilities for blinding and complete elimination of bias. Double-blinding may be possible with drugs, but hardly fits in the contextual reality of acupuncture therapy. Single-blind studies are a compromise and their worth requires assessment for each study protocol. **c)** While medication is directed increasingly toward specific mechanisms generating pain, we continue to study acupuncture within the diagnostic categories of pain and that, as suggested, increases the uncontrolled variables of each study. 'Low back pain' or 'chronic neck and shoulder pain' is often categorised for a study cohort, and even with the strictest entry criteria diverse mechanisms for individual pain will confound the outcome. Whatever the protocol for controls, the best studies of patients in diagnostic categories when treated with either an anti-inflammatory drug or with acupuncture may not necessarily show outcomes in each study invariably satisfying an outright conclusion for effectiveness, and certainly it is less likely with acupuncture because the response variables to this stimulus are greater. Randomisation when patient numbers are small will not ensure ironing out variables or an evenness to stimulus response characteristics. **d)** In the present state of uncertainty about the mechanisms underlying pain, especially that of neurogenic origin, even large cohorts in a study are unlikely to provide stable results.

A wide range of complementary therapies including acupuncture are finding increasing favour in the West with the clinician, and more so with a public[ix]. The reasons for increasing clinician support are diverse but certainly include the evidence of clinical studies. The public's information systems ranges from the anecdotal, a neighbour's experience, to the traditional therapist weaving erudite spells of metaphysical theory, or to a public sold on blurbs promoting the new found commerce for 'nature' cures. The clinician/acupuncturist explains his own version of acupuncture, information built around a staple of empiricism. It may well be that accepting the "wild and variable" results there still is a fall-back to the empirical usefulness of acupuncture which appears to go beyond the evidence for an adequacy for managing patient pain.

The studies of acupuncture as Evidence Based Medicine (EBM) continue. Finding evidence with protocols of acupuncture therapy as a hands-on mode is less often attempted. This is a methodological problem, involving the design of suitable and convincing controls. So far studies compromise on basic therapeutic features to suit the requirements of the methodology of EBM. We are yet to discover whether acupuncture is effective when conducted within its traditional epistemology, and whether culture or ethnicity contribute substantially to results. Could the contradiction between the increasing resort to acupuncture and the uncertainty for its effects as seen from available studies be because the latter do not reflect the reality of the clinic, whether the therapy is traditional or from among the many variants for its present practice. The evidence from RCTs do not depict the reality of acupuncture therapy in clinical practice.

The present evidence for the clinical value of acupuncture or its neurophysiological mechanisms allows conjecture, controversy or interpretation. That is not to deny acupuncture as a therapeutic mode. Evidence must be pursued by improving the tools and following more inclusive methods for clinical study. No allowance can be made for the proposition that evidence is not necessary by subscribing to the argument that we have always 'known' that traditional therapies work.

Neurophysiology of Inhibitory Controls

From the Sixties there has been evidence of the inhibition of nociceptive neurons at the spinal cord level and the possibility of inhibition of those neurons by stimulating afferents from the periphery. Kolmodin and Skoglund[x] demonstrated that tactile stimulation which activated large diameter afferents excited interneurones at the dorsal horn, and subsequently inhibited cells transmitting nociceptive impulses. The functional implications were consolidated into a theory of pain modulation by Melzack and Wall along with other important findings a little later. The report of descending inhibition by the stimulation of supra-medullary sites was identified to the central midbrain; stimulation specifically of the periaqueductal grey causing a potent analgesia in rats sufficient for abdominal surgery without any resource to chemical anaesthetics[xi]. The Reynolds findings were followed by a further discovery of major significance in pain research. Specific receptors at some of these central sites where electrical stimulation had caused analgesia were discovered to have opiate binding properties, and this in turn led to the search for possible endogenous or naturally occurring ligands—substances with opioid-like activity to explain the analgesia caused by stimulation. By 1975 certain hitherto unknown endogenous neuropeptides, the enkephalins and endorphins, were implicated in the inhibition of pain transmission and in physiological conditions of stress or fear.

Significantly the endogenous opioid system was also implicated in the analgesia, resulting in conditioning experiments on animals, such as when a light cue is made to precede a noxious stimulus then the exposure to the light cue alone produced analgesia. An important experimental tool in research to establish opioids as responsible for analgesia is the use of naloxone, a specific antagonist to certain endogenously released opioids. Naloxone is an antagonist very specifically to met-enkephalin. Conditioning cues which cause analgesia implicate met-enkephalin release which is substantiated by the analgesia reversal following naloxone.

What was to be understood from these pioneering efforts was that two interrelated physiological mechanisms are available for the control of pain. An afferent stimulus of sufficient intensity from the periphery could initiate nociceptive inhibition at spinal cord levels. Secondly there is a descending inhibition from brainstem and supramedullary levels. At spinal cord levels the action is upon neurons of the substantia gelatinosa (SG)

175

of the dorsal horn. The neurons of the SG function as a gate, shutting off excitatory impulses resulting from nociceptive stimulation at a pre-synaptic level. Environmental threats, as when flight is a perquisite for an animal's survival, show also profound post-synaptic inhibition. These mechanisms for pain inhibition are available in acupuncture analgesia. Supraspinal inhibition is a direct stimulus effect evoked by acupuncture but it is also a component of the clinical conditioning in therapy, especially of hands-on therapies which include acupuncture. Supraspinal inhibition can also be mobilised with other sensory modalities like the application of warmth and cold or massage, and importantly by cues.

Experimental studies on acupuncture and a few clinical studies also demonstrated a correlation to the release of neuro-peptides including the endorphins, which had implications for the inhibition of nociceptive impulses in animals and the relief of patients in pain. The use of naloxone has been mentioned, the opioid antagonist with ligand properties at specific met-enkephalin receptor sites, and since naloxone reversed the analgesia obtained from the use of acupuncture a strong central opioid link was suggested, at least for some of its effects[xii]. Electro-acupuncture with endogenous opioid release has been established experimentally in the normal animal, but these mechanisms are likely to differ from those of traditional manual stimulation acupuncture techniques and the analgesia that follows from its therapeutic use.

The Gate Control Theory

The major development in pain research and the possibility of inhibiting pain was experimentally demonstrated in the nineteen-sixties. Clinical possibilities of pain inhibition by utilising techniques of mechanical stimuli at peripheral and central levels of the nervous system, and the further unfolding of neurotransmitter substances and their modulators at specific receptor sites have produced, apart from their importance for the fundamentals of pain, research, drugs for pain with better localisation at their sites of action.

It was the publication by Melzack and Wall of The Gate Control Theory in 1965 that consolidated the emerging evidence and proved a significant development for the future of pain research. It has had very wide and far reaching implications for experimental work in the field as well as for the treatment and management of patients in pain. From a clinical perspective it explained the failures of surgical approaches to treating localised pain, the questions which were exercising clinical scientists and surgeons[xiii]. Pain had its previous explanations and was thought to be mediated by the hard-wired and specific neural anatomy of a system commencing with afferent nerves from the periphery progressing through the spinal cord to the highest centres of the central nervous system. The Gate Control demonstrated the possibility of modulating the excitation resulting from nociceptive stimuli of pain at synapses of the dorsal horn of the spinal cord by other peripheral afferent nerves responding to noxious or non-noxious stimuli. The entire structure of its theory was reviewed once again, after early criticisms by Nathan in 1976 who maintained that the Theory ignored known facts about stimulus-specificity of nerve fibres eliciting pain, and that while fibres, the majority non-myelinated, could be excited by various stimuli thermal, chemical or mechanical, they had in common the fact that they were nociceptors—fibres excited by high intensity stimuli that might cause tissue damage.

Nathan's criticisms were built around two fundamental concepts which any theory, he maintained, needed to account for. Nociceptive fibres were specific in responding only to nociceptive stimuli and they demonstrated the singular quality of transmitting only that information. Secondly that there were other Aδ and C fibres with the capacity to respond to different stimuli. Wall[xiv], however, pointed to the distinction; non-myelinated fibres could be prognostic in that they had predictive possibilities dependent on the stimulus, or that they were diagnostic. Certain Aδ (myelinated) and C fibres transmit impulses only when exposed to a particular quality of stimulus. Nociception and none other, therefore, follow a stimulus of sufficient intensity among some fibres while others alter sensation with the stimulus intensity. The end result varied depending on the intensity of stimulation and impulse transmission. The response of some afferent receptors to stimulus intensities would be (if the number of + symbols indicate grades of stimulus intensity) as following:

A thermal stimulus of intensity grade results in:

+	++	++++
Warmth	Heat	Pain

A mechanical stimulus results in:

++   ++++

Pressure   Pain

But certain mechanoreceptors respond only at high stimulus intensities and only with

++++

Pain

P D Wall re-stated his proposal of the "Gate Control Theory" in 1978 accounting for the criticisms of Nathan and others, and made three conclusive points in his restatement which he summarised as follows.

"(1) Information about the presence of injury is transmitted to the central nervous system by peripheral nerves. Certain small diameter fibres (Aδ and C) respond only to injury while others with lower thresholds increase their discharge frequency if the stimulus reaches noxious levels.

(2) Cells in the spinal cord or fifth nerve nucleus which are excited by these injury signals are also facilitated or inhibited by other peripheral nerve fibres which carry information about innocuous events.

(3) Descending control systems originating in the brain modulate the excitability of the cells which transmit information about injury".

In summary, "Therefore the brain receives messages about injury by way of a gate controlled system which is influenced by (1) injury signals, (2) other types of afferent impulse and (3) descending control".

ACUPUNCTURE MECHANISMS.

Application of heat or cold and massage have been mentioned as having a pain relieving effect, but the mechanisms explaining it were consolidated in the proposals of the Gate Control Theory of Melzack and Wall. It was also obvious that a few basic features of analgesia from acupuncture and related techniques did find an explanation in the theory. Later research findings provide greater detail of the two basic inhibitory mechanisms involved in analgesia, the peripheral and central descending inhibition of cells of the dorsal horn.

Dorsal horn cells of the spinal cord or trigeminal nucleus level, excited by a stimulus of injury for example, may also be inhibited by afferent peripheral stimulation. Such stimulation conveys sensations related to a needle insertion into skin and underlying tissue, which may be perceived by an individual as ranging from the innocuous to tolerable or momentary pain, or as other innocuous sensations (as with moxibustion, the controlled warmth applied at acupuncture points). It is possible, therefore, to elicit various grades of sensation within the many acupuncture techniques in vogue. At the level of the dorsal horn, acupuncture stimulation is augmented by descending inhibition as well.

Acupuncture analgesia (AA) has been extensively studied in both subjects and animals. Peripheral stimulation with the needle is able to either inhibit or reduce the sensation of pain or, in animals, the response to nocuous stimuli. The evidence has been demonstrated in animal studies of the neural pathways involved, from the periphery to central neurones in the spinal cord and at defined areas of brainstem, midbrain, sub-cortical and cortical levels using techniques akin to acupuncture.

As to the mechanisms offering long term improvement following acupuncture for more chronic pain, the evidence is largely speculative.

A) It is most likely that, at least, the initiating mechanisms of pain control in chronic clinical pain commences in mechanisms similar to AA.

B) The discovery of opiate receptors and the further isolation of the opioid peptide groups, such as the enkephalins and endorphins which are naturally released endogenous ligands to these receptors, are effective mechanisms in pain control and also demonstrated with acupuncture. A part of the explanation for the durable mitigating effects of acupuncture on chronic pain may lie in the developing complexity in evolution of these receptors.

C) There is increasing evidence of specific brain areas involved in the descending controls on pain and more, specifically, the intricate network at these levels may also be activated by acupuncture.

A system for descending controls, as previously mentioned, was identified as early as 1954 by Reynolds. He demonstrated the inhibition of nociceptive withdrawal reflexes in the rat after stimulation of the brainstem reticular formation. Withdrawal reflexes are the involuntary movements in response to a noxious stimulus; for example in humans a spontaneous withdrawal of a hand or limb away from an accidentally touched hot pan or, in the rat, shown as a tail flick when exposed to a noxious stimulus. In the experimental animal it was postulated that a system of descending inhibition to transmission occurred at spinal cord levels on the neurons excited by nociceptive activity. If the pain following injury is not in conformity to the extent of traumatised tissue, or apparently absent in certain circumstances of fear, attention or anxiety, it could be explained by the inhibiting activity of the system involving a neural connectivity from specific cells in brainstem areas such as the periaqueductal grey (PAG) to cells of the dorsal horn in the spinal cord or trigeminal nucleus. In particular environmental contexts, the activation of these descending inhibitory controls is for survival. But environmental factors such as the evocation of intense attention or anxiety for the organism and, in a clinic situation, patients receiving a specific therapy or procedure intensified by the expectation of benefit, experience pain modulation through the mobilisation of these central mechanisms; sometimes so powerfully that it is sufficient for the complete inhibition or suppression of pain (references are available in the chapters following).

Components of the sensory response to the inserted needle: DeQi.

The manipulation of acupuncture needles inserted into tissues, usually muscle, should evoke a further sensation, known as the DeQi, when the technique is used traditionally. It offers a manual control over the stimulus and is of low intensity and of a low frequency. DeQi is understood best in its own therapeutic culture. The classic description in the previous chapter underscores both its subjective nature for the patient and is an objective aid for the therapist. A therapist's skill lies in part in his ability to rapidly elicit Deqi from the patient.

In the terms of research 'pain threshold' is close to quantifying the extent to which an individual will submit to the above graded stimulus before he experiences the qualitative change of sensation as definitive pain. When a needle is rotated at an acupuncture point it rapidly arrives at a pain threshold. DeQi may be considered to be the response from the patient of a sensation short of the pain threshold. However, its perception by patients within its culture signifies the arrival of Qi, an energy form depicting all that therapy can achieve from that expectation. The therapeutic significance of DeQi must be stressed and not written off either as a placebo effect or cultural conditioning. We have some indication of the importance of culture and ethnicity on the perception of pain, but not as yet to distinguish one man's sensation from another's DeQi in any definitive study.

Culture and inbuilt learning are amongst further variables on the perception of pain. As an objective study, "—Carragee and colleagues compared patients who had fixation of femoral fractures within 1 week of injury in two U.S. hospitals with a matched group of patients in three urban hospitals in Vietnam. Over a 15-day period, the Vietnamese patients were given, on average, 0.9 mg of morphine equivalent units as compared to 30.2 mg given to those in the United States. Interestingly, only 8% of the Vietnamese patients reported that their pain control had been inadequate, whereas 80% of the American patients did so—"[xv].

As for the quality of sensation, Deqi can only be described as the change in sensation from the time of a needle insertion to that when the needle is twirled. Often there is a sudden increase in the intensity from a much localised perception of this fine needle in the tissue to a substantial and sudden fullness around the point—a localised tension or a lightning radiation, short lived but uncomfortable. As mentioned, it may occasionally be painful, or an equivalence to a sub-pain threshold. Continued manipulation of the needle for a length of time results in frank pain, and any further stimulation in pain that is intolerable. Syncope has also been noted in individual sensitivities.

For therapist and patient, however, DeQi conveys important attributes of therapy. The accuracy of the location of the acupuncture point is related to the rapidity with which the sensation appeared, and a mastery of technique for obtaining Qi is conveyed in the proficiency of the therapists needle manipulation. These hands-on requirements are part of traditional acupuncture to its best practice. A placebo pursuit for this aspect of acupuncture therapy may even be in acknowledging the difficulties of fashioning one, to say the least, to be problematic.

It is difficult to relate the reasons for the sensory experience to specific mechanisms in terms of the afferents involved, and in all likelihood DeQi in its subjective variety would involve individual differences to those mechanisms as well. fMRI is an investigatory tool as of now. With manual acupuncture eliciting 'Deqi' sensation a correlation has been established with thin afferent fibre excitation, in fibres also specifically responsive to bradykinin. It has been demonstrated by Japanese research groups, who lay emphasis on gentle manipulation techniques with fine needles for immediate therapeutic effects as opposed to the slower induction of analgesia with electro-acupuncture. What is interesting from their research is that moxibustion, the use of mild heat over acupuncture points from lighted moxa candles (Artemisia moxa) has a history older than even Chinese meridians and needle stimulation. DeQi sensations may also involve polymodal receptors and C fibre afferents. In recent years manual acupuncture in human subjects has been noted to produce signal responses at limbic and paralimbic structures of the cortex as well as at other sub-cortical and brainstem and cerebellar levels. An acupuncture point, well known in tradition for an easily elicited 'Deqi' by manual stimulation, was chosen, in fMRI studies, to demonstrate significant signal changes at the various levels of these supraspinal structures[xvi].

It could be that the manipulation initiates fast c-fibre pain (nociceptor specific) as some consider it to be. However, single fibre micro-stimulation of a c-fibre afferent has demonstrated the sensation of burning pain and that only at high frequencies and not at low frequency manual stimulation. Burning pain does not relate to the type of Deqi patient response which is often described as a localised but heavy muscle sensation, restricted to a time length of seconds in an area surrounding the inserted needle. However, Deqi must be appreciated for what it is—a sensory perception which, however, is not abolished by anaesthetising a cutaneous nerve. That was shown to be possible only if a muscle nerve bundle at a specific point is anaesthetised. In clinical practice propagated sensations i.e., a radiation, is often discerned by subjects, especially at extra-sensitive acupuncture points, e.g. Zusanli, Stomach 36. This sensation too is considered DeQi by the therapist.

Zusanli is located with the knee in semi-flexion and the breadth of the terminal phalanx of the index finger (compared with the patient's and hence more modular and not a metric measure) lateral to the lower margin of the tibial tubercle, a palpable crest. It lies in the tibialis anterior muscle at a similar depth of the needle from the skin surface. The sensation may be rapidly elicited at the 'point', with the needle in the tibialis anterior muscle near its origin, and with a gentle rotary movement eliciting the occasional radiation along L4, 5, nerve radicles (peroneal nerve). The point is often a 'trigger point'.

Therapeutic technique requires the localisation of 'points': the details relating to their position in surface anatomy, angles and depth for needle insertion, and specifying the tissues penetrated, the innervation and blood supply in the region of 'points'. In other words, the morphological features of traditional Chinese Acupuncture 'points' should promote an awareness which would prevent regional or systemic hazards likely in ignoring the regulations to their clinical use. From the elements of Chinese literature and anatomical studies this author had compiled in 1991 the uniform detail for a list of acupuncture points for a teaching manual. It has since been translated into Swedish[xvii] as a Compendium for courses for the modern student of medical acupuncture, making for the safer practice of acupuncture in the knowledge of 'point' anatomy. Apart from traditional localisation of points this information should be available for anybody practising acupuncture today.

The clinical equivalent of a noxious peripheral stimulus in the cat and rat, appear to consistently excite nuclei in specific areas of brain stem, signified by signal increases, for instance in the rostral ventral medulla. Well-structured recent studies on human volunteers suggest that Deqi stimulation correlates to widespread signal decreases in the cerebro-cerebellar complex, while increases are seen if Deqi is perceptibly painful.

It adds to possibilities that the stimulus of acupuncture may mediate many more pathways via spinal cord neurons to substrates of the higher centres and that more than one afferent type is involved in multiple reflex pathways of both autonomic and somatic systems. The clinical use of acupuncture, it must be stressed, uses techniques of stimulation at undefined ('ah shi') points as well as the defined sites, and with varying intensities and frequencies. 'Ah shi' relate to 'trigger' points and usually respond with pain on needle puncture. Even DeQi stimulation stresses the importance of varying the sensory perceptions of the patient by techniques of manipulation for differing traditional diagnoses. A host of vivid adjectives define a multitude of the techniques in classical literature but it is unlikely that these variants of technique evoke separate neural mechanisms. One or other circuitry may predominate in the varying techniques. Since they finally reflect a subjective quality of response in individual and in species, exact neural mechanisms are not predictable in the state of our present knowledge of functional neural networks.

Much of the experimental work began in the recognition of acupuncture analgesia, and the evidence in this area was soon established. Bridging the distinction between analgesia as an experimental effect and the pain reduction that results from its clinical use is a research project of some magnitude. There are innumerable clinical studies but a systematic approach with a view to clarifying results from the many techniques used in acupuncture is wanting. This would entail comparison of traditional acupuncture with many other modes of use in vogue at present. Each innovator has his own interpretation for explaining the function of his particular technique.

Dorsal Horn Cells. Segmental Effects of Acupuncture stimulation

The cells of the dorsal horn are, functionally, projection neurons which carry inputs to higher brain centres, excitatory neurons relaying input to projection cells, motor neurons in the spinal reflex circuitry, or other interneurons. Finally, there are inhibitory interneurons, which modulate and control inputs to other cells.

Primary afferent nerves are neurons with cell bodies in the dorsal root ganglion, and from there its axon in the dorsal root synapses onto the cells of the dorsal horn in the spinal cord. The smaller diameter myelinated and unmyelinated axons segregate toward the ventrolateral part of the root and form the Tract of Lissauer at the dorso-lateral corner of the spinal cord. Amongst them are the nociceptor unmyelinated C-fibres and Aδ fibres, some exclusively responding to nociceptive stimuli, and most polymodal which respond to other stimuli as well as, for instance, innocuous thermal stimuli. The fibres divide caudally, and rostrally eventually terminate in the upper part of the substantia gelatinosa (SG) (Lamina I and II). Some of the larger of the Aα fibres in the dorsal root enter the dorsal columns of the spinal cord medially, and then their ascending and descending branches synapse with the neurons of the dorsal horn. Their axons synapse with cells in the deeper layers of the dorsal horn and from there to 'tracts' ascending in the columns of the spinal cord and thence to the higher brain centres. Shorter interneurons connect to neighbouring segments of the spinal cord.

The processes of the inhibitory control at this level of the spinal cord are descending inhibition from medullospinal axons to the spinothalamic cells of lamina I directly and through further synaptic ramifications. The inhibitory synaptic action is mediated by serotonin or enkephalin, depending on the position of incoming afferent nerve synapse on the dorsal horn cell. The descending axons may inhibit the spinothalamic cell post-synaptically in reference to the incoming afferent nerve. Post synaptic inhibition could also be mediated by an intermediary T-cell neurone. There is pre-synaptic inhibition also with reference to the afferent nerve synapse mediated by opioid action on nociceptor afferent activity. It must be emphasised that this outline of inhibitory function at dorsal horn level is amongst many possible synaptic structural variants, diverse receptors and their specific transmitter substances.

Aβ fibres carry touch (skin) sensation. Some small myelinated Aδ fibres carry muscle pain, and also possibly signal a part of the needle sensations described above[xviii], although Kawakita et al[xix] consider that the precise receptors and afferent fibres responsible for Deqi, have not been precisely identified. Mention has been made of the possibility of thinner polymodal afferents responsive to bradykinin as likely mediators. However, in proposing the importance of DeQi there seems to be an inconsistency in the further suggestion that, since certain trigger point locations tally with some acupuncture points, it would answer to the quality of sensory response to the needle with common mechanisms for both trigger point stimulation and acupuncture point needling. Needling the former is a painful response and felt as such by the patient. Proper DeQi responses from 'point' stimulation ought not reach threshold levels of pain, and only momentarily if they do.

Synaptic excitation or inhibition is possible following a peripheral stimulus or injury, and hence inhibition may be provoked either by the latter or by different applications of peripheral sensory stimuli. The Gate Control Theory in its original conception offered both possibilities. One inhibitory possibility occurs when low threshold fibres of touch are activated. An inhibitory synapse within the spinal cord mediates inhibition of the nociceptive afferent input. The reduction of pain by stroking or gentle massage is one example within an unfolding array of inhibitory mechanisms by peripheral stimuli.

The site of action for the 'gating', whether pre-synaptic or post-synaptic, of the neurons of SG has been much debated. They appear less important although some evidence is available of their differing receptor actions especially as now opiate function is better understood for its role in pain inhibition. Unlike the higher centres of the periaqueductal gray (PAG) and rostroventral medulla (RVM) where endogenous opioids, met-enkephalin and B-endorphin, activate descending neurons, at the level of the spinal cord postsynaptic enkephalin inhibition of nociceptive neurons is a likelier mechanism[xx]. Bowsher[xxi] in his chapter specifically postulates evidence in the small stalked cells, demonstrated in the cat and humans, which can release enkephalin when stimulated. This mechanism of stalked cell excitation is inhibitory to SG cells and can prevent further transmission of nociceptive information at this level. They react at frequencies of stimulation of about 3 Hz, which is that of manual acupuncture.

Thin myelinated Aδ afferents, high threshold mechano-receptors conveying pain including sensation of pinprick are excitatory on SG cells and, through their synapses, on the wide dynamic range (WDR) cells of lamina V. SG cells also receive polymodal unmyelinated C afferents. Evidence of an opioid mediated presynaptic inhibition by primary afferents is also present, but is unlikely to be a direct enkephalin action as is mediated by postsynaptic terminals contacting neurons of the Spinothalamic tract (Stt). Presynaptic inhibition may not be direct, possibly an opioid suppression of the inflammatory mediator, substance P, released by nociceptive afferents.

Endophinergic opioid receptors are the mu (μ) delta (δ) and kappa (κ) receptors, and activated by the release of met-enkephalin, beta endorphin and dynorphin at the respective receptor sites. At the spinal cord level there is evidence for the activation of receptors presenting enkephalin and dynorphin, peptides at the μ and κ receptors. The frequency of stimulation determines peptide inhibition, and in animal studies met-enkephalin receptors are found to be predominantly active with lower frequencies, and dynorphin at frequencies between 20-100Hz.

It may be that acupuncture mediates stimulus activity at differing receptors in varying frequencies of electrical stimulation when needles are coupled to machines designed to provide them. This in turn may involve different afferent fibre diameters and their cells in the spinal cord. Despite uncertainties at the present time, the sensation of 'deqi' can be correlated to excitation of thin afferent fibres with polymodal receptors. Manual acupuncture, which is a low frequency of stimulation possibly below 3 Hz. may account for it. Thick myelinated afferents' (Aβ) activation, as possibly with moxibustion—localised warmth not amounting to heat at acupuncture points, may also induce analgesic effects at segmental levels and could involve concepts of gating. TENS (transcutaneous electrical stimulation) or electrical stimulation effected through needles of low intensity and high frequencies (100 Hz) are Aβ fibre mediated, possibly involving kappa receptors and dynorphin; while high intensities resulting in muscle fibre contractions with low frequencies of about 2 Hz electro acupuncture are mu receptor and Aδ fibre mediated[xxii]. The evidence from clinical studies gives an indication of the parameters of stimulation that can best achieve relief in certain diagnostic categories of pain (Ch. VII), though stimulation parameters in those studies appear to have greater relevance to the pathophysiology of pain rather than the anatomical 'head and neck pain', 'low back ache'—the gross diagnostic categories of Pain.

The inhibition at the dorsal horn, both at SG and lamina V (WDR) cells responding to painful stimuli, is thus possible by segmental activation of different afferent fibres using varying frequencies of stimulation. The WDR cells are convergent cells, being excited by most stimuli from peripheral afferents in a graded manner. Manual stimulation at low frequencies, perceived as Deqi, inhibits painful stimuli at this level by involving polymodal receptors (PMRs). The involvement of these receptors is suggested in their sensitisation. They then respond with tenderness as 'trigger points' do. Some trigger points correlate to certain acupuncture points, but in traditional literature the 'ashi' points are observed without any relationship to acupuncture points. Trigger points may also appear anywhere on the body surface without the strictly described localisations of acupuncture points. Such attributes to PMRs require clarification in further studies, but their likely relevance to each other has been considered previously. The activation of WDR cells, lamina V and deeper layers of the dorsal horn convey painful impulses and their further projections through the spinoreticular tracts to the higher centres. At segmental levels via the circuitry described they may thus be initially inhibited through stimulation of PMRs at acupuncture points.

Nonsegmental Effects of Acupuncture and evidence for its mechanisms

Apart from segmental nerve stimulation and the response of their neurons and cells at the dorsal horn levels, more widespread effects may occur and not confined to the regional distribution of segmental nerves. The most likely neurophysiological basis for acupuncture therapy may become clarified as we unravel such mechanisms. At present we lack explanations for its longer term benefits. Here again a multiplicity of mechanisms are likely. The neural circuitry at higher levels of the central nervous system and their transmitter substances are involved in analgesia. At least two further experimental models other than that involving the peptide β-endorphin have been well documented in studies over recent decades. But it must be stressed that, while separate mechanisms are postulated, functionally they may present together, with one or other predominating and further dependent on the environmental circumstance.

Descending Pathways

There are two descending inhibitory pathways involving a) transmitter substance serotinin and b) adrenalin. Another non-segmental model, convincingly shown in the rat and put forward by the LeBars group in 1979, was Diffuse Noxious Inhibitory Control (DNIC). The impressive experimental analgesia by PAG stimulation, demonstrated in the rat by Reynolds in 1968, may involve these systems since the descending neural circuitry in the dorsolateral funiculus converge on to SG cells of the spinal cord and inhibit pain. Some or all of these mechanisms may well be available for the analgesia obtained with acupuncture. Explanations for the longer term alleviation of clinical pain must be conjectural at present but are likely to commence from these mechanisms.

The candidate cells for inhibition are the high firing WDR cells present in lamina V and in deeper layers of the dorsal horn. WDR cells are polysynaptic receiving interneuronal relays from multiple afferents both excitatory and inhibitory. The cells send axons to the opposite side of the spinal cord then ascend in the spinoreticular tracts. Nociceptive information from the spinoreticular tract is carried to the reticular formation, the interlaminar hypothalamus and hypothalamus. The spinothalamic is again a crossed tract conveying information from Aδ fibres to the cells of the marginal zones of lamina I. It is the collateral connections of this pathway and the release of two inhibitory transmitter substances, serotonin (5-hydroxytryptamine or 5-HT) and noradrenaline which could be responsible for some of the non-segmental effects of acupuncture.

The serotenergic System

The periaqueductal grey (PAG) of the mid brain receives collaterals from the spinothalamic tract conveying axons of cells originating in Lamina I. The descending pathways from PAG relay in the nucleus raphe magnus (NRM) in the medulla oblongata. Further, the descending pathway is conveyed in the dorsolateral funiculus from the NRM to the stalked cells of the spinal cord. Apart from non-segmental effects that may result from acupuncture stimulation, initiated by transmitter substance serotonin along this pathway, its collateral synapses in PAG are powerfully enkephalinergic as is their final destination on the stalked cells in the spinal cord. Effects beyond pain inhibition are involved in the activation of the serotenergic system. The PAG itself receives fibres from the prefrontal cortex via the hypothalamus, which in turn connects with the PAG. The pathway is also endorphinergic, and in humans the cortico-hypothalamic relay plays a role in homeostasis as well as a few psychic functions. It can hence be hypothesised that non segmental acupuncture effects on pain, including its longer term alleviation, may involve this extended circuitry as well.

The noradrenergic system

In some animals, including some primates, lamina I cells projecting to PAG send further collaterals to the locus coeruleus lying in the pons at the junction with the medulla oblongata. This area is a mainstay of noradrenergic axons. Noradrenaline (NAD) acts directly to inhibit the cells of the SG and others cells in the spinal cord which are excited by nociceptors. The nucleus paragigantocellular reticular nucleus has been implicated in the noradrenergic system but indirectly through the locus coeruleus. The control of this system may be from prefrontal cortex and the arcuate nucleus in the hypothalamus.

Neurotransmitter release is related to the homeostatic and metabolic requirements of an organism. Both serotonin and noradrenaline as neurotransmitters are a part of systems with their neuroanatomical connections in the prefrontal cortex, ventromedial and lateral hypothalamus and the cerebellum. The systems are implicated in the control of many metabolic functions, for instance, in hunger and the timing of the desire to eat, and in feelings of satiety. Dysfunctional release of these particular transmitters have a bearing on obesity, hypertension etc.

Neurotransmitters and neuromodulators, demonstrated as important in an area of pathophysiology, are obviously a part of neural circuitry involved in maintaining normal bodily function, its homeostasis and metabolism. There is experimental confirmation of their metabolic role as well as the possibility that they are mediators of the pain inhibitory neural circuitry.

Acupuncture stimulation, it should not be forgotten, while mobilising the pain inhibitory circuitry for pain alleviation in clinical conditions, finds a rationale for its use in many metabolic disorders that have not progressed to established pathology. Appetite regulation and hunger, obesity, benign hypertension and anorexia nervosa have been studied and suggest that acupuncture may be an alternative to drug control in these conditions.

The cannabinoid system.

One outcome of recent research is the isolation of the active substance of that ancient narcotic drug marihuana. It has been termed anandamide, the word derived from the Sanskrit is presumably an acknowledgement of the use of marihuana in the pharmacopias of Traditional Indian Medical systems, especially in Ayurveda; or perhaps from its narcotic attribute 'anandam' or happiness. Endogenous cannabinoids and their receptors have since been discovered and these involve particular CNS sites and a system with its own neural pathways. Certain metabolic processes which determine weight loss or gain have recently been implicated this neural pathway. It is likely that, as with the serotonergic and noradrenergic, the cannabinoid system impacts pain. Acupuncture use for appetite suppression (weight control protocols) and as anti-addiction therapy is being employed in the practices of European clinics, and is gaining in importance. The hypothesis of acupuncture mechanisms involving the endophinergic cannabinoid system as the basis for anti-addiction and appetite suppressant effects, or as a parallel implication for reducing pain, need further exploration, basic and clinical research.

Diffuse Noxious Inhibitory Controls (DNIC)

In distinguishing likely mechanisms for acupuncture techniques one can look at two distinct possibilities that relate to the intensity of needle stimulus. With low intensities and at low frequencies, as when obtaining

DeQi sensation through the manual application of needles, segmental and non-segmental mechanisms are involved and likely neural pathways outlined. While rotating needles for DeQi, the manipulation may result in frank pain but this is not usually a requirement for therapeutic effect. However, pain need not negate effect either; for certain patient problems acupuncturists may use the method of applying the needles to elicit pain. For centuries, variants on methods producing localised pain have been known to suppress pain experienced in other areas of the body. From Greece (electric eels) to China, and through many other parts of the Eastern and Southern world, the possibility has been used for therapy as well as ritual display or black magic, which would ordinarily be painful. Counter irritation is a recognised technique for suppressing pain.

DNIC[xxiii] is a possible front runner for the neural mechanism explaining the clinical relief for forms of musculo-skeletal pains, especially those associated with muscle spasm. The mechanism has so far been demonstrated in experiments by Le Bars and his group. Following painful acupuncture, therapeutic effects on human pain could be possible, in a way similar to their demonstration of effects using noxious non-segmental stimuli in animal experiments. In a series of studies they initially applied a noxious stimulus on the peripheral receptive field of the animal generating impulses centrally in WDR cells of the spinal cord or its homologue in the trigeminal nucleus of the medulla. The pattern of the amplitude of these impulses was considerably reduced if the animal was subjected to a further noxious stimulus applied at a widely separate receptive field. For instance, applying a noxious pinch to the hind paw of the animal initiates the electro-physiological record at WDR cells of the convergent neurons in the cord. The amplitude then reduced when the second stimulus was applied by a forceps pinch to the face or tail, sufficient in intensity for the animal to vocalise at the noxious nature of the stimulus. A noxious stimulus repeated with bradykinin injected into the viscus had a similar result. Considerable importance lay in finding that the inhibition of baseline neural activity outlasted the duration of the application of the second stimulus by hours.

A series of further experiments confirm that these effects are seen only on the convergent neurones of WDR cells and not on purely nociceptive neurones. They are triggered through myelinated Aδ afferents or Aδ and C afferent fibres. A series of synaptic loops are involved in carrying the impulses to supraspinal structures in the ventrolateral tracts of the spinal cord. The descending fibres are carried back to the spinal cord in the dorso-lateral funiculus. There is now evidence of cortical structures in this inhibitory circuitry, but a major location that has been identified for the descending fibres is in the caudal part of the medulla, an area quite separate from other areas involved in other non-segmental inhibitory effects. This is the Subnucleus Reticularis Dorsalis (SRD), and lesions in this area of the medulla strongly reduced the effect of diffuse noxious inhibitory control. The SRD seems fairly unique for its property of responding to only nociceptive stimuli and a further special feature is that the nucleus carries on it the representation of the entire parts of the body.

Acupuncture utilising momentary pain—above the pain threshold—is a well-documented method of clinical practice[xxiv]. Felix Mann was a recognised proponent of the method in the West, but for patient pathology his methods had further parameters in the use of acupuncture not only for conditions of chronic pain but for systemic ailments as well. His methods included strict anatomical localisation of the point to be stimulated, and his teaching required acquaintance of the basic knowledge that doctors learn in the medical sciences.

DNIC as experimentally demonstrated explains immediate pain relief in clinical conditions and, to an extent, the longer lasting relief often seen with the painful DeQi modes of acupuncture. Extrapolations from the experimental DNIC relate effect for conditions of acute pain; e.g. the relief from an acute state of trismus and pain resulting from pathology of the temperomandibular joint; the neck muscle spasm in acute torticollis (wry neck), and in low back-ache with the intense pain and board like rigidity resulting from muscle spasm. Neurophysiological explanations for therapeutic benefit with painful stimulation in other ailments can only be tentative at present. The example below closely follows experimental DNIC effect in its immediacy as well as in the longer term relief which follows. However, it does not explain the non-recurrence of pain and spasm long after neural inhibition from the needle stimulus ceased. In the clinical purview of most therapists involved with acupuncture pathology with a satisfactory outcome is in treating chronic pain overlaid by such acute episodes.

In traditional acupuncture certain specified acupuncture points are recognised as painful to needle. Shenmen, on the meridian of Small Intestine VI, is approached at the junction of ulnar styloid process with its head. The point is situated in ligamentous tissue beneath and caudal to a palpable styloid and a needle twirled there can elicit exquisite pain on stimulation necessitating stimulation to be momentary but repetitive.

Following a long interstate car ride in the US and the fortunate company of a young Swiss doctor who was also a trainee at our Chinese course, treatment described above relieved me of that commonly known condition of acute 'lumbago' intense pain and rigidity of the the lower back as lumbar erector spinae and psoas muscles go into acute spasm and appropriately described as the 'locked' back. Attempted movement merely increases muscle spasm and pain. These acute episodes of pain are superimposed on chronic pathology[20].

Summary of the evidence of neurotransmitters and pathways involved in acupuncture analgesia

Various neurotransmitters, bio-chemicals involved in transmission of nerve impulses, have been mentioned as involved in acupuncture analgesia at various levels of the central nervous system, and they along with others were demonstrated to be implicated in the mechanism of analgesia in a study by a Chinese group[xxv]. Their evidence showed correlations of neurochemical changes in the CNS following acupuncture and its modification by

---

[20] Therapy with acupuncture for the type of pathology can produce a quality of relief that is remarkable but may be beyond the possibility of a study with standard protocols. We are left with evidence admittedly anecdotal. I had seen the effect of needling in this manner on at least 3 patients in in the Beijing clinic for acute states of pain To those of China were added my later personal experience related above. In the clinic the decision made for a patient was for the needles to be located bilaterally at the Shenmen point, followed by their simultaneous twirling for a few seconds until a pain threshold was crossed. Stimulation was then stopped before the process was resumed again. All the while the patient was asked to try and move his back, which after about fifteen minutes of treatment became possible. That terminated the treatment session. The patient was reasonably mobile with much reduced but tolerable pain on leaving the department. More remarkable was, after a period of rest and within twenty four hours, recovery from pain and spasm was virtually complete. The patient was a member of the Beijing Opera Company. Two days later he greeted us backstage with many bows and beaming smiles with others of the company. He was apparently fit and free of pain, not only at that evening's performance but had been so a while after the single session of treatment.

pharmacological manipulation. The studies were based on experimental data from rats and rabbits.

Serotonin (5-HT) and Opiate-like Substances (OLS) are demonstrably at high levels in rat brain, and correlated to excellent analgesia following acupuncture. Moderate analgesia after acupuncture showed when only one or the other of these substances was tested, while lack of analgesia or its marked diminution correlated in the absence of either substance. Similar reductions of acupuncture-mediated analgesia could be demonstrated when blocking acetylcholine synthesis at their muscarine receptors by atropine in rabbits. It suggests that acetylcholine is yet another important substrate in the mechanism of analgesia by acupuncture.

Evidences of Cortical and Subcortical signal alteration following acupuncture using Brain Imaging Techniques and its functional implications.

Metaphysical explanations in most traditions of medicine, and certainly in TCM, involved the heart as the ultimate arbiter of physiological function. Science in medicine now offers constituents of the central nervous system as the mediator and the brain as the final determinant of sensation and cognition with control over the somatic motor system and influencing reflex autonomic functions. The tools are constantly being improved for the investigation of specific structures in cortical and sub-cortical areas. Positron Emission Tomography (PET) and fMRI have enabled the techniques for scanning blood flow and offer a means of assessing the change that occurs when the organism is subject to a variety of environmental inputs. The inputs are many but others, like acupuncture and including other peripheral sensory techniques, offer much towards controlling pain pathology.

Lewith et al have reviewed studies reporting brain activation when acupuncture points, traditionally ascribed to have other specificities of function, were stimulated. UB (urinary bladder) 67 is used for aspects of visual dysfunction. Activation of the visual area of the occipital cortex was noted in small numbers of subjects by some workers, although others have demonstrated that it is not a consistent finding. Another functionally specific point for nausea and vomiting is PC (pericardium) 6. Studies suggest that acupuncture stimulation at this point for nauseous subjects selectively activates neural substrates in the left superior frontal gyrus, the anterior cingulate gyrus, the dorso medial nucleus of the thalamus as well as the nausea-specific substrates of the cerebellum, and relate those findings to clinical effectiveness The activation did not occur with sham (non-acupuncture point) needle penetration.

Brain substrates in acupuncture modulation of pain.

Inhibitory mechanisms following stimulation at peripheral levels occur at the spinal cord, but the process further involves the higher centres of the brain and their potent descending inhibitory systems. The pain inhibitory system was experimentally considered to function in the organised neural networks at the levels of the dorsal horn of the spinal cord, the brainstem and the midbrain and their descending modulatory systems.

Studies directly aimed at clarifying the role of specific acupuncture point stimulation with modern neuro-imaging techniques in volunteer subjects provide evidence of additional effects on the limbic, paralimbic and subcortical gray, i.e. at multiple levels of the cerebro-cerbellar complex, with modulatory implications on pain, inflammation and, possibly within an extension of that complex, on stress. From imaging studies it is apparent that the complex has a feed-forward and feedback loop. The feed-forward loop comprises the sensorimotor cortices with limbic and paralimbic structures to the brainstem, the reticular formation, periquductal gray, the pontine nucleus, and thence via the ponto-cerebellar tract to a feedback system through the ponto-thalamic to a thalamo-cortical projection.

It can presently be postulated that controlled sensory stimuli like acupuncture and other environmental stimuli, by means of this complex extend a role for the autonomic system and related immuno-humoral systems, toward the modulation of inflammation and pain. The modulatory processes of acupuncture mediate neurogenic response in somatic systems and signals via the vagus nerve responses of the autonomic systems.

Other workers (Wu et al) implicate the pain-related matrix following studies on healthy volunteers. fMRI was used to evaluate the effects of modes of acupuncture, namely mock and electro-acupuncture, minimal acupuncture on specific or non-specific acupuncture points. Significant activation occurred of hypothalamic areas, primary somato-sensory cortex and rostral anterior cingulate cortex. However, they did not report specific acupuncture points as especially functionally relevant in analgesia.

A more recent study (Hui et al) has fairly convincingly demonstrated that deqi (non-painful) evocation, traditionally considered essential for clinical effects, on St 36 reduced signals in the limbic system. While the system plays a role in the regulation and integration of sensorimotor, autonomic, endocrine and immunological function, and in cognition and effect, its feed forward connections through fibre bundles to the PAG, reticular formation, raphe nuclei and midline structures are, as previously noted, a part of the pain inhibitory circuitry. Thus the structures of the limbic system, comprising, amongst others, the amygdala, hippocampus, anterior thalamus and the cingulate gyrus, form, through interconnecting fibres with the midbrain structures, a limbic system-midbrain composite circuitry.

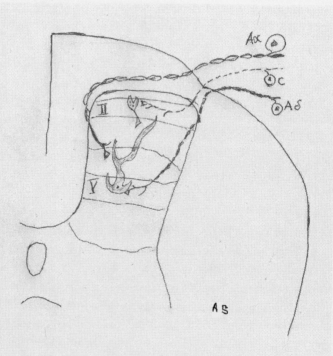

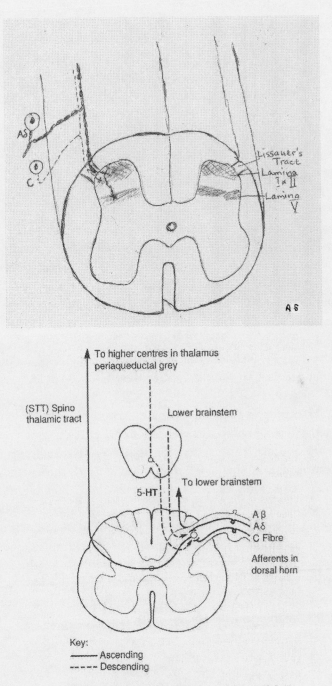

Labels in figure (top):

Aδ

C

Lissauer's
Tract

Lamina
I x II

Lamina
V

A δ

Labels in figure (bottom):

To higher centres in thalamus
periaqueductal grey

(STT) Spino
thalamic tract

Lower brainstem

To lower brainstem

5-HT

A β

A δ

C Fibre

Afferents in
dorsal horn

Key:
——— Ascending
- - - - Descending

Spinal and supraspinal mechanisms in pain modulation.

CHAPTER VI

PAIN PHYSIOLOGY

Living things have material composition, are made up finally of units, molecules, atoms and electrons, as surely as any non-living matter. Like all forms in nature they have chemical structure and physical properties, are physico-chemical systems. As such they obey laws of physics and chemistry. Would one deny this fact, one would thereby deny the possibility of any scientific investigation of living things.

Ernest Everett Just, biologist and embryologist, 1883-1951, quoted from the essay by Stephen Jay Gould, 'Just in the Middle'

The chapter introduces the science of pain: an outline of the morphology of pain systems that convey the sensation from periphery, through peripheral nerves to the central nervous system; the spinal cord and higher centres, and the generation of neurophysiological pain mechanisms. The repetitions from the previous chapter into the present may make for tedium but the hope is for some readers unfamiliar with the subject, that it is easier to follow. The modulation and inhibition of pain is surveyed in the cyto-architecture of the pathways, partly with a view to explain specific therapeutic possibility. It attempts a basic understanding of the mechanisms for the control of clinical pain by peripheral sensory stimulation (PSS) through techniques including acupuncture, but without attempting to present constantly updated information on neurology and neural mechanisms relating to Pain.

Recent developments in Medicine and Pain

It is undeniable that industry is a major participant responsible for developments in medicine, the products of bio-technology, pharmaceuticals; and in genome research we see also the less savoury evidence of commerce and profits consolidating in Medicine and its practice. The social sciences suggest that commerce alone is unlikely if not inimical to the total goal of populations being sustained in better health, and policies directed towards that goal are for the State in its awareness that maintaining the Health needs of a nation should not depend on an ability to pay but should be available without such discrimination to all. The State is the major player to manage and be accountable for the economics of Health Welfare. There are contradictions as Corporates enter the field for Health delivery and in a world where the purchasing power of its citizens is so disparate the abysmal quality evident in the many indices to measuring the Health of a Nation is the indicator that Health management as a State enterprise offers better results. The better and the best achievers are the countries having planned delivery systems for Health Care irrespective of the Nation's wealth.

We turn to an ethos of about 70 years ago when clinical scientists had both feet—one for research and the other for patient care—planted in the clinic. The impetus was for the suffering of patients to be considered as a problem for research; the efforts for its solution are an example of Medicine's frontiers expanding in the emerging Science of Pain. The pioneers defined research which led to discovery, rephrased theory and changed the emphasis to the problem, even including physician attitudes to Pain. Though they continue to suffer chronic pain patients have more choice and prospects for relief in surgical, anaesthetic and manipulative procedures, and in the development of pharmaceuticals in the constantly expanding research for the understanding and control of Pain.

While a heuristic process is implied in the methods of the clinic, overburdened routines of practice often hamper introspection and speculation. The tendency is to overlook or write off untoward results or unexpected outcomes. Where sometimes the circumstance of an uncommon patient response requires to be more closely examined, it may just be ignored. A recurring complication requires discernment of failure and questioning the therapeutic procedure. It may be that the therapy itself prolongs or increases the distress of the patient. However, specialists are inclined to dismiss patient distress as unlikely to relate to therapeutic procedure and today in the routines of parametric investigations the clinician's own specialised cognitive capabilities are increasingly set in abeyance.

The idea that certain problems and sufferings of patients in pain could be better dealt with by that age-old derivative, namely morphine, started another look at a drug which had gone into disfavour for its addictive properties. A series of research initiatives as striking as any in the lore of biological science followed, not least was to reconsider reasons for the intriguing persistence of certain pains in patients after surgical ablation of a presumed site of pain. That posed a possibility of pain being more complex in its neural connectivity than a dedicated track of neurons from periphery to the cortex leading to its perception. One programme of basic research questioned the standard explanations, and a major reorientation of theory followed. Another emphasis to the treatment of pain was suggested. Much debate was to follow but that only mobilised the intellectual resources of many groups of scientists internationally and an ever widening range of implications. Pain, hitherto reduced to being a symptom of disease, now has many constructions in a pathology of its own.

Pain could be either physiological, an immediate response to the stimulus or, else if persistent, a symptom of other pathology or a malfunctioning relating directly to the pain sensory system whose neurons when stimulated have the variable attribute of leading to either excitation or inhibition, and spontaneously modulate the sensation. In that process we now recognise the system to be more dynamic than previously thought. Repeated exposure of central neurons to stimulation is not an unusual environmental occurrence, and can cause their *sensitisation*. That state will generate more pain than warranted. Advances have also resulted from clinical observations of patients with intractable pain which persisted after blocking inputs from injured tissues, or after surgical ablation at various levels of the pathways, once thought to be conveying pain.

A subjective description of a patient's pain may relate to a specific lesion or other pathology. The relationship may sometimes be obscure, though its ultimate reality for the patient may not be denied in its subjectivity. Noordenbos, a neurosurgeon and an early influence on changing the approaches to the problem of pain, quotes Kipling in the Introduction to his book 'Pain' published in 1959, "Chela, know this. There are a great many lies in the world and not a few liars, but there are no liars like our bodies, except it be the sensations of our bodies" (in 'Kim').

Derbyshire[i] recognises that patient reality, biologically and specifically, in his statement: "In addition to the noxious event, the bio-psychosocial model introduces psychological and social factors that may mitigate or increase the final experience of pain. Thus a given stimulus might be experienced as *more or less painful* because of hormonal fluctuation, criterion effects, differences in body size, skin thickness, blood pressure, social expectations, cognitive variation, quality of stimulation and in psychological traits such as anxiety or depression. Given the many sources of variation, it is perhaps unsurprising that gender differences in response to noxious stimulation are generally small and are *swamped by the variation between individuals*" (my italics and refer also to the discussion in Placebo on Mas Related Genes)

There is a maze of age-old cultural and religious superimposition to suffering pain. While clinicians respond to a patient's suffering they previously have accepted its necessity and some inevitability. Another attitude in the clinic was that persistence of patient pain, when beyond somatic explanation, was psychogenic. Western societies by and large progressed to a non-acceptance of the metaphysical reasons for pain. The equivocal philosophy behind it has largely been transformed by scientific research; a collaborative effort of workers in many fields of medicine now finding that some reasons for pain initiated better methods for its control. Collaborations such as the International Association for the Study of Pain (IASP), have fostered the much needed consolidation of many biological disciplines towards that control. Anaesthesiology was in the forefront of the clinical disciplines involved.

World populations now have increased life expectancy, but are also prone to greater degenerative and neoplastic tissue change. The survival rates of patients from disease have markedly improved, but their quality of life is often undermined by chronic pain which is often worse in the elderly. There are unprecedented numbers surviving the trauma of combat plus large scale civilian casualties in the indiscriminate violence of war and civil strife. These add up to greater numbers of a world population living with pain, increased numbers with disabilities following injury or prolonged pain after surgical procedure, and younger patients with pain following uncontrolled infections like HIV. Survival rates improve with better medication, techniques in surgery and patchy health care, but chronic pain takes its toll on the quality of life of many who survive.

Another aspect to the consideration of pain as unnecessary suffering lies in a change in social ethics. Pain and suffering have been, and still sometimes are, regarded as retribution for transgression against God or his fellow man. Atonement through pain[21], imbibed even today in many cultures, transcends religious identities, running through societies not only of a Christian West but of many in the East. Science, in regarding pain as a disease, may have helped disassociate the issue from religion and engendered a secular appreciation of the problem of pain in society. In this instance it was initiated by motivated medical scientists investigating pain who were intensely aware of avoidable suffering and campaigning for available drugs like morphine which previously had been met even with organised resistance to its use.

Physiological function of pain.

The perception of human pain is regarded as a response to injury or a protective response to incipient injury. While organisms have evolved these physiological mechanisms for their protection, clinicians are more generally concerned with how best to overcome the often unnecessary consequences of pain which outlast primary usefulness in the process of tissue repair.

There are individuals with a congenital inability to perceive pain. They suffer from a mutation of a nerve growth factor—the tyrosine kinase receptor—which results in a deficiency of this receptor function in high threshold sensory neurons, i.e. those responding only to intense stimuli. The loss of pain sensation means stimuli with a potential to injure cannot be recognised and consequently cannot be avoided. Such people are in danger of constant injury, exposed as they are in daily life to repetitive trauma which normal individuals, because of their pain, have the capacity to avoid.

---

[21] Christopher Hitchens has this story as told to Malcolm Muggeridge by Mother Teresa who seemed in relating it able to appreciate the problem, but it underscores a tenacity to beliefs about pain. An exemplary personality in her intense concern for the derelicts and destitute, Mother Teresa maintained that prayer was to be the preference for assuaging the sufferings of those in her 'ashram' at Calcutta. During routine rounds to help and give encouragement to them, one pleaded to be given something for his pain. Her response was kindly but firm in offering him comfort. 'Dear man, you will be better if you remember that Jesus is kissing you where you have pain'! The intensity of the man's pain was such he promptly suggested that it be far better if Jesus would immediately stop kissing him and he be given some medicine instead.

The acquired disease, Leprosy, presents a similar problem but with a different etiology. Paul Brandt the eminent reconstructive and plastic surgeon spent a lifetime working with leprosy in India. He titles his autobiographical book, "The Gift of Pain", with possibly a 'Giver' in view, but, of course, in the context of his work is reference to the invaluable function of the sensation of pain—an indubitable evolutionary trait developed to protect the organism from injury. Leprosy, a bacillary disease, gradually destroys specific peripheral nerves, e.g. as frequent examples, the ulnar and posterior tibial. When treatment is neglected patients with leprosy have a disassociated loss of sensation progressing to complete loss of sensation within the receptive fields served by those nerves, and hence of pain also. The normal reflexes, avoidance responses to injury, are absent from the peripheral fields of limbs innervated by those nerves. Trauma is unrecognised. Injury follows, and then infection. Progressive inflammation and ulceration, again painless, lead to tissue loss. This could involve the digits and, increasingly, parts of the limbs, hands or feet—the well-known stigmata of the patient with leprosy. The result of the patient's unawareness of pain is a disastrous liability, the inability to avoid the hazards of repetitive trauma.

Some qualification is required to the above statements with regard to insensitivity to pain in leprosy. These patients are not absolutely devoid of pain within receptive fields of the nerves destroyed, which are no longer served by normal sensory responses. They do report pain. Its nature is disoriented, often spontaneous, and not necessarily a response to a stimulus. Essentially, pain of that nature is not a protective response. It is difficult to speculate on how this neuropathic pain originates.

A personal communication from a friend and former director of the Central Leprosy Research Institute in India is illustrative of some bizarre consequences of leprosy in relation to pain. A patient with a lesion of the posterior tibial nerve had lost sensation over the area of its supply and, after years of living with a foot without pain and consequently ravaged by infections and trophic ulcers, the man requested its amputation which was duly done. Months later he came along, and reported that he now understood what it was to feel pain in his foot. He had developed and described in the missing foot a very typical 'phantom pain'! Phantom pain can be a harrowing experience for many patients, and for clinicians, when it presents in its insolubility, is a sobering enigma of science. Pain in leprosy has still not been persistently investigated. Here we may have,

203

fortunately in diminishing numbers, still a ready-made possibility of studying a progressive peripheral nerve lesion in patients.

The above patient history is a rare instance of pain in leprosy. Following lesions of ulnar or posterior tibial nerves, and despite complete loss of sensory modalities and motor disabilities in its receptive field, this neuropathic entity retains paradoxical complaints of pain. Studies of pain in leprosy could offer more information on the nature of pain in the receptive field of a nerve that has been destroyed by the bacilli. Diabetic pains and other peripheral neuropathies are more distressing, and with limited possibility for adequate control are as yet much more of a clinical problem than pain in leprosy—a disease that may well be a part medical history.

Pain pathophysiology

Up to five decades ago human pain was a 'symptom' and not considered as having pathophysiological causes as separate from the pathology of the underlying condition. Research in that space of time has been discovering many neurobiological factors involved in human pain. Pain could be perceived in the activity of neural pathways following stimulation. Peripheral afferent nerves have their cell bodies in the dorsal ganglia of the nerve roots to the spinal cord, and its axons synapse at the dorsal horn of the cord to project from there in the tracts to the higher centres of the nervous system. The excitatory effect of a stimulus may be modulated by other inhibitory circuits at synapses at various levels of the system. The perception of pain, therefore, is an outcome of inhibitory and excitatory effects.

There are pains which play a protective role in its perceived immediacy in reflexes initiated by the stimulus. That role also applies to longer term *nociceptive pain* (pain essentially due to nociceptor activity) following inflammatory processes—such pain usually resolving as healing takes place. Some inflammatory pains, as in rheumatoid arthritis, persist in the pathology of the disease. Post inflammatory pain is an adaptive pain evolved for survival. The post-operative pain of surgery should be adaptive, although one is aware that some post-surgical pain, in its occasional persistence over a longer period, is maladaptive and pathological.

Maladaptive pains do not appear to serve that primary function: *Neuropathic pain,* where the pathology lies in the peripheral nervous system or elements of it as in diabetic neuropathy and the radiculopathy, following lesions of the vertebral column, are examples of pains usually felt in an extremity when pathology is at the level of the nerve root. Maladaptive pains may manifest abnormal activity in the *autonomic* (sympathetic) nervous system, the various syndromes most often restricted to regions of the body. *Functional pain* (clinical pain also defined here, in Chapter VII, as Idiopathic pain) is another wide pathophysiological canopy. These pains show no neurological deficits. While there may be signs of pathology these may not relate to any specific anatomical site, structure, tissue or organ. Functional pain results from a hypersensitivity of the nervous system which amplifies pain and no cause is found attributable for it. Certain kinds of headache and fibromyalgia may be considered as functional pain. Clinically, elements of one pain category often present with another. Migraine headaches are often initiated in hormonal shifts, provoking an abnormal sensory processing of cerebrovascular nerves.

The plasticity of the nociceptive system generally allows responses depending on functional demands upon it. Molecular and ionic changes occur at the cellular and the neuronal synapses of the system signalling pain but, when deviant, are likely markers of pain pathophysiology. Some may be common to synaptic transmission at other sites of the nervous system in other sensory functions or in the function of memory. Understanding the pathophysiology of pain in relation to genetic variability and drug responses has increased the potential for its greater control.

Improved experimental techniques and technological developments for localising lesions, including those of the nervous system, have provided a better understanding of the mechanisms that maintain pain. Changes in molecular biology and abnormal gene expression are known to be accompaniments that signal the onset of pain. They presently only outline possibilities and offer prospects of better pharmacological control directed at a molecular level of pathology. Pharmacology of that order aimed at individual rather than standard medication or therapy is another possibility[ii]. At present the clinician supervises an algorithmic cycle of medication for pain, a trial in the clinic but hit or miss *in application*. In the future such approaches may be replaced by more targeted therapy at molecular levels as they become better defined and lead to medication and dosages which take account of the individual. Variability is increasingly seen in the individual beyond general mechanisms that maintain pain.

It is within the developments of the neurophysiology of pain and progress in the immunohormonal background to disease that a traditional modality of treatment such as acupuncture may find the possibility to advance. Most traditional therapies epistemologically accept uniqueness, and fashion treatment to fit the individual. While individual therapies or a holistic approach sound feasible, within its epistemology there is a considerable divergence in definition to variability. The science of pain may find experimental evidence for variability at the molecular levels of causative mechanisms. Basic research is unravelling them, for instance, pain sustained in changed gene expression recognises an individual patient is more likely to respond to pain therapy if the degrees of molecular variability can be pharmacologically addressed. Whether there may be some consonance to molecular variability and observed differences to individuals, as far as it relates to treatment methods with acupuncture is an option possible for study.

Investigatory tools and techniques

The account presented here of the mechanisms that involve pain will not be exhaustive but, hopefully, will be sufficient to explain a few of their basic biological implications. The neuro-anatomical pathways for the transmission of sensory impulses up to spinal cord levels in the dorsal horn are well established and, to a lesser extent, their further connectivity to the higher centres in the brain. Less well understood is how and at which level the transmission of impulses finally translates into perception. Exhaustive data are available on neural pathways and mechanisms that modulate or inhibit the perception of pain, but theoretically there are divergent interpretations of the research. As for the fairly intractable clinical problems that collect under Complex Regional Pain Syndrome (CRPS)[iii] the tentative nature to proffered solutions suggest that many patients continue in pain. There are more bridges to cross to explain experimental mechanisms for pain in clinical pain syndromes before the answers can be found toward more specific therapies to deal with the latter.

The mechanisms for sensation are normally initiated through a *high-threshold sensory system*. Nociceptive studies on animals also provide the information towards understanding pain. There is considerable work on healthy human volunteers and increasing clinical material which substantiates the mechanisms of pain forthcoming from research on animals. Tissue damaging stimuli in selected species of inbred animal groups (inbreeding securing some genetic uniformity) or genetic manipulations on them, by the technique of 'knockouts', that delete specific receptors help to identify particular molecules involved in nociceptive responses in those animals. What we know of neuropathic pain and the likely mechanisms for its establishment are extrapolated from those studies. The influence of particular genes on pain as observed in animals may not transfer to humans. Gene knockout is not a naturally occurring process in any species. The proteins that genes encode are too valuable for the over-all survival of the organism.

In man, data on single nerve fibres relating to the transmission of sensory impulses of pain from the periphery are available using micro-electrodes. Electrical neurograms provide much of the theoretical reasoning for pain perception by neuronal excitation and inhibition. Positron emission tomography (PET) and other scanning methods—fMRI more recently in vogue, have added valuable information on the location of impulses reaching the brain, and its possible role in processing the information. Experimental evidence about the morphology and molecular level organisation for the transmission of afferent impulses from peripheral tissues to central neurons in the CNS is available, as well as that on descending inhibitory systems from the brainstem which also finally focus on the dorsal horn of the spinal cord. From experimental studies, details of synaptic neuroanatomy and molecular pathology following noxious stimuli and tissue damage are also forthcoming.

The molecular biology[iv] of peripheral nociceptor activity shows alteration of transducer function at many levels along these neural pathways, leading to changes in the distribution of existing proteins or the expression of novel ones following altered gene regulation in the central neurons. After injury and cell damage there is a release of, or alterations to, chemical transmitter substances and molecular level activity, causing trains of electrical potentials which precede nociception. These types of altered activity offer new and innovative targets for the pharmacological alleviation of pain. If the neuro-physiological mechanisms are proving to be a rich field for attempting better drug control of pain, the role of older drugs like the opioids[v], now better understood, continue to be invaluable as they are still the least likely to cause untoward effects on other systems—a hazard which accompanies the more recent medication against intractable pains and even postoperative pain.

Pain Measurement

Human pain can be assessed although it is a subjective expression of a sensory modality. Measurement of human pain, while limited to the experiential-emotional, is invaluable for its clinical investigation although there are limitations to the methods of its assessment. Numerous scales of measurement are in vogue. They have a high degree of robustness for a subject or a patient, but are restricted *to the time of assessment and the context in which it is made.* The memory of Pain is a different matter. It is well to keep in mind Kipling's caveat. A classical novelist whose authoritative observance of the nature of human response are pertinent for the scientist.

A stimulus of graded intensity is experimentally used to quantify pain thresholds by assessing the level at which the preliminary sensation becomes distinctly painful. High thresholds of stimulation, individually variable of course, are required before the sensation is perceived as pain. Threshold assessment produces comparatively more stable readings in healthy subjects than for patients with pain. Again, it needs be stressed that measurements on any scale are an account of subjective quality: variations to individual perceptions or gender cohorts[vi], ethnic groups and so on, in Clinical Study base their analyses on data presented by Pain Scales. Statistical analyses of measurements of human pain are valid, as are also the measurements from animal experiments which involve their nociceptive behaviour, but the analyses of pain scales must find further support in other measures of outcome.

An elementary outline of a a few basic concepts of the biology of pain, often referred to as nociception, the behavioural content of pain in animals, is outlined here. Pain can only be defined in terms of a human experience whereas, *nociception is a response to the excitation of nociceptors, which gives rise to particularised patterns of behaviour in the animal.* The patterns of behaviour are sufficient in higher species of animal to differentiate progressive states of discomfort, panic, pain and suffering. Restricted to human sensation, pain is a term whose intensity can be conveyed in nuances of language and thus differentiated. Excitation of nociceptors can occur without pain as when the inhibitory pathways within the system of pain transmission are subject to effective environmental activation.

Morphology of Pain Transmission Primary afferent nerves

The awareness of pain is a normal response to a high threshold stimulus. Normally the 'threshold' before perceiving pain is a measurable stimulus intensity. To the individual in the environmental context the stimulus causing pain would be, incipient to injury, frank trauma and in inflammation and repair following injury. The response may be more than one of merely eliciting pain. The sensory afferent may initiate a cycle with an efferent component, a motor reflex such as the withdrawal of a limb from fire heat. In the normal subject when the stimulus is of sufficient intensity to be *noxious* or damaging to tissue a chain of neural events is initiated in those afferent nerve endings which respond to a noxious stimulus. An intact network of the nervous system is required, from the nerve endings of peripheral nerves to their neurons in the posterior horn of the spinal cord, and the relay system of ascending neurons from spinal cord to brain stem, thalamus and up to the cerebral cortex. Innumerable subsidiary relays exist at many levels from and to the neurons of the spinal cord which are a part of this neural network serving further excitation or inhibition and modulating the sensation before culminating in the perception of pain.

Peripheral nerves are comprised of the afferent sensory and proprioceptive, as well as efferent motor (somatic) and post ganglionic nerves of the autonomic nervous system. Thus the mixed population of nerves characterise various functions in their morphological differentiation, for example, nerves myelinated or not, or differing in their axon diameters. The axons of primary *afferent* nerves are grouped depending on axon diameters. The action potential is the resultant electrical activity generated by the constituent axons of the nerve as a whole when the stimulus is of an intensity sufficient to initiate it. Conduction velocities relate to axon diameter. The major groups are Aα, Aδ, and C fibres having respective axon diameters of 6-22 μm, 2-5 μm and 0.3-3 μm (α δ C). Aα and Aδ are myelinated while C fibres are not. Sympathetic post ganglionic fibres serving autonomic function also fall within the diameter range of the latter and are non-myelinated. Tissues have specific receptors that respond to noxious stimuli and these are nociceptors.

In the skin

Only the nociceptor signals an increase in frequency of discharges when the stimulus reaches noxious levels. Although some Aδ afferents signal warmth at non-noxious thresholds they may respond as a nociceptor afferent when that heat is sufficient to cause tissue damage. Afferents that respond selectively to warmth, touch or cold do not signal an increased impulse frequency if the stimuli attain a degree sufficient to be damaging to tissue. Nociceptive primary afferents are mostly to be found amongst those of Aδ, and C ranges. Most C fibres have their cell bodies in the dorsal root ganglia, but about 20% are post ganglionic fibres with their cell bodies in the paraspinal ganglia of the sympathetic chain. When stimulated in alert human beings and the intensity of the stimulus moves from the innocuous to the noxious range, Aδ, and C afferents respond with an increase in electrical discharge to signal pain while the Aα afferents continue their steady discharge *without any increase* in firing rate[vii]. Even if the intensity of the heat is sufficient to cause damage Aα afferents continue to signal sensations other than pain, and so the majority of Aα afferents do not function as nociceptors. Only C afferents are nociceptors plus a proportion of the myelinated Aδ which are responsive to high thresholds of *mechanical* stimulation, such as shearing forces. Others are unresponsive to mechanical stimuli. Myelinated Aα afferents are mechanoreceptors, sensitive to mechanical stimuli but, as mentioned above, do not signal a change even if those stimuli have attained intensities that are noxious. On the other hand some Aδ fibres can respond to mechanical stimuli at low thresholds, but when it is of sufficient intensity as to be tissue-damaging they fire maximally—which defines their function as nociceptor afferents. Similarly when the stimulus is of an intensity to produce erythema of the skin some Aδ fibres increase electrical discharge rates, signalling pain. Aδ nociceptors that also signal heat are mechanothermal nociceptors while some Aδ are High-Threshold Mechano-receptors (HTM). Myelinated nociceptors have receptive fields of about 5mm^2 in human hairy skin[viii].

Further qualities of the fibres that mediate pain may be described. Aδ pain is distinct, sharp, well localised: it is comparatively immediate, rapidity related to the speed of impulse transmission in these larger diameter fibres. Slow pain mediated by the thinner C fibres is diffuse, unpleasant, sometimes unbearable, and is the type of pain that, when persistent, could bring a patient to the clinic. C fibres constitute the majority of peripheral nerve afferents. Their receptive field is smaller than of myelinated nerves. In the skin the modalities of sensation to which a major proportion of them respond are noxious thermal, mechanical and chemical stimuli. This class of C-fibre is the C-polymodal nociceptor (C-PMN). Systematic studies, though, show responses mainly to mechanical and thermal stimuli.

The axons of nociceptors primary afferent nerves are normally found amongst unmyelinated, C fibres or myelinated, small diameter Aδ fibres. However, in some species, evidence has been presented of Aβ fibres (diameter thickness between that of Aα and Aδ, 5-12 μm) which normally only respond to innocuous stimuli, respond to touch but have a role in nociception with inflammation or tissue damage[ix].

While some of the evidence on nociceptor activity is from studies on primate skin, corroborative evidence is forthcoming in humans. The insertion of microelectrodes into a fibre of superficial nerves in awake human subjects goes some way to demonstrate and delineate the afferent function of a peripheral nerve. Data of afferent nociceptor activity in other primates confirms evidence derived from single fibre microelectrode stimulation in the human, with a proviso that it may be a response elicited from the stimulation of more than a single fibre. No naturally occurring stimulus on a responsive primate system, whether mechanical, thermal or chemical can be restricted to single fibre activity.

CENTRAL CELLS AND PATHWAYS CONTRIBUTING TO PAIN TRANSMISSION

The Spinal Cord. The cytoarchitecture of the dorsal horn. Functional attributes in development

The gray matter of the spinal cord in section is a dumb-bell shaped configuration, with its handle around the central neural tube. Roof and floor plates of the developing spinal cord are made up of non-nervous, ependymal and glial tissue which do not give rise to neuroblasts. A narrow marginal zone becomes a pathway for commissural fibres. It is the alar and basal lamina that, by differentiation, gives rise in the posterior horns to neuroblasts of receptor cells (afferent) and those of the motor cells in the anterior horns, respectively. The cells differentiating in the alar lamina are afferent second neurons; the first afferents have their cell bodies in posterior root ganglion, derived from the neural crest. Hence, native to the dorsal horn are the intrinsic dorsal horn neurons, and later constituents in development, the extensive branching central terminals of primary afferents and other inputs and outputs to the CNS.

Small diameter afferents and lamina I neurons are developmentally associated and to be differentiated at that stage from the large diameter afferents that project deep into the dorsal horn (Altman & Bayer 1984). The lamina I afferents from small dorsal root ganglion cells co-ordinate their arrival in the spinal cord with the inception of native lamina I neurons. Those cells developmentally arising from autonomic interneurons of the lateral horns, associate with the afferents as they arrive during the developmental process of rotation of the dorsal horn. On this view there appears to be support for the small diameter afferents and lamina I neurons constituting a physiological homeostatic sensory system separate in function from the deeper large diameter afferents essentially serving exteroceptive function—a perception of the body in positional relationship to the exterior. Pain sensations in this model traverse specific pathways, including the spinothalamic tract, to integrative pathways at higher centres which process perception, while discriminative touch and positional senses in the model are a function of the deeper layers of the dorsal horn. Such specificity, `labelled lines´ is a point of contention. Wall and others (1973) state that neurons of lamina V are involved in the persistent and referred pain experienced by patients through stimuli that are normally non-painful (allodynia). Cells in Lamina I and, predominantly, Lamina V can in some circumstances be enabled to respond to low as well as high threshold stimuli. These are the wide dynamic range (WDR) neurons which also have a larger receptive field than nociceptive-specific (NS) cells.

Views on functional significance of the Laminar organisation of spinal gray

Nathan's[x] stated views on laminar construction and connectivity were arguments which challenged Melzack and Wall's Gate Control Theory, leading to the 'Restatement', a comprehensive game changer to former theories about Pain. In the context of acupuncture and allied techniques the mechanisms of pain inhibition can be understood in aspects of The Gate Control Theory.

Potent inhibitory effects for clinical pain inhibition follow from neural sequences to peripheral stimuli at dorsal horn levels and involve the higher centres as well. The neural components of inhibition, its descending circuitry and synapses on the neurons of the spinal cord, are outlined in the chapter on acupuncture mechanisms. However, no convincing neurophysiology explains the long-lasting pain mitigation, sometimes clinically evident in the use of stimulation techniques for selected pain pathology[xi].

The theory as stated by Wall in 1978[xii] is important for understanding the analgesia that follows from peripheral sensory stimulation techniques (PSS). It is also necessary to follow a few of the controversies which continue around the theory, and a background appreciation of the impetus that research into pain neurophysiology has achieved since its enunciation. PSS may have other physiological attributes, and some have been explored and stated. Acupuncture effects and the mechanism of longer pain relief require further explanation. Controlled peripheral sensory stimuli as, for instance, when repetitive low frequency electrical stimulation of skeletal muscle activates the release of endogenous opioids by specific ergoreceptors of muscle tissue, as suggested by Sven Andersson et al, may be pursued. Presently the evidence demonstrated by Le Bars et al shows that diffuse noxious inhibitory control (DNIC), a painful peripheral stimulation at a separate site, can reduce nociception. This was further correlated to persistent and lasting diminution of signal size at the dorsal horn neurons serving the site of reduced nociception, well after stimulation initiating DNIC had ceased.

The organisation of the dorsal horn and sensory processing

The dorsal horn and its homologue in the medulla, the spinal nucleus of the trigeminal serve as the preliminary station for the processing of neural inputs. Noxious stimuli at the primary sensory neurons need initially to be converted by transduction into electrical activity before it can be further transmitted. While much is known about the intricate structure of the dorsal horn, an important junction of sensory and nociceptive activity, making sense of it in terms of the connective units and the processing of that activity is an issue of complexity not fully resolved.

Explanatory models of pain have in common certain basic features of sensory neural structure. They commence in a primary afferent nerve, but at the periphery the receptors respond to nociceptive stimuli. The primary afferent is a peripheral axon with its cell body situated in the dorsal root ganglion and its peripheral terminals in skin or other tissues. Peripheral afferent terminals that are sensitive to nociceptive stimuli are nociceptors. The cell body in the dorsal root ganglion receives no synaptic connections. Hence, apart from transmission, the neuron may not play a part in further sensory processing of nociceptive signals. From the dorsal root ganglion the majority of dorsal root axons project through the dorsal root of the spinal cord. The dorsal root comprises about two thirds of unmyelinated axons, while the remaining third are myelinated. The axons also relay ascending and descending branches which extend to one or two segments beyond the entry of the parent axon. The smaller diameter axons tend to segregate to a ventrolateral position in the dorsal root as it approaches the spinal cord, and the larger are positioned medially. The larger medial fibres entering the dorsal columns of the spinal cord bifurcate into ascending and descending columns and its collaterals also penetrate the dorsal horn. The smaller diameter axons by and large constitute Lissauer's tract, a majority of nociceptor elements entering the dorsolateral edge of the dorsal horn. From here their terminals enter the gray matter of the spinal cord.

In outline, Rexed's architectonics of the spinal cord of the cat described ten histologically distinguishable laminae in its gray matter, a scheme generally accepted. There are, of course, differences within mammalian species, though this is the fundamental pattern of the neuronal organisation of spinal cord gray matter. The laminar pattern of the spinal gray proceeding dorsal to ventral comes about from the differentiation of neural tissue, the nature of the intrinsic or migrating neurons and the respective densities of their axons and synapses within enveloping glial tissue. Lamina I; mention has already been made of its content of cells and further functional detail is given below. Lamina II, also known as the substantia gelatinosa has tightly packed small neurons. Lamina III is considered part of the former lamina by some workers (Nathan). The neurons here are less densely packed than in Lamina II. Lamina IV contains large neurons and their dendrites spread diffusely into other layers of the dorsal horn. It is the thickest layer of the dorsal horn. Lamina V has smaller cells, and in the cat is situated medially within the dorsal horn from cervical through to lumbar segments of the spinal cord. Lamina X is in the vicinity of the central neural canal while Laminae VI to IX are variably distributed in the more ventral parts of the dorsal horn. When mentioning the functional significance of the contents of each of these laminae, even if there is no uniformity of acceptance in the details, a clearer picture of their organisation may emerge.

Functional Morphology

Lamina I receives myelinated Aδ fibres as well as non-myelinated C fibres—the latter via synapses of interneurons from Lamina II. Both types of afferents excite high threshold cutaneous nociceptor neurons. There are some cells which respond to low threshold mechanical as well as high threshold noxious stimuli, and thus are enabled by a 'wide dynamic range' (WDR) of stimulus intensities. Cells supplied by non-myelinated afferents also respond to high temperatures applied to skin and to irritant chemicals, these polymodal nociceptors responding to a variety of noxious stimuli. The latter, slow conducting fibres once activated show prolonged activity, as for instance, heat at 50^0 C applied to skin continues to cause pain well after the stimulus is removed and the skin has cooled. An equivalent experience, from an environmental stimulus, is sunburn. Polymodal nociceptors are also responsive to chemical substances such as bradykinin, serotonin and nor-adrenaline. Nociceptor-specific cells may be restricted in numbers and are to be found within a population of cells which are generally subject to modulation by the convergent projections of other afferents of descending systems, as well as from neurons from other segments of the cord. The synaptic projections onto a single nociceptor-specific neuron will have the effect of enlarging considerably its cutaneous receptive field. In fact, certain Lamina I cells have inputs from low threshold mechanoreceptors, and with increasing intensity of stimulus they respond as nociceptors. They have the capability to respond to stimuli of varying intensities, from non-noxious to noxious, and are therefore wide dynamic range neurons. The polymodal nociceptor neurons of Lamina I, the spinothalamic fibres, send their axons to the thalamus.

Lamina II comprises the substantia gelatinosa. Some consider Lamina III to be an inclusive part. The axons of its fine intrinsic neurons run into Lissauer's tract in the lateral column. At any particular spinal cord segment many of the neurons of Lamina II synaptically connect to further segments, but by no more than a couple onward from the location of its cell body. Its cells are excited by noxious stimuli. Synaptic connections with other Lamina II neurons are the rule but, as mentioned before, a certain class of Lamina II neuron have axon synapses to neurons of Lamina I and relay nociceptive inputs. These stalk or 'T' cells are excitatory relay points for nociceptive inputs. The neural network of Lamina II is also made up of the innumerable dendrites from cells in Laminae I, III, IV and V and comprises of predominantly inhibitory neurons.

The neurons of Lamina IV receive descending contributions from the brain. Those of Lamina III and IV respond to innocuous stimuli, but their projections to wide dynamic range neurons increase the range of responses. Fields and Nathan favour the view that the cells of Lamina V respond maximally, but not necessarily only, to noxious stimuli. They are wide dynamic range neurons and have a great degree of convergence, their receptive fields being generally larger than Lamina I neurons. The density of neurons in this layer is less than of Lamina I or II, but interconnections between these laminae and Lamina IV provide a convergence of inputs and further projections to brainstem and thalamus.

Neurons of Lamina VI in the main respond to exteroceptive stimuli and are seen in the spinal cord at their cervical and lumbar enlargements. These neurons provide for the sensations that relate the body position to the environment, from muscle, joint and tendon. Lamina VII and VIII have somewhat complex systems of nociceptor neurons providing ill-defined receptors for muscle and viscera. These cells too project to the thalamus and reticular formation of the brain stem, as do the nociceptive neurons of Lamina X.

The above description of the anatomical organisation of gray matter is generally accepted, although the physiological responses to nocuous and innocuous stimuli are subject to debate in their on-going detail. Consideration of the convergence of primary sensory afferents onto dorsal horn cells and recording their response is unlikely to entirely reflect or confirm their part in human sensory function. *In the main, dorsal horn cells demonstrate plasticity of responses to stimuli depending on their intensity, excepting a few of them.* But, then, nor does plasticity of dorsal horn response define an equivalence in a change to sensation[xiii]

Ascending spinal cord pathways for pain

In humans, the major pathway is the column of the white matter of the spinal cord within its anterolateral quadrant. This has been confirmed in studies dating back to Brown-Sequard in his 1860 Lectures. Pain can be well localised, even if all other spinal cord fibres are interrupted, provided one anterolateral quadrant is intact: this is sufficient for the perception of pain. However, the experimental resections, cordotomies, involving this area do not result in permanent analgesia. Pain recurrence after a time, though not invariable, is often the case, and repetition on a second occasion may still not produce analgesia. This suggests that there are other pathways by which nociceptive information can be transmitted to the higher centres. They may not ordinarily provide that function, and their plasticity for processing nociceptive information may well take time to be established[xiv]

From primate and clinical studies it is seen that the predominant pathway involving normal nociception follows the projections from dorsal horn neurons to the brain via the opposite spinothalamic tract (STT) situated in the anterolateral quadrant of the spinal cord. Its neuronal connectivity to the cells in the grey matter, especially laminae I and V, has been referred to above. Most STT fibres cross over to reach the contralateral nuclei in the reticular formation of the medulla and from there, having reached the medial thalamic nuclei, project into specific areas of the cortex. Another component of the STT reaches the lateral thalamic nuclei and then proceeds to further separate cortical projections. An ipsilateral component is directed to the intralaminar sector of the thalamus. More specifically the projections of the medial division are to the central lateral nucleus of the thalamus and of the lateral division to the lateral part of the ventrobasal (VB) nucleus, as well as the posterior (PO) nuclear group. The significance of thalamic connectivity and cortical projections are taken up elsewhere.

The excitatory responses of STT cells to nociceptive stimuli are demonstrated in studies using noxious mechanical and thermal stimulation of skin, noxious chemical stimulation of muscle or noxious mechanical, thermal or chemical stimulation of viscera, but excitation of these cells to a lesser degree is noted even with innocuous stimuli. There is, therefore, a convergent input onto the same cells from both peripheral nociceptors and mechanoreceptors. This feature of STT cells assumes significance in descending inhibitory responses. While cells whose receptive fields on body surface or face generally show an excitatory response when stimulated, they could also be inhibited in certain circumstances. An inhibitory reaction has been noted in response to noxious stimuli. Whether or not this is due an increased signal-to-noise ratio of ascending information and not direct suppression of nociceptive transmission, the response assumes significance for therapeutic measures with peripheral sensory stimulation. Most acupuncture techniques in vogue today tend toward noxious intensities and the inhibitory pathways of pain and its control have been discussed.

Another ascending pathway associated with pain is the spinoreticular tract (SRT). Its origins from deeper laminae V, VI, VII and VIII project to both sides of brainstem in the main to the reticular formation. From here there are projections to the intralaminar part of the thalamus. Ipsilateral projections of this tract are also seen. The reticular formation receives axons from STT and thus, finally, it is a spinoreticulo thalamic pathway by its overlap to the medial spinothalamic projection

From cells in laminae I and V there are also projections in the spinomesencephalic tract to the reticular formation, the lateral periaqueductal gray of the mesencephalon. So far the evidence for the involvement of this tract in nociception is meagre. It is a working assumption, however, that recurrence of pain after anterior cordotomies can involve these tracts as well as the spinocervical and the post synaptic dorsal column pathways ascending in the dorsal funiculus of the spinal cord. While it is assumed that the ipsilateral tracts provide a pathway for conveying nociceptive information in the above circumstance, it may not exhaust the possibilities for such transmission as other multisynaptic interneuronal chains may well be available. The pathways described, in addition to conveying nociceptive information to the brain, are also involved in the modulation of pain through their control over descending systems. This essential feature of the pain network naturally determines its immediate perception, but it must function for the perception over a period of time as well.

A phylogenetic reading of these tracts shows that the spinoreticular tract is a feature of all vertebrates, including fish. In lower species it is the major pathway for nociceptive transmission. When the spinothalamic tract makes its appearance amongst lower vertebrates it initially has much in common with its precursor, the spinoreticular tract. As the paleospinothalamic pathway on the vertebrate scale its cephalic projection is to the *medial* thalamus. Increased encephalisation in higher vertebrates is a feature of primates, and the spinothalamic tract reflects additions to nociceptive function by the lateralisation of its neurons in the ventrobasal nucleus of the thalamus. Within the context of extending nociceptive connectivity to the higher centres it is referred to as the neospinothalamic tract. and an enhancement of primate capacity for affective expression and motivational behaviour (Melzack and Casey, ref. In Fields Chapt 3).

The original paleospinothalamic tract conveying sensory nociceptive information thus has in the primate another dimension to pain perception. The evaluative and motivational-affective aspect of pain is morphologically a reflection of increased encephalisation in humans. But caution is due, as that attribute can only be studied in man through his improved cognitive ability and verbalisation. Cognitive evaluation of the sensory aspect of pain being a reflection of pain threshold is more stable than the affective-motivational aspects which are a factor of tolerance, and variable even for an individual in context dependence. Clinical research requires the totality of a pain experience, but measurement is semantic dependent. Standard questionnaires prepared for one language has limitations in another, another aspect of cultures on the perception of pain.

Affect and sensory discrimination are parcelled together in human pain experience. They are an expression in words and even corroborated for similarity do not necessarily convey the same connotation in translation. Transposition of word-dependent tools require caution in interpretation and the more so if they are used to evaluate as a scaled measure. To a lesser extent, even sensory discrimination may not convey the meaning in literal translation to another language. The pattern to the word arrangement of 'The McGill Pain questionnaire' was developed from expressions used by patients in pain: standard words nuanced affect and were given scaled values as grouped words for analysis in clinical research. The design may not convey its intended meaning for an entire population with a common language. The groups derived from a markedly different ethnic identity may regard pain and and the expression of affect in some cultural variety. Any assessor listening to a patient in pain must be struck by standard expressions related to their culture but that variety in the languages of civilisational spaces possibly in itself making for a worthwhile study of semantic subjectivity and the pain experience. Formulae of verbally analysable pain questionnaires constructed in the English speaking world must consider the different population cohorts which answer them. Standardisations of groups of words offered to patients for clinical measurement of their pain experience do not necessarily translate or offer the given ratings in translation.

The recent studies of cortical connectivity from the thalamus assume importance with the use of scanning techniques such as Positron Emission Tomography (PET) and functional Magnetic Resonance Imaging (fMRI). It has become possible to visualise areas of the human cortex involved in some painful clinical conditions. Experimental methodology of the many studies offers reasonably consistent evidence of nociceptive cortical connectivity, but the functional processing of nociception may not be attributed exclusively to a cortical area. The different methodological approaches in the assessment of cortical function may account for discrepancies or else, within small patient populations, there is the greater likelihood of heterogeneity in the processing of nociceptive activity at the highest levels of neural function. To detect variability greater methodological sophistication in the future may provide some conclusive answers.

Sites for further nociceptive projections from the dorsal horn. Thalamus and Cortex

Following the nociceptive process from the dorsal horn, the second order projections are predominantly in the opposite ascending pathway of the STT of the spinal cord to the brain stem. Cells of the of lateral and medial thalamus nuclei carry brainstem projections to the limbic system and to the cortex in further projections[xv]. Essentially projections from the thalamic nuclei to the cortex maintain the nociceptive neuronal pattern of a lateral and medial system. Anatomically the neurons of nociception in their rostral passage are not discrete as neurons with other properties intermingle with those of nociception.

The lateral thalamic nuclei, ventral posterior inferior (VPI) ventral posterior medial (VPM) and ventral posterior lateral (VPL) receive input from lamina I as well as from lamina V nociceptive neurons. The nociceptive process from the latter is largely served by WDR neurons. They are not exclusive to the lateral thalamic nuclei as these laminae also contribute to medial thalamic nuclei, as in the posterior part of the ventromedial nucleus. However, division into lateral and medial systems of cortical connectivity suggest respective functional distinctions of pain. For the lateral system cortical representation is in the primary and secondary somatosensory cortex (S, I and S, II). Within its anatomical limits functions of sensory discrimination, specifically stimulus localisation and sensory integrative function may be served.

The medial system is in the anterior cingulate cortex. The insula, while receiving a major input from the lateral system, itself projects into the limbic system and serves as an intermediate relay. The proportionate contribution of nociceptive inputs is not clear from the spinothalamic tract to this latter distribution. Additional to the cortical projections mentioned, there may also be inputs into the prefrontal cortex with further inter-cortical connectivity. The primary and secondary sensory cortex and the anterior cingulate have shown single cell responses to nociceptive specific neurons as well as to WDR neurons with their convergent afferent inputs from nociceptive and other sensory modalities. Functionally the system involves widespread sensory integration mediated in the limbic connectivity from the insula, while attention and affect are directed in anterior cingulate connectivity. The prefrontal cortex involves aspects of pain, its affect, emotional concomitant and memory (ibid. Treede RD et al:).

Peripheral and Central Nociceptor processing signalling or inhibiting Pain.

The signalling process of transduction commences the conversion of the stimulus into electrochemical energy, when a stimulus, coded for a nociceptor, converts to an electro-chemical impulse. The conversion is achieved by the expression of ion channel receptors by nociceptors and normally occurs at high threshold levels of activity. Ion channel receptors are generally non-selective Na or Ca channels, but they remain gated until the stimuli are appropriate. Noxious heat, chemicals or mechanical forces capable of tissue damage open up the channels for the flow of Na or Ca ions to the nociceptor terminal. It sets up an inward current which depolarises the nociceptor membrane. If the depolarising current is sufficient to cause greater action potential in the nociceptor, then further voltage gated channels will open. The extent of activity is reflected in the intensity and duration of the noxious stimulus. Unimodal nociceptors respond to one form of stimulus only, like noxious heat. Excitatory potentials are mediated at post-synaptic membranes of central neurones by an amino acid glutamate at the ligand gated membrane receptors. Much of the activity is expended at the spinal cord neurones though evoked action potential may relay into the thalamus and cortex.

The action of opioids, cannabinoids γ-aminobutyric acid (GABA) and the anticonvulsant gabapentin is situated at the receptors of the presynaptic axonal central terminals of the nociceptor where transmitter release is reduced by their ligand action. Post-synaptic inhibition is through a hyperpolarisng action potential at dorsal horn neuronal sites. The reduction of transmitter release at presysnaptic sites on voltage-gated calcium channels, and at the postsynaptic sites through the opening of potassium or chloride channels is by an inhibitory hyperpolarising potential. Effective sites of inhibition, while the same for opioids and their ligands, are not restricted to the nervous system. Medication aimed at ligands of the μ opioid receptors will obtain an inhibitory effect on pain, but the action on sites outside of the neurons and receptors of the pain system may result in side effects. Gabapentin, given for pain, may demonstrate unsuitability in patients because of this.

Sensory processing of pain involves facilitation and inhibitory mechanisms controlled by many spinal cord circuits. A perceived threat to an animal, or for the human aware of an environmental threat, may provide pain reduction in the inhibitory processing mechanism. For example, pain inhibition may be evoked should that response aid survival. In a given environmental situation suppressing pain, even in the face of severe injury, could ensure survival and hence would be the appropriate response. The chapter on Placebo discusses more fully responses to battle injuries and the process of the placebo; vital evolutionary extensions of the sensorial facility for pain inhibition in the human as increased complexities are perceived regarding the environment.

Acupuncture is a stimulus which evokes an inhibitory response, but the input has been fashioned for therapeutic quality beyond the mere stimulus input of the needle. The agent, the acupuncturist, and his methods of particularised needle practice make the basic needle usage a stimulus with more empirical complexities as used for patient pain. The 'ritual' or the context equated with the placebo ignores empirical content. However immediate analgesia is viewed, longer term effects of this therapy, when they occur, cannot be explained in the molecular mechanisms just discussed.

The sensory-discriminative component of Pain

Functional criteria of nociception are provided from physiological studies. The identified properties for primary afferent neurons are: a high threshold for response, intensity coding in the noxious range, its polymodality and, following injury, primary hyperalgesia signifying sensitisation. Second order nociceptive neurons in the cord have properties like receptive field changes following secondary hyperalgesia. Single cell recordings from primary and secondary somato-sensory cortex and the anterior cingulate cortex have shown responses to noxious stimuli when applied to nociceptive specific neurons as well as wide dynamic range neurons (WDR), having convergent inputs from both nociceptive and other afferents.

The clinical answer to the spatial query 'where does it hurt?', as a stimulus localisation or in an experimental context, features a somatotopic organisation at the dorsal horn levels for nociceptive inputs as well as at the lateral thalamus and the S,1 area of the primary somatosensory cortex. Nociceptive specific afferents with receptive fields of limited size, which could include tactile sensation, provide peripheral neuronal connectivity to the different levels mentioned. Localisation is the most precise for skin, less so with deeper tissues of joints and muscles, and well known to be unreliable with viscera.

Stimulus localisation and intensity discrimination are two properties of the sensory-discriminative component of pain which may relate to separate nociceptive pathways. There is evidence from a patient with a lesion that involved the lateral thalamic system, where spatial localisation but not pain intensity discrimination was considerably affected[xvi]. WDR neurons with large receptive fields may better encode stimulus intensities than nociceptive specific neurons.

The affective-motivational component of pain

The paramedian reticular formation in the brainstem is classically associated with escape behaviour from noxious sensory stimuli (Melzack and Casey 1968); thence, to the medial thalamic nuclei, the pathways have a further diffuse projection into the limbic system of the cortex. The anterior cingulate cortex of that system has been largely implicated for the affective-motivational component of pain (Treede et al). Recent studies on humans demonstrate the anterior cingulate cortex to be widely recruited, along with the prefrontal cortex, in the affective-motivational component to pain perception. It possibly forms the evolved counterpart to more basic escape behaviour. Escape behaviour has been well established in the brainstem reticular formation of, for example, the nucleus gigantocellularis and its interlaminar thalamic connectivity. The evidence suggests that cortical sites are implicated with emotive qualities, repulse or other motivational motor programmes, which can be factored in should that be the required survival response.

Evidence of cortical activation from chronic clinical conditions has been forthcoming, though only in a few studies. Interestingly, in the burning mouth syndrome the activation of some sites described above is generally less, as compared to controls, when noxious heat is applied to one side of the face. Areas of the anterior cingulate cortex show hyperactivity in at least two studies with chronic facial pain. It is difficult to derive any definite conclusion from these findings, but one suggestion is that habitual pain may reduce the responses of sites in the brain normally involved in pain inhibition, thus rendering the condition, burning mouth disorder, chronic and more intractable.

Setting out components of the central nervous system as pathways for the transmission of nociceptive inputs from the periphery to the spinal cord has been achieved with fair certainty, though in certain pathological states it is also known that these may be carried by alternative pathways. From the spinal cord to the brainstem we see a number of pathways transmitting nociceptive impulses. From the brainstem there are pathways to nuclei of the thalamus, on to the anterior cingulate and insula (the limbic system), and the cortex. These extensions and later nociceptive projections provide greater certainty about cortical representation in pain perception. It is now known that these centres signal pain and modulate it through their descending pathways to the nociceptive neurones of the spinal cord, although there is uncertainty as to functional specificity. It was established in primate studies that the somatosensory cortex receives projections from nociceptive pathways. Positron emission tomography (PET) and improved techniques have achieved further localisation in recent controlled clinical studies, and advanced the importance of cortex function in the totality of pain. Previous to these studies the projections to the thalamus were considered finally sufficient to mediate pain perception and it was doubted that cortical centres were involved.

Peripheral Nociceptor and central pathological processing.

Cell disruption results in release of K^+ ions and a lowered pH. Cellular voltage-gated depolarisation and a release of a variety of chemicals capable of further nociceptor activation follow injury or inflammation. Some of these chemicals are called *algogens* as they signal pain. These endogenous chemicals activate the nociceptor, either resulting in immediate pain or else in nociceptor sensitisation which increases their excitability and lowers pain thresholds. The release of adenosine triphosphatase, for example, activates a purinoreceptor to signal pain. The vanilloid receptor-I (VRI) is a transducer of C-fibre nociceptors. Capsaicin may be an activator of the VRI receptor or activation may be heat induced, suggesting that the receptor is a physiological transducer of noxious heat[xvii]. Other inflammatory substances like bradykinin, prostaglandins, leukotrines, serotonin, histamine, N growth factor octapeptide (NGF-OP) and substance P are released dependent on the intensities of stimuli which slowly build up, enabling trains of action potentials followed by cellular sensitisation.

Sensitisation is the increased sensitivity of a nociceptor or its synaptic neurones following repetitive application of the noxious stimulus. The heightened receptor response to repetitive heat stimuli is a notable feature of high threshold mechano-receptors (HTM),. Clinically, sensitisation is signified in hyperalgesia, the exaggerated response to a persistent noxious stimulus and a common experience following inflammation or tissue injury. The feature need not be restricted to the area involving the inflammatory process or injury as hyperalgesia may be perceptible in surrounding cutaneous tissue fields. Sensitisation can show in three variations from the normal: as a decreased threshold to the stimulus-response function of the nociceptor, as an on-going spontaneous activity, or an increased response to supra-threshold stimuli. The two former changes in nociceptor activity effectively result in a distinctly uncomfortable if not painful sensation when as, for example, stroking the skin with cotton wool produces an altered manifestation of sensitisation, clinically termed *allodynia*. It is the unpleasant response to a stimulus normally not uncomfortable or painful. Allodynia is usual in post-herpes pain where even ordinarily worn clothing causes friction discomfort or pain. Hyperalgesia to punctate stimuli is another form of hypersensitivity due to injury or inflammation, where small diameter afferents may be involved.

Trains of action potentials can be initiated in nociceptors by sustaining intense stimulus activity. They release neuropeptides, substance P, N growth factor and glutamate. At rest potential N-methyl-D-aspartic acid (NMDA) receptor channel activity is blocked by the magnesium ion. It is activated by glutamate which releases the block by depolarisation. This is another sensitisation feature and an activity-dependent increase to neuronal output at dorsal horn levels by closely timed repetitive inputs. The plasticity to neuron function is determined by their levels of activity, and here a form of sensitisation develops known as *wind-up,* which is the amplification of pain experienced to the repeated application of noxious heat.

Innumerable sensitising agents, some already noted, are inducted at the peripheral and central sites of neuronal activity. They are the result of natural stimuli like tissue injury and/or inflammation. Damage to cells releases neuropeptides like substance P which contributes to sustained activity at nociceptor receptor sites and, following their sensitisation, results in hyperalgesia. It also produces vasodilatation and oedema. Specific prostaglandins result from inflammation: prostaglandin E_2 is derived from the expression of cyclooxygenase-2 (COX-2) and its action is on arachidonic acid, in turn derived from the action of an enzyme in inflamed tissue on membrane phospholipids. Arachidonic acid derivatives lead to a reduction in the threshold of peripheral nociceptors, and accounts for the hypersensitivity to normally non-noxious stimuli. The exquisite tenderness to touch after sunburn is a case in point.

Electrical activity resulting from the transduction of stimuli at the peripheral nociceptor is conducted via the dorsal root ganglia to the neurons of the spinal cord and brain stem. If stimulus intensity is sufficient to relay action potentials to the post synaptic dorsal horn neurons of the spinal cord, to synapses at thalamic and suprathalamic levels of the brain and onwards to the cortex, transcriptional changes will occur along synapses of this neural network. The resultant changes, some facilitatory and some inhibitory, are mediated either along monosynaptic pathways or at multisynaptic interneurons. The functional properties and excitability of neurons that feature in these pathways are not fixed, their sensitivities and responses change depending on the nature of the stimulus and resultant expression of proteins at the periphery, and to the extent of the peripheral sensitisation of nociceptors. Nerve growth factor and substance P, produced at site of inflammation and transported to dorsal horn neurones, increase sensitisation and amplify the excitation of these nociceptor central terminals. Exogenous stimuli of sufficient intensity, as with tissues incised in surgery, inflammation or ectopically generated activity of injured nerves will all result in persisting peripheral nociceptor activity leading to on-going pain. Such stimuli sustain transcriptional conversions to existing proteins and alter the character of the normal molecular machinery of the cell. A hypersensitive state to subsequent stimuli, the result of sensitisation, thus follows inflammation or injury and sustains the activity of nociceptors leading to intense central inputs.

Glutamate (excitatory amino acid) released at post synaptic sites of dorsal horn neurones mediates the excitation of these neurones, although only a fraction of them relays to the thalamus and cortex. At the dorsal horn much of the action potential spends itself in local processing or modulation as also toward controls for its transfer. Presynaptic receptors on the central terminals of nociceptors may play a part in post synaptic inhibition via specific voltage gated channels by reducing the release of neuro transmitter substances. The sites for the ligand based action of cannabinoids, γ-aminobutyric acid (GABA) receptor ligands, and the anticonvulsant gabapentin for opioids, have been mentioned. Dorsal horn processing, as we see, is a context-dependent dynamic function, and extend descending controls from suprapinal and cortical levels to the chains of facilitatory or inhibitory return relays to dorsal horn neurones.

Changed proteins show altered function and distribution, and influence gene regulation at central neurons. These may be limited to the parts of the nervous system that receive the inputs of injury. A localised up-regulation of an endogenous opioid peptide, dynorphin, is one example. Other genes may be widely activated, even after a local peripheral tissue injury. The mechanism for the expression of COX-2 is the result of a circulating humoral factor released by inflammatory cells and its action on cerebral vascular endothelium to produce interleukin-1β. On entering the cerebrospinal fluid interleukin-1β acts on extensive pre and post synaptic sites expressing its receptor interleukin-1, COX-2 expression and consequent cascades of prostaglandin E_2 result in generalised neuronal excitability. There is a diffuse central sensitisation seen in later phases of inflammation which causes widespread aches and pains as well as other systemic disturbances of impaired appetite and disturbed sleep cycles. Such pain patterns characterise certain chronic inflammatory diseases as well as postoperative pain syndromes.

The possibility of targeting newer drugs for the management of pain is directed at those mechanisms maintaining pain in the evidence of on-going studies, especially those responsible for its chronicity. Targeting specific mechanisms also raises a host of related issues. Considering an end product like COX-2, for instance, may not deal with the intermediate factors which allowed widespread sensitisation. The fashioning of therapeutic agents requires a closer consideration of the processes involved rather than the final target. Therapy directed at widespread neural pain mechanisms is even more difficult to secure because of the systemic side effects.

Therapeutics, presently directed wholly towards developing and improving drugs for targeting pain, could perhaps be usefully combined with techniques of sensory stimulation, including acupuncture. Sufficient work has not been done toward combining drug therapy with such practices, and is unlikely to be of interest to a pharmaceutical industry. Techniques like acupuncture suffer from a) the unevenness in patient response seen in clinical trials and interpreted as a lack of neurophysiological evidence for its clinical application, b) Unwarranted assumptions follow from studies which cannot not produce incontrovertible evidence for the use of techniques or therapies in methods designed for therapeutic products that have evolved far later; in general a trial on patients with the prefix of 'placebo controlled' for an acupuncture study is an oxymoron.

Peripheral nerve injury

Axonal injury to peripheral nerves may alter the distribution of K and Na ion channels and result in increased membrane excitability leading to ectopic impulses arising in the nerve axon without peripheral inputs. It explains the spontaneous pains following even minimal nerve injury when normal inhibitory mechanisms are disrupted. Peripheral nerve injury increases the expression of $\alpha_2\delta$ voltage-gated calcium-channel receptors and reduces μ opiate receptors at the neuronal cell membrane, thereby diminishing responses to morphine following nerve injury[xviii].

The down-regulation of μ opiate receptors may partly explain the diminished effectiveness of acupuncture and possibly of transcutaneous electrical stimulation (TENS) at low frequencies in neuropathic pains. There is evidence that the analgesia following these modes of peripheral stimulation is partly mediated by the release of endogenous opioid peptides. With low frequency TENS and acupuncture, the analgesia obtained has been reversed by naloxone. This has been demonstrated in human subjects in a few studies, and further corroborated in animal studies[xix]. The sites of action of ß-endorphin a potent endogenous opioid peptide and its antagonist, naloxone, are the μ opiate receptors.

Microglia and peripheral nerve injury

Evidence of the involvement of dorsal horn microglia in peripheral nerve injury has been presented in studies. They are macrophage-like cells which are normally quiescent but, after nerve injury, are activated to be the source of cytokines and chemokines which then alter gene transcription. Microglia constitutes only a small percentage of the complex of tissues of the central nervous system, but the evidence is that they act as sensors for maintaining homeostasis. Once activated by trauma or ischaemia, there are changes in glial cell morphology, their numbers increase leading to the expression of new cell surface molecules which then produce chemical mediators like cytokines or immuno-molecules. Models of peripheral nerve injury using such as ligation or the transection of sciatic or spinal nerves, demonstrate this type of glial activation which is followed by changes in the animal behaviour. Touch and other normally innocuous stimuli are now followed by the limb withdrawal reflex in the animal, where the corresponding human expression might be allodynia. Increased microglial activity causes direct increments to the pain processing activities of neurones in this network, and plays a role, not only in their sensitisation, but also in the long term amplification of neuronal responses[xx].

The sympathetic nervous system and pain

Another differentiated pathophysiology of pain seen in patients with inflammatory change following injury or nerve damage is an increase of activity in the anatomically and functionally associated systems of the nociceptive network. The systems associated with the nociception involve the endogenous modulatory systems, the somatomotor, the neuroendocrine and the autonomic nervous system.

Heightened sympathetic activity in some patients produces a fairly characteristic syndrome. The pain is on-going, and assumed to occur after long term central changes have taken place, not only in the spinal cord, but in the brainstem, thalamus and forebrain. While peripheral nerve injury may feature prominently in some, the syndrome of on-going pain, hyperalgesia and allodynia, coupled with oedema, abnormal blood flow, sweating and other trophic changes may occur without obvious nerve injury. The many signs and symptoms of this syndrome may affect an extremity, its deep somatic tissues, or extend to viscera and even a region.

The sympathetic component of the autonomic system may sustain nociceptor activity in certain circumstances, usually following injury. Chronic pain in this instance is a syndrome described as sympathetically maintained pain (SMP), previously referred to, amongst others, as causalgia and reflex sympathetic dystrophies (RSD). Sudek's atrophy was another, an osteodystrophy and a diagnostic entity with symptoms and signs maintained in sympathetic over-activity which sometimes followed minor trauma and immobilisation. Complex Regional Pain Syndrome, (CRPS I or CRPS II), includes the former diagnoses, and now forms two fairly distinct groups of neuropathies.

CRPS I is the more common and develops with minor nerve injury, or sometimes even without, while usually CRPS II is associated with a distinct peripheral nerve lesion. The presence of nerve injury allows for the distinction between the two. The pain in both is attributable to sympathetic system activity. Following trauma to deep seated tissues or viscera or following exaggerated inflammatory responses in an extremity, patients may display associated SMP symptoms. Without distinct signs of a peripheral nerve lesion they are considered within the CRPS I category. The overlap of signs and symptoms in both categories, however, are considerable and responses to sympathetic blocks, once assumed to have diagnostic significance are equivocal.

Abnormal sweating and swelling of an affected extremity along with changes in reflex vasoconstrictor activity clinically manifest amongst the list of symptoms and signs of sympathetic involvement. Reduced motor power and joint movement in a limb, with progressive wasting, are further signs. Widespread hypoasthesia is sometimes seen. In some CRPS I patients this group of symptoms responds to sympathetic blocks with a reduction in pain intensity which often outlasts the local anaesthetic blockade and sensory conduction.

This brief survey of pains especially relating to CRPS does not convey the extent of the distress to some patients which for the physician is again significant towards the diagnosis. Patients are referred onwards to the round of specialities, including the surgeon, and when not updated in the advances in pain science, with their interventions they are likely to make patient distress intractable.

Pain, Neurophysiology and pitfalls to treatment

The past 50 years have seen phenomenal advance to understanding pain and its pathophysiology, and that progress has been outlined in another chapter. Prior to the pioneering research initiated about about that time Cartesian models of sensory transmission comprised accepted physiology, having a long innings despite the clinical mishaps that followed with adherence to that doctrine. Noordenbos in his concluding chapter quotes French from his 1958 review[xxi], "Knowledge concerning the primary sensory system is well established and part of neurological orthodoxy—". That physiology was essentially of receptors at the periphery conveying specific sensory impulses along their dedicated neural pathways to the cortical centres of the brain and leading to a particular sensation; a neurology that applied as much to the sensation of pain.

Noordenbos had noted, that the surgical extirpations, excision of neuromas, cordotomies designed to prevent or interrupt pain transmission along those pathways, did not control pain, or if it did for a while, recurrence was frequent. He initiated studies and stated the possibility of both excitation and inhibition at central levels evoked by peripheral stimuli. Impulses conveyed through multisynaptic afferent systems of pain at spinal cord levels formed intermediary loops capable of reinforcing or modulating pain. He maintained that such a system would account for the failure of surgical interference to specified pathways as the remedy for intractable pain. Kolmodin and Skoglund[xxii] in 1960 further demonstrated that large diameter afferents which conveyed tactile sensation, in fact, did evoke nociceptive inhibition at central levels.

Wall and Melzack with their 'Gate Control Theory' in 1965, questioned the entire Cartesian concept of pain causality, its perception and 'dedicated' anatomical neural pathways for pain. Their studies maintained that pain following injury was subject to a functional dynamism of the many neural pathways. Diverse inputs on the neurons of the spinal cord follow from both the periphery and from descending pathways from higher centres which were capable of modulating pain perception. Their studies reinforced the clinical appreciation of Bonica and others, and laid the foundations for later studies in pain pathophysiology; a research effort with a distinctive multidisciplinary character that has resulted in far greater progress to understanding mechanisms of pain, and its therapeutic control within the space of a few decades.

Understanding was extended as to why the experience of pain is less intense than it should be in relation to the reality of tissue injury, disability and gross damage. Pain perception may be modified in the neural system dependent on cognitive evaluation of the environment in its threats or its security. Neural pathways up to cortical levels, responsible for transmitting and modulating pain impulses following injury, are thus capable of creating 'virtual realities', as when analgesia is an appropriate behavioural aid to escape. In another human experience, as with an injury sustained in competitive sports activities, analgesia results in an ordinarily painful bone fracture, when the subject's attention has been intensely focussed to allow him to continue the game. Beecher's works on placebo were pioneering studies and are considered further in the next chapter. Pain alleviation amongst patients is often through their expectations of therapy, a cognitive feature which clinical research equates to artefact. There may be degrees of disconnectedness with the reality as the situation warrants for animal or subject in such reduced pain experiences.

Its obverse can be seen after an amputation, with the limb still in pain, the 'phantom' of a virtual limb being sustained in neural mechanisms[xxiii]. The extent of the problem suggested in innumerable studies amongst amputees manifesting phantom limb pain varies from a minority to considerable highs of over 80%. Homeostasis, those physiological adjustments appear impossible for some patients to achieve; in this instance disturbing, often painful or bizarre perceptions replace the reality.

CHAPTER VII

TRADITION TO BIOLOGY

Traditional acupuncture. Historical Excerpts & Venerable skills.

Professional physicians developed theories even while practising acupuncture as a craft. Theirs was often a hereditary occupation. Empirical observations were incorporated into a body of metaphysical Chinese Theory. The examination of patients for a diagnostic decision was within its logic and so was the treatment that followed. Theories were elaborate and essential to be thoroughly imbibed as the only guide to facilitate good practice; if well understood and adhered to the results demonstrated it.

Shih Sung, the physician, is quoted below from his preface to The Chen Ching section of the Manual, 'The Huang Ti Nei Ching' written around 1100 CE. The Chen Ching, or the Needle Manual, was one section which had been preserved in Korea when previously thought lost during the turmoil of earlier wars and destruction in China. It had been recovered a hundred years earlier and presented to the Chinese court by the Korean ambassador. The author considered the importance of the manual in the following passage. *"Unfortunately this work has been almost lost and very rare for a long time past, so that hardly anyone has studied it. Medical practitioners who study medical books can be effective in their therapeutics, but never was there one who could accomplish this without such reading. As for those who try to practice without it, and without having served their apprenticeship in good medical families, they harm and kill (their patients) more severely than if they took a knife and stuck it into them. That is why there is an old saying that scholars who do not study medical books (to help their parents) may be considered unfilial—"* (quoted from from Celestial Lancets)

The historical growth of TCM has uncertainties yet is worth pursuing. While tracing it one must make allowance for a lineage that reaches so far into the past that it becomes part of the mythology of healing of a particular geographic area and its unique culture. Ancient myths have identifiable similarities over neighbouring land areas and further afield, as they transmit through peoples' migrations, trade and the consequent exchanges of special knowledge. The skills of personages who enhanced healing had their special value which converted occasionally in antiquity to mystical powers.

TCM was and still is a system of therapeutics which incorporates herbal medicine, moxibustion, acupuncture and massage. Moxa and thermal applications over certain points on the body can be traced back to at least the period around BCE 500. The concept approximates to cautery, though the heat generated by tinder cones of artemesia placed on the body is mild in comparison. Acupuncture was by needle insertion, its special effects in scrupulous localisation of the hsueh, 'points' and the depths of insertion of equal importance. Again, astute physicians over the centuries, observant of special effects, brought increases to the numbers of points and possible therapeutic enhancement. To these, over time was added elaborate sophistication in the qualitative methods of stimulation.

The major compendium of acupuncture was the Nei Ching or rather the Huang Ti Nei Ching, which roughly translates to 'The Yellow Emperor's Manual of Corporeal Medicine. Its format in its first part, the Su Wên, relates to the human body in health and disease, and the therapeutics of acupuncture in particular. It is set out as a series of questions and answers, an exchange between the Emperor and his three expert physicians. The Yellow Emperor, Huangti was a renowned and reputed intellectual of the Han, the Dynasty commencing circa 200 BCE.

Well before and apart from the attestation of the Nei Ching certain sculptural reliefs at a temple in Shantung province reveal the almost supernatural awe in which physicians were held. The depiction of Pien Chhio, possibly of another famous physician in antiquity, shows the figure of a man with the head and beak of a bird, a pointed instrument in his hand, standing over a kneeling woman and holding her wrist; in another he is with a patient and others behind waiting for treatment. Liu Tun-Yuan who discovered these reliefs (see J N., Celestial Lancets, Chapt. Historical growth p 87-90) believes their origins to be from Wei-shan Hsien, the birthplace of Pien Chhio, and the bird-headed human figure to be that physician, his name meaning the 'Magpie'. Later writings suggest Pien Chhio to have been aware of the locations of points, some indeed with a specially potent therapeutic property such as Baihui, Du 20. This nomenclature is as used in 'Essentials of Chinese Acupuncture, Foreign Languages Press, Beijing. 1980, while Needham's historical accounts refer to the point as Pai-Hui[22] (TM 19). One may make allowance in interpreting

---

22 Into the nineteen sixties the U.K. had problems with residues of tuberculosis and its occasional meningeal manifestation. A specialist treatment, and often rather futile in retrospect, was to instil streptomycin into the cerebrospinal fluid (CSF) at the lumbo-sacral level. Those were early days for that antibiotic and the injectible formulations then available did not permeate cerebrospinal fluid (CSF). The mode of entry for streptomycin delivery in meningitis to CSF was therefore directly via the spinal route into the sub-arachnoid space. Unfortunately the pathogen-antigen reaction led to protein filaments forming in the CSF and subsequent blockage of the spinal canal. The streptomycin was then delivered routinely at a progressively higher level. The cisterna magna (cerebello-medullary) was the space that was entered as a last resort to instil streptomycin bypassing the lower level blockage.

To revert to acupuncture point usage amongst the ancients there is one, Yamen, today described on the Du channel mid-line channel terminating in the point, Baihui. These points are numbered Du 15 and Du 20 respectively. Needham assumes the latter point to have been used from ancient writings. If so, one assumes the remarkable recovery in the legends was from needling them for patients in coma or, following epileptic fits.

The *surface anatomy for the location of Yamen, however, was the point of entry to the cisterna magna in the procedure used at Black Notley Hospital in Essex, England for instilling Streptomycin, and a procedure I have repeatedly used on patients in the early sixties.* The chief of the unit who taught me the procedure had no knowledge whatsoever of Acupuncture. I noticed an anatomical correlation at the Beijing course in 1983.

Acupuncture point localising over the centuries today have their anatomical landmarks and this point could have shown some remarkable effects on occasion. However, one suspects only in its more heroic use—should the fine point of the needle, penetrate beyond the cisterna—to stimulate neural tissue of the medulla oblongata itself. Present day acupuncturists of any hue are discouraged from using this point, certainly not to a depth where it could penetrate neural medullary tissue. In Sweden the point, Du 15, was *off* the teaching list.

The Du channel, (Sinarteria Regens, TU-MO of Porkett) who describes it as originating "at the perineum and follows the spine straight to the indentation between atlas and the occipital bone, *where it penetrates into the brain, emerges again on the top of the skull*—". I make their anatomical locations as described, to correspond to the two points, Du 15 and Du 20. Their traditional use amongst others is also for epileptiform symptoms and meningitis or encephalitis.

stories in the ancient literature of patient treatment and recovery conveyed sometimes in considerable hyperbole. However, their awareness of the potency of certain points in stories associated with legendary figures like Pien Chhio from China could be supported in evidence, although eye-witness accounts transcribed a millennium later into the literature of acupuncture could hardly be vouched for accuracy.

The motif of the bird with a human head appears in Aryan myth, again a possible recurrence of in mythologies from Egypt; or the sirens of Greece in India become apsaras, the figures are continuity but their roles transform in the respective civilisations. The Gandharva figures in the Vedic story are the male counterpart of the apsara. They have their abode in the heavens, fly, make music and play their roles, celestial or earthly in conception and healing. Liu Tun-Yuan's interpretations take the reliefs to the Han period and the exchanges with the Indian subcontinent undoubtedly as inspiration. There was a fruitful commerce in visitors, trade and ideas between these civilisations in former transactions, as is seen in the Buddhist cave sites of China. Ideas of the respective therapeutic systems were mutually examined, but it would seem that each was largely content to function within its own epistemological superiority.

Returning briefly to the Huangti Nei Ching we find an idea of how the needles were to be used in acupuncture therapy. Huangti petitions Chhi Po, "I would like to know the Tao of acupuncture" and his reply, quoted in The Celestial Lancets p, 90, 91 "The first thing in this art and mystery is to concentrate the mind (on the patient as a whole) then, once you have decided on the state of his five viscera, whether Xu (*deficiency, asthenic*) or Shi (*excessive, plethoric*) as indicated by the nine pulse observations, you can take the needle in hand. If you have felt no death-like pulse, and heard no inauspicious sound, then the inner and outer signs are in correspondence. You must not rely on the external appearances (symptoms) only, and you must fully understand the coming and going (of the chhi in the tracts); then alone can you perform acupuncture on the patient. Patients are either of Xu or Shi constitution. In the five former do not lightly apply the needles, in the five latter do not delay to do so. When the Chhi has arrived the needle must be withdrawn as quickly as possible. The twisting of the needle must be done in an even and regular way, quietly and attentively watching the patient to observe any minute changes when the chhi arrives; such changes are so obscure they can hardly be seen. When the chhi arrives it is like a flock of birds, or the breeze in the waving millet—only too easily can one miss the fleeting moment. The physician must be like a crossbowman, pressing his trigger not an instant too soon, not an instant too late". (The interpretation within the above brackets is mine)

Literary cadences apart, this ancient descriptive fragment captures the quality of a sensation for the patient which the traditional practitioner must appreciate for a successful treatment as he hones his techniques to required sophistication in acupuncture. There is need for the closest patient observation and variation of stimulation intensities, and the arrival of chhi (an energy transfer) can be gauged by a changing expression or verbal response, signs that those well-versed in the metaphysics of acupuncture must decipher for good treatment.

Acupuncture therapy, biological attributes and clinical studies

The neuro-physiological developments were considered in previous Chapters. The experimental research on the biological effects of acupuncture is an on-going subject with progress in molecular biology process of sensory transmission. Understandably, though the clinical possibilities get more research attention. The subject constitutes another paradigm for development quite separate from traditional precepts, although many clinical studies still subscribe to the use of acupuncture points described in tradition. There are many definitions to the practice of acupuncture today, and their exponents certainly make claims for their own methods of clinical use. At present acupuncture may present as anything from traditional practice on the one hand to insertions of needles into peripheral tissues in a variety of ways and each non-traditional mode of clinical acupuncture explained in a scientism, but insufficiently supported in scientific research. I use scientism, when exponents resort to scientific terminology for explanation without adhering to the important corollary of validating the explanation by a method before it is science. The references in this paragraph below underscore the science; studies based within comprehensive programmes to understand Peripheral Sensory Stimulation (PSS), a variant acupuncture, its biological effects[i] examined by research method extends their possibilities in further clinical studies. Those programmes involve experimental research and clinical studies with acupuncture[ii] [iii] [iv] although in the largely PSS variant.

Medical traditions in Europe have moved to this other paradigm but there are no historical parallels of such shifts in Traditional Chinese

Medicine (TCM). While modern and up-to-date medical care is standard practice in China, TCM continues to offer its therapies as a social utility. In Europe the change to the medical system that followed was gradual in that it contained previous functional therapies, a few forms of folk medicine and their 'cures', and certain Paracelsian innovations—metallic derivatives for therapeutic use etc[v]. But in time the change to the culture of modern medicine was complete, and residues of older practices were shed, largely in the scientific modernisation required by the system. This entailed discarding insufficiencies in observations or experiential statements and the theoretical explanations of previous practices. A statement of theory with an empirical content would lend itself to an appropriate hypothesis which then could be subjected to experiment and verified. Verification contains an inductive principle to the extent that what has been verified has universal emphasis. The Popperian dimension[vi], however, insists on the *demarcation*; a statement if experimentally falsifiable defines the empirical. This emphasis allows progress and development from the empirical, not the stasis and immutability seen in the Chinese epistemology of Acupuncture Theory. Many of its statements require reinterpretation to discern its empiricism. *Demarcation* here refers to the line between statements which further scientific discourse and others of a kind eminently not falsifiable as the metaphysical tends to be.

The theory of The Five Elements is a case in point; their order and system of correspondences, extended to organs and TCM pathology, are logically derived philosophical assertions. Medical science, however, in its tendency to devalue other epistemology, loses sight of empirical derivation in the content of ancient medical theory. Chinese physicians' observations stemmed from the empirical and were formalised. As with perception of 'Chhi' which may pass the Rubicon of 'demarcation' in science method provided it were considered as the subject to be tested rather than dismissed in the regulations of controlled group trials. 'Chhi', as a necessary perception to sustain the validity of an acupuncture point when needled, was thought to be essential for sound treatment. Today's studies barely account for the relevance of an empirical tradition. The skill of the hand in inserting a needle into tissue and its follow-through sensation was claimed to be essential therapeutics, but to consider its validity in evidence based medicine requires innovative controlled clinical trials. A randomised study of patients, one group allowed the entire gamut of a traditional physician's acupuncture attentions against a similar treated

treated by an acupuncturist with modern competence. The latter control may not necessarily test a claimed empirical skill but a single blind study is possible for the purpose. Innovations have resulted in other 'hands-on' disciplines like surgery[vii]. For the present Chhi is yet to be considered as having therapeutic content. But, only in a dismissive disinterest of the present scientist, an exclusion which rarely concedes therapeutic possibility in a demonstrable skill, hence, hardly examined in scientific study.

Biology in acupuncture development today, but not its practice, is essentially an endeavour in the newer paradigm, neither related to the tradition nor aiming to derive the value necessarily contained in its history. Experimentation was not the norm, but was not unknown either, in Chinese tradition. It was of another order, directed to solving a specific problem rather than pursuing an empirical generality. The prelude to Chinese innovation and improvements to their medical heritage and some experimentation in medicine were demonstrated in examples such as the introduction of the concept of tracts (meridians) and pulse diagnostics in acupuncture. TCM went much further afield in improvising forms of variolation for small pox and had experimental 'answers' for many diseases in the use of medicinal herbs.

Introducing biology to acupuncture at present is largely to account for *the needle effect*. That too was available in tradition in translation as the 'pricking' therapy of acupuncture, a variant mode without 'chhi'. Biology is satisfied to consider acupuncture effects attributable to the sensory effect of a needle insertion into tissues, and as such the rest of a system of therapeutics and traditional theory is largely superfluous[viii]. Peripheral sensory stimulation and its somatic sensory effects (see Chapt-DNIC effects etc) is the content of acupuncture, and tenets for its traditional use are barely considered, including a major one—that treatment differs as it is selected for each patient problem. Such a proposition is almost untenable for a research protocol. Further, as a disease runs its course, individual responses alter, requiring constant adjustments of treatment.

Reasons for not attempting traditional precepts are that they generally present incompatibility to the regulations of medical experimentation and clinical trials. Pulse diagnostics is a good example. Methods of investigation cannot take on board the variety of individual physiology when the trial participants are reduced to the classified pathology of the group. Much of the empiricism contained in TCM refers to individual variation and not to the variables of a group. In their contrasting paradigms, traditional practices do not translate in science and hence scientific methodology and the protocols of a clinical trial are barely applicable. Whatever the merits of a well-controlled clinical trial, we are left with its positive or negative results for a 'cohort', and evidence of whether cohort behaviour would explain an individual response is absent. In the present design of trial protocols, clinical investigations on acupuncture can hardly subscribe to the precepts of TCM. There are elements of traditional acupuncture that are functional and useful for the patient despite the incongruities of their presentation. But the negative evidence in clinical trials confirms the view of the sceptics: evidence derived from a rigid methodology designed to assess a 'product' and not for 'hands-on' practices like acupuncture. We have not arrived at convincing methods for the latter, while a few scientists, in their implacable opposition to acupuncture, seem often to convey prejudice rather than due scientific scepticism[ix].

Pursuing acupuncture requires modern biology to examine TCM statements for an empiricism that is discernible though necessarily stated within its own knowledge systems. TCM theory has principles which have found modern physiological explanation. The mere idea that a needle puncturing the skin and setting in train a series of responses with therapeutic effects such as analgesia, was a discovery with its own explanation in TCM. Naturally, the statements of concepts about human functions and across millennia and in respective epistemologies make for incomprehension as physiology. But a bridge across them in this instance lies in the application of the observations of older therapeutic knowledge which produce virtual response. Some of that knowledge has been tested and developed in the epistemology of science, providing insights for the present. Since over the ages there have been hardly any changes to human physiology in the particular statements of an ancient therapeutic procedure, claims to correct abnormal function in a patient could provide a hypothesis for exploration.

We may be reaching the position that only the practice of acupuncture denuded of its tradition can allow for validation in the evidence-based medicine of our time. That assumption is unwarranted without more variants attempted in protocols for clinical study. Within their ancient terms of learning traditional therapists still provide patients substantial relief. Clinical study protocols with a little ingenuity may find means to accommodate the apparent irreconcilabilities in traditional practice, or at least attempt its investigation as a control against other modalities in investigating acupuncture. The totality of traditional practice is rarely attempted on the presumption that it does not fulfil the norms for clinical investigations. Prior discoveries in TCM find only the barest acknowledgement, while attempting the most rigorous applications of clinical study regulations. If an adaptation to method is not possible for the therapeutic modality under investigation, the position suggests a methodological insufficiency of Clinical research. That being so acupuncture studies conducted in protocols that satisfy regulations of method without an understanding of its necessary practices are inconclusive in equivocal outcomes. We have repeatedly taken up the regulatory need for a placebo control which bears repeating. Further on the chapter, one study specifically directed to acupuncture and 'placebo' demonstrates the inadequacy of a placebo for acupuncture as contrasted with a true placebo for a drug when both were used for for pain relief. Many studies in satisfying the standards of 'evidence based medicine' show acupuncture as no more effective than its placebo. But, for acupuncture a placebo is feeble as a control, and displaying the merit of a study using a placebo control group cannot provide the conviction suggested. However, the placebo continues to be the standard bearer of evidence-based medicine. Invariably results reviewed in another context with placebo acupuncture offer different evidence. Replicable protocols fail to recognise the immense variability involved in individual patient responses or their gross pathology. A clinical study with acupuncture is often not convincing as a replicable exercise, and even simulating protocol cannot contend with the variability. Studies in diagnostically categorised patients with pain can be repeated but different outcomes are likely since beyond the diagnoses individual responses pertaining to pain present great objective and subjective variety.

These exercises have paradigmatic constraints and have not taken on board traditional concepts of practice. Use of pulse diagnostics is entirely overlooked. The evidence of any correlation between an individual's pulse variation and a pathological diagnosis is not apparent to the medical investigator. In tradition the pulse comprises part of other examinations including the patient's appearance, features of the tongue etc., but often pulse readings are conclusive in clinching the therapist's decision on treatment. Pulse variations refer directly to epistemological diagnostics which are a distant cry from pathology in the present culture of medicine.

The acuity of detecting pulse variations is both individual and subjective, and described in qualities of the examiner's acuity, the specialised perception at his fingertips. The process does strain the credulity of physicians today and certainly his grosser responses at his fingertips! Yet, before laughing it off stage we are left not merely with anecdotes, but also caveats from substantial mandarins like Needham, and his "—word to the wise in due season"[23].

Traditional therapists claim this faculty, and in many Eastern cultures diagnostics are through pulse readings. Amongst such practitioners a few have outstanding reputations in pulse diagnosis. To train finger-tip sensitivities during the years of traditional apprenticeship and to learn to perceive pulse variability in such detail as to be able register a change of a patient's condition is an art. We may regret its obsolescence, but present patient pathology to confirm diagnosis is a tremendous advance and depends on other investigatory tools.

Meridians, Acupuncture Points and Biological Significance

Meridians or the Channels and Collaterals continue a relevance to practice. From the Chinese concept of conduits that convey forms of energy a physiological importance emerges. Acupuncture meridians were

---

[23] This position does not accord with Needham's (see text p 12. Introduction: Celestial Lancets, Lu Gwei-djen & Joseph Needham). "Not everyone with a modern-Western medical qualification can immediately perform all the traditional-Chinese therapeutic feats. Pulse diagnosis, for example, as well as a very organicist psycho-somatic approach, is a fundamental feature of the traditional art, which after all depends on much subtle theorising, not of course in the modern style, but not non-sense either. We offer, therefore, a word to the wise in due season."
Non-traditional performers of a variant practice could be aware of the possible. But I must also point out that today's non-traditional training produces therapists with a considerable function who are relevant to modern medical disciplines. Since the mid-eighties Sweden, for example, has trained ancillary workers-a few thousand physiotherapists, nurses, midwives and doctors and dentists within a syllabus of physiological lectures and practical training for use of a non-traditional variant of acupuncture. In the field of chronic pain alleviation they are a part of the health delivery system where many pain clinics or physiotherapy establishments have a resource for the use of these 'qualified' and certified practitioners. That it has therapeutic relevance is recognised by the Swedish Socialsyrenssen (Medical Council) by certification for practice as an ancillary resource of its health delivery system. For a traditional therapy to remain on the scene of modern medicine requires training in both systems in order to contribute health delivery safely and effectively. Acupuncture, it should not need stressing, must find scientific revival and without dismissing the 'feats' of its traditional practice.

elaborately worked out to fit many other concepts in TCM. While about 160 points on the body surface were known, around the first century BCE they were expanded to 365, satisfying the theoretical structure and as a part of a reticulate circulation contained in 12 meridians. The empiricism was essentially attributable to the 'points' and their localisation. Their later distribution along the meridians was a formalisation of acupuncture theory in the knowledge of the constellations, celestial circles and calendrical cycles which appear in the configuration of meridians. Originally they were named after China's great rivers. Further details worked theoretical concepts to convey the essential effects of the points along them. The Lo was a Yang vital force of energy, and the Mo was Yin and substantial blood. The two forms of energy were in contact at vital points, also known as junctional points. Later development to the theories was that the blood furnished pulses which could determine variants from normal body functions, and its flow provided a circulation for the delivery of nourishment and clearance of waste products through its smallest pores, which indeed amounted to rudiments of a capillary system. These theories were fitted into the philosophy and culture of the time, of macrocosmic effects on an earthly microcosm.

Meridians in TCM have been considered by medical science from various viewpoints and finally found to be without any morphological support; they lacked evidence to warrant their configuration. The transformation of an ancient practice into peripheral neural stimulation has its origins in Chinese acupuncture. The points on the Meridians of TCM emerge in medical science, but stated differently in kindred concepts and some similar functional applicability. Relating to sensory perception, in particular of pain, such examples are contained in present concepts of trigger points, referred pain, and dermatomes, myotomes and sclerotomes. Head's dermatomes have their physiological relevance in diagrammatically marking the likeliest area of a cutaneous nerve supply. The same can be projected for the concepts contained in meridians. Both are representations, but the former can be understood as of anatomical relevance while the ancient merdian of TCM suggests an empirical kinship to Heads later observations. Trigger point therapy consists of applications of the needle expounded in great detail by Travell and Symonds. The points are usually myofascial, intensely sensitive and painful to palpation and not stable in their distribution, but they too are apparent as the 'ah-shi' points of tradition.

Consider effects on specific organs when needles on the meridian of the Bladder were inserted at their specified 'point' locations. There is confusion, insufficient appreciation of organs in TCM, as well as of many translations which ignore semantics. Organs in ancient Chinese literature do not transform to anatomical organs, but the six organs in its theories elaborate to a further functional role. However while those functions are untenable, points on the Bladder Meridian are prefixed with the names of organs in the Chinese nomenclature as used in the 'Essentials'[x] which appear functionally relevant. A part of the course of the Meridian of the Bladder is drawn bilaterally on the back (see fig. Chapter III) where it runs on either side of the spinal spinuous process at a distance of two finger breadths from the midline (index and middle finger measures one and a half chun, the modular Chinese measure. The named points, for example, at the levels of the spinuous process of Thoracic 5, Lumbar 2, and sacral 2 foramen are, respectively: Xinshu or Bladder 5, where Xin names the heart; Shenshu or Bladder 23, Shen being the kidney; and Panguanshu or Bladder 32, Panguan, the bladder. Hence, we should note the distinct possibility of reflex efferent stimulatory effects from the needles inserted on these acupuncture points, effects which could be regional, on a dermatome, a myotome, or a sclerotome which includes the organ; embryological development being segmentally oriented from the spinal nerves which makes them a functional unit. Peripheral stimulation evokes both somatic and autonomic responses. Acupuncture on the 'Bladder' meridian stimulates the points at serial levels of the sensory dorsal branches along the range of spinal nerves and will elicit segmental somatic reflexes while the rami communicantes' link to the sympathetic and parasympathetic autonomic chains evoke responses from those systems as well.

An example of rapid benefit by point stimulation on the bladder meridian at lower lumbar levels is found in the relief of the intensely painful and acute spasm, a board-like rigidity of paravertebral spinal muscles and intra-abdominal muscles—the psoasquadratus lumborum—'lumbago' in popular parlance. Rapid reflex myotomal, both somatic and the likelier general autonomic responses, would account for such effects. Sclerotomal and longer lasting systemic corrections are the documented effects in the use of this invaluable meridian of TCM: there are many acute conditions where dramatic corrections are possible from an adequate acupuncture therapist and availed of by patients. They should provoke a pause before traditional theory is dispensed with as of little consequence or, worse, as an irrelevance for science.

Stimulating acupuncture points elicits reflex effects to correct acute or chronic pathology. The named point locations on the back of the trunk relate to the levels of sclerotomes and myotomes, making their stimulatory function neurologically rational. Meridian sketches of the Gall Bladder on the head and neck show a remarkable resemblance to dermatomal maps; the latter depicting figuratively the demarcation of the nerve supply to the head, neck and face by the occipital, maxillary and mandibular nerves

Many acute or chronic problems of this region respond to treatment using those points. Rapid relief is possible with acupuncture for trismus, a muscle spasm of the jaw due to motor disturbances of the trigeminal nerve, as well as incipient migraine headaches, allergic rhinnorhoea and torticollis, commonly known as 'wry neck'. Relief of muscle spasm relies on the judicious selection of points on that meridian, along with equally important techniques to control the intensity of stimulation. Over-stimulation can make an acute problem worse.

The viability of the meridians in tradition was demonstrated on treating the patient. The anatomical arrangement of their configuration and sensory responses has since been demonstrated experimentally. TCM subscribed to the transfer of energy to the ching lo from the ching mo or blood circulation. In such theorising, bizarre as it is to medical science, functional effects of point stimulation on the meridians prioritised the experimental findings of Head, Sherrington and Kellgren by a couple of thousand years. Their experimental demonstrations showed reversal of the response—as we understand clinical peripheral pain referred to the deltoid region from lesions involving the diaphragm (Spinal cervical segments, 3,4,5)[xi]. TCM however produced a therapeutic function, while later neural connectivity explained the reason underlying referred pain. Acknowledgement in priority once again has been overdue.

Traditional precepts have undoubtedly benefited patients in chronic pain but explanations for its use for today's practising professional have to relate to physiology. We face a basic problem in elucidating acupuncture through research protocols. The individuality of the patient is a self-evident factor for the traditionalist as it is to a great extent at the modern clinic. But the designs of therapeutic studies of acupuncture lose the individual to the group in the usual protocols of evidence-based medicine and clinical trials.

Biological Acupuncture

Clinical studies over some decades suggest that the sensory stimulus elicited with a needle insertion through the skin is Peripheral Sensory Stimulation (PSS), a biological adaptation of acupuncture therapy. That a traditionalist using acupuncture has advantages denied to PSS cannot be contradicted or confirmed, essentially for a lack of methodological evidence. However to assume from the criticisms in this monogram that PSS is 'the parson's egg' is not a valid interpretation either. It certainly has proved relevant for patients treated in variant practices of PSS, even without using the many precepts of the past. Apart from therapeutic practice, PSS is invaluable for investigating the science of acupuncture. Having brought acupuncture into the arena of modern medicine in the empirical practices presently in vogue, many patients have found benefit from it while its development has been in very substantial experimental[xii], and clinical research[xiii].

Innumerable experimental investigations and clinical studies have been on patients with chronic or acute pain. Analgesia or pain reduction is mediated by an afferent stimulus through neural pathways that control the input to systems mediating pain, and the insertion of an acupuncture needle is basically one such peripheral stimulus. But practitioners using needle insertions also prescribe parameters for its use. Studies sometimes describe points on the meridians as though without the further requisites of tradition. Varying stimulation intensities by certain manipulations of the needle, or altering points in on-going treatment is traditional practice for effectiveness, but difficult to accommodate within a study's protocols. Biological studies of acupuncture within such methodological restraints furnish validated evidence for use. For many reasons that possibility is presently denied to traditional acupuncture. These are the paradoxical challenges that the scientist interested in acupuncture must try and unravel. Many studies with acupuncture are available to demonstrate its use for patient pathology and a few studies of the many of conducted by colleagues at the Karolinska, Gottenburg University and other Swedish groups have been acknowledged in the notes and references.

SIX STUDIES[XIV].

Features of Pain pathology which determine outcome to Acupuncture treatment.

Our group at the Karolinska Institute, Stockholm, in one series of clinical trials found that the differentiation of pain pathophysiology amongst patient groups offered fair clarification for the extent or lack of benefit using acupuncture. The discrimination of pain in this manner goes further than considering it as a symptom of pathology; it differentiates pain by its own pathology, and is clarified further in the previous Chapter. Aetiological factors of the somatosensory complex are the cause of pain pathology and its continuity must be accounted for by changes within that complex. Persisting inflammation of tissues involving specific pain receptors, the nociceptors of the neural pathways conducting pain, distinguishes a chronic nociceptive pain from other patient pains, where aetiology is again referable along that pathway but to other foci.

In five of the six studies in the series reviewed below we used Meridians and their described acupuncture points. Point selection was not based on traditional practice or precepts but on their location for the likely somatic stimulatory effect referred to the tissue or organ of pathology. They were supplemented with points chosen on the limbs as previous experimental studies had suggested that these could reinforce stimulation effects. The studies were reasonably conclusive within their limitations. They make no claims to providing standards for investigation but may convey adaptability to methods for a complex practice such as acupuncture which is unlike investigating a singular therapeutic or pharmacological entity.

The present studies, in using acupuncture for patients in pain categorised by such pathophysiological aetiology, provided better indications to its use. A prevailing attitude that acupuncture could be tried when much else fails in chronic pain may be justified to an extent if we regard its chronicity as having different reasons within the pathophysiolology of neurones that transmit pain. A summary of those trials is presented as an example for the use of acupuncture largely shorn of traditional theory but not entirely without a few of the practical applications of traditional acupuncture.

The six studies enrolled a total of 412 patients with chronic or acute pain into smaller groups to examine the factors which influence the outcome of treatment with acupuncture? The methodology and protocols kept therapists separate from the evaluators, and to that extent blinding was possible. Controls in one trial used 'placebo acupuncture' but the five others compared different treatments in the patient groups. Validated pain scales were used to assess pain. Four of the studies had long term follow-ups and five randomised patients to the different trial groups.

STUDY I

Acupuncture in Head and Neck Pain. (Paper in Thesis) The initial trial was on 177 patients within a regional category of head and neck pain. The specific diagnostic groups amongst the 177 patients were:, 30 with Secondary trigeminal neuralgia; 16, Chronic sinus pain; following tooth extraction or facial trauma; 7, Temperomandibular joint pain; 39, Scalp muscle contraction headaches; 6, Central Pain (CP), which was referable to lesions along the spinothalamocortical pathways); 43, Suboccipital and cervical musculoskeletal pain; 36, Head and neck pain associated with psychological distress (**Table V in Study I p 25 in Thesis**) summarises the progress, with treatment up to a 2 year follow-up of results from acupuncture. This study with the separate diagnostic groups above considered possible parameters of acupuncture in 10 initial treatments within a twice weekly schedule. Those parameters with the best outcomes were continued as the optimal ones for later studies if the protocol required them.

The parameters for study

a) <u>the sites for needle insertions</u>. Segmentally, on points on Chinese Meridians. Segmental selection in this context refers to the perceptive area of pain, a dermatome; the area over skin supplied by an afferent of a cranial or a spinal nerve marks the segments. Three groups were tested with this parameter, a segmental selection alone, or extrasegmental points alone or thirdly with a combination of segmental and extrasegmental points. The largest number of patients with immediate relief was among those where segmental points alone were used. The most effective parameter, however, where the longest lasting relief was obtained in more patients was by the combination of segmental points along with distal points, or extrasegmental points on the same or another meridian. It must be noted that in the trials on patients with secondary trigeminal neuralgia only 17 of the 30 patients enrolled benefited sufficiently to go on to longer term treatment.

b) Stimulation Intensity. 16 patients with chronic sinus pain were randomly allocated to two groups to assess the effect of superficial insertion of needles compared with deep insertions at the prescribed traditionally recommended depths. A heightened sensation following insertion was procured by a twirl of the needle back and forth for a few seconds till it was deemed by the patient as having reached a limit of tolerance, or was distinctly (amounting to pain) perceived in comparison with the initial insertion. This may emulate the sensation known as the DeQi (Chhi) in tradition and while it signified amongst much else in its theory, for the therapist it marked a correctness of point localisation if rapidly elicited. The trial's outcome was that superficial intradermal insertions of needles were less effective than the procedure with deep insertion into subcutaneous tissues; 5 and 10 of 16 patients responding in the two respective groups after the 10 treatments.

c) Duration of treatment. Another parameter tested on 43 patients with cervical or suboccipital musculo skeletal pain was to arrive at the most effective length of time for a single treatment schedule. 30 minutes at each session was found to be optimal in comparison to shorter or longer periods. 24 of 43 responded with less pain in the 30 and 60 minute sessions whereas only 14 showed a similar result over 1 minute and 5 minute sessions.

d) Stimulation modes. 52 patients, 7 with temperomandibular joint pain (TM), 6 with Central Pain (CP) and 39 with Scalp Muscle Tension (SMT) headaches were tested with 4 different modes of acupuncture: **Manual** stimulation—needle insertion to prescribed depths followed by DeQi; **Superficial**—the insertion of needles with a minimal sensation if any; **High** frequency—80 Hz electrical stimulation by an appropriate apparatus whose leads were attached to 3 pairs of needles, and **Low** frequency—the same with 2 Hz electrical stimulation. High frequencies caused a tingling sensation akin to paraesthesia and with low frequencies, depending on the intensity of the voltage, there were perceptible muscle or muscle fibre contractions. Voltages were adjusted to intensities according to patients' comfort during treatment.

50%-100% pain reduction on a Visual Analogue Scale was seen in 10 patients treated with the Superficial Mode of acupuncture and 17, 20, and 19 patients using respectively, Manual, and Low and High frequency stimulation.

The 177 patients referred to us for treatment with the above diagnoses were from various clinics: physical medicine, medical rehabilitation, medicine, neurology, orthopaedic surgery, Ear, Nose and Throat, General Surgery and neurosurgery. After the treatment schedules a retrospective assessment was possible in terms of the differing outcomes of the diagnostic groups. The analyses strongly suggested that patients with specific diagnoses broadly differentiated by pathophysiology (see below) had more consistent outcomes from acupuncture treatment. Further studies paid attention to this indication. Neuropathic Pain following nerve injury to or pathology involving neural tissues is identifiable by clinical symptoms and signs which can be confirmed by tests for neural involvement. In the first study the results of patients with Secondary trigeminal neuralgia and CP suggested that these pains were only minimally responsive to a modality like acupuncture and we did not pursue any further trials for these categories. In the preliminary trial for suboccipital and cervical musculoskeletal pain, 43 patients responded very differently from 36 others with head and neck pain associated with psychological distress. In the latter group 7 patients only benefited from long term acupuncture treatment, though none was free of pain

Pathophysiological Differentiation of Pain

In four trials that followed, patient pathology was differentiated to Nociceptive Pain and patient groups and controls were studied for response to acupuncture. The groups were made up of patients post dental surgery (molar tooth extraction); those suffering chronic pains from trauma and degenerative musculo-skeletal pathology of the lower back; and a group of women with the periodic chronic visceral pain of dysmenorrhoea. Continuous nociceptor activity causing pain can be a functional response associated with healing as in the acute pain following a tooth extraction; or protective, preventing further trauma when the inflammatory process is maintained by chronic factors, for example the lesions of skeletal and paravertebral tissue resulting in chronic pain.

Since it was apparent from a retrospective analyses of Study I that Neuropathic pain was least responsive to acupuncture, patients whose pain was due to damage to peripheral nerves or attributable to lesions along the neural pathway for pain were excluded from the later trials. These are, however, patients that present the clinician with almost intractable problems. Other protocols and more comprehensive trials featuring traditional therapists may suggest methods of acupuncture use for these patients but need to be confirmed in evidence. Clinical studies on strictly demarcated neuropathic pains, using traditional therapists in one group and possibly medication in another, should make this possible. At present anecdotal evidence may be a reason for the continued referral of these patients for acupuncture treatment.

In another differentiated category of chronic pain are patients with no clinical or investigatory evidence of pathology whose condition can be distinguished as an Idiopathic Pain Disorder (IPD). Their pain is chronic and intractable. These patients were examined for responses to acupuncture in a separate study (III), in this series of trials. The diagnosis had been suggested by Williams and Spitzer who separately defined and distinguished their pain from that of Pain Prone Disorder, which is pain distinctly psychogenic in origin or with a history of depressive disease[xv]. IPD patients have pains that are long lasting but pain is not referable to any anatomy—neural, visceral or tissue. While the distribution of pain may be related to a region or a visceral site, no demonstrable pathology could account for it. Yet, it is important to distinguish patients in this category. Clinicians tend to find a psychogenic reason for chronic pain that presents in the above patterns. Williams and Spitzer find sufficient reasons to distinguish IPD from pains associated with neuroses and depressive disease: patients with the latter are often able to somatise their pains to an organ or specific site. They also suggest other markers for the distinction between idiopathic pain disorder and psychogenic pain. The latter may resolve if the patient's psychiatric problem is controlled.

STUDY II

Comparative Study of Diazepam and Acupuncture (Paper in Thesis)
Patients with Cervical Osteoarthritis made up the groups in this trial. An antidepressant, diazepam has its use for pain even if depression is not a concomitant problem. The trials on 44 patients were not a long term

study but a comparison of their immediate responses to treatments with acupuncture or diazepam and their respective placebos. The entry to each mode was randomised and followed through with the other modes also randomly. Acupuncture needling was at described TCM points on the head and neck plus a bilateral point on the dorsum of the hand. Elicited sensations following the insertion and further rotation were as confirmed by the patient. The 'placebo' for acupuncture in this study was intradermal insertion of needles at the same points but without further rotation. In this method the initial insertion was sensed but the sensation was not of the same intensity as the true acupuncture modality nor was there any repetition of the sensation as with true acupuncture during the schedule of treatment. However, this 'placebo' is still a modified form of acupuncture, far from the pharmacological concept of placebo as an inert substance.

Summary of outcomes

Diazepam, acupuncture and sham acupuncture all produced *significant pain reduction* and only the placebo for diazepam failed to elicit this response. In this study the placebo for diazepam in identical tablet form and the assumed placebo for acupuncture produced very different responses: the latter showing significant reduction of pain both on a sensory scale and on one determining the degree of unpleasantness (affect). The placebo for diazepam did show some reduction of patients' pain on the latter, but not on the sensory scale. This trial featured under the label of a placebo controlled study. But questions remain, not least about the appropriateness of any placebo contrivance for acupuncture. A possible conclusion would be to accept that the study compared two separate acupuncture groups. In the opinion of this writer the issue is unresolved even after two further decades of attempts at fashioning a suitable 'placebo' control for acupuncture studies.

STUDY III

Acupuncture for Idiopathic Pain Disorder (IPD) (Paper in Thesis)
The above diagnosis was established on twelve patients at the Karolinska Hospital's Pain Clinic at the Dept. of Anaesthesiology, who were then referred to our group at the Institute for treatment with acupuncture. These

patients had pains lasting for years. The average duration was 12.6 years—the shortest period of pain being 2 years in one patient, and the longest 38 years. The Pain Clinic had excluded anyone with evident pathology and followed up with stringent examination and tests for somatosensory involvement. No pain could be attributed to an affective or psychiatric illness; hence the diagnosis of IPD according to the definition of Williams and Spitzer. Of course, the duration of pain affected patients' quality of life. Excepting one, they were unable to do a full days work and required periods of rest during the day. Mood changes were apparent and naturally admitted to, but none was neurotic within the diagnostic definition of the term. These were patients who had previously had various forms of physical therapies and medication

Further examination of the patients charted the location of their pain. In all studies pain was rated on visual analogue scales, the ends representing worst pain possible and no pain at either end of the scale. In this study those end points were used to maintain a daily graph sheet, and at regular intervals the patients marked their evaluation of pain experience. These daily scales were maintained for two weeks prior to beginning treatment and again after finishing the schedules, offering a comparison between pre-treatment status and that following acupuncture. The treatment schedules were usually at 2-3 week intervals and since 10 treatments were recommended the survey extended over months.

Needles were inserted at sites of bony prominence to the depths of periosteum and bone, one in the proximity of pain and another at a distal point also included in this therapy. Acupuncture used in this way reduced the number of insertions, but exploration and manipulation of the needle over two periosteal points elicits a momentarily painful sensation more intense than other methods of acupuncture. The entry point for the needle is most often a traditionally named point. The parameters for periosteal needle techniques for clinical acupuncture are recommended by Felix Mann[xvi], its best known exponent. The possible mechanisms of its action, Diffuse Noxious Inhibitory Control (DNIC) have been experimentally demonstrated by the LeBars group and discussed further in other chapters. Acupuncture delivered at brief though painful intensities was used on these patients as they had undergone many diverse forms of treatment over previous years, including other modes of acupuncture.

Summary

Results of treatment

Ten patients had brief reduction in the intensity of their pain, mostly following each treatment, but relapsed to their usual levels of pain and did not improve in the long term. The periods of improvement were sufficient reason to continue treatment schedules. Two patients obtained substantial improvement in this group after 7 treatments. The graphs confirmed the responses of four patients over the weeks and months. The first and second chart are indicative of the general response to treatment amongst the majority: a reduction of pain for brief periods and a lack of any consistent pain relief denoted a response trend which patients could not consider as an improvement to their condition. The other two graphs are specific to each of the two patients who did benefit from the treatment. It was mainly a long term reduction to pain, with one patient practically free of pain after her seventh treatment

In this differentiated category of Pain, two 2 patients had sufficient improvement to their chronic pain for prolonged periods, enabling an improved quality of life. For at least 3 years in one patient, and 19 years in the other, they had suffered chronic pain and its many daily limitations. Ten patients out of twelve having no benefit are undoubtedly of statistical significance and is usual evidence for drawing a negative conclusion for acupuncture therapy for this specific category of pain. The benefit for two patients should not be dismissed within that conclusion. These patients had run the gamut of attendance and treatment by diverse methods in many clinics. That must be taken account of in the otherwise negative evidence of the study.

The study is constrained by its regulations. At a Pain clinic, there would be better opportunity to vary treatment modalities or even acupuncture modes for the patients with long lasting pain and some amongst them who may be diagnosed as IPD. From the evidence of the study, acupuncture obviously was not an alternative as treatment. In the climate of 'best practices' as routines for the clinic, its inclusion on that list is unlikely. 'Best practice' features in Health Services like the newly initiated programmes recommended by US Government Agencies and financed partly through Private Insurance for Universal Health Care[xvii]. 'Best practice' offers clinical discrimination for the physician, but for patients 'evidence based medicine',

PAIN CHARTS

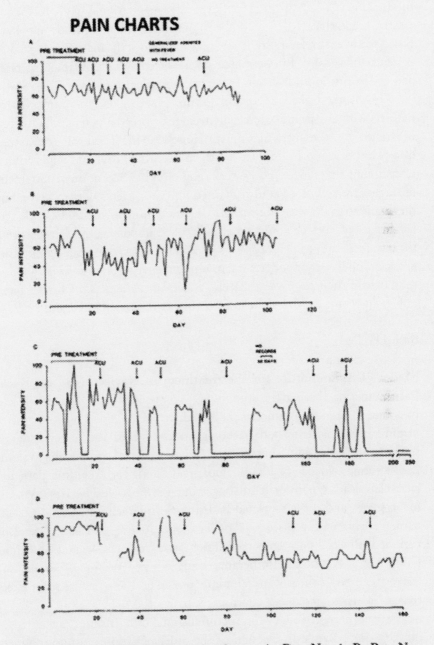

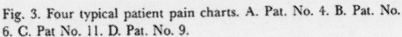

Fig. 3. Four typical patient pain charts. A. Pat. No. 4. B. Pat. No. 6. C. Pat No. 11. D. Pat. No. 9.

in limiting choice through policy recommendation, may preclude a treatment alternative that could be found effective. In the study above we find a ready example of physicians retaining a discriminative approach to patients and therapy. But here again we are faced by a scientism, its sceptics and the institutions for profit in the realm of Health Care.

This study lacked a control group, placebo or any other. These patients with persistent pain on an average of over 12 years and a history of attendance at many clinics must themselves offer a control. The virtues of a placebo group in context for them are unrealistic and superfluous. Consistent pain reduction over weeks and months without the requirement of further treatment was only obtained for two patients of the twelve, but the quality of relief was substantial. The study protocols could be critiqued for the lack of a placebo only if method is more important than the context: the nature of the problem, patients in pain for years, the general responses of the group to treatment etc. If two out of twelve responding with a long-term ease to their pain was a placebo effect, the patient as the final arbiter of benefit is entitled to it. The issue is further discussed in Chapter VIII

STUDY IV

Modes of Acupuncture for the treatment of Nociceptive Low Back Pain (Paper in Thesis). The study was on patients with chronic low back pain but selected from amongst those where the pain was of nociceptive origin. These patients had pathological change to the lower lumbar spine or sacroiliac joint but with a functionally intact nervous system and without evidence of a radiculopathy. Criteria for excluding patients were claudicating pain or pain suggesting a sympathetic nervous system involvement and those who had had surgical intervention for their back pain. Patients with a history of major depressions or neurosis were also excluded. Referral points for recruitment and treatment were a Research Clinic and a Private Physiotherapy Clinic. 43 patients were selected for trials, 10 amongst them were randomly placed on the waiting list for later treatment. They served as a control group.

Patients accepted that acupuncture using 3 different modes would be initially tried. Random selection of the order of exposure to each mode was followed by patients' choice of the mode they thought best to continue treatment in. 3 patients dropped out of the study without completing the trials. The modes of acupuncture to be tried after needle insertion on the selected points were: Manual Stimulation (MS) and electrical stimulation at Low (LF) and High (HF) Frequencies. These modes of acupuncture using electrical stimulation are now in fairly common use but depend on therapist preferences. A few studies amongst Swedish groups on subjects with experimental pain had suggested the effectiveness of LF stimulation but at intensities producing muscle contractions[xviii], but therapy with intensities producing repetitive muscle contractions as rule are uncomfortable for patients.

Needles were inserted over Traditional points on named meridians. They were selected on the basis of their likely myotome and sclerotome effects. Usually 3 pairs of paraspinal points were selected, plus two or more distal points. The methods of stimulation and optimum parameters followed were the results of Study I.

Assessment procedure

The outcomes from treatment were on nominal pain scales and other measures which were a) patient assessments of Activities of Daily Life (ADL), b) pain scales and descriptors of pain, c) measurements of mobility.

<u>ADL.</u> Routine daily activities related the extent of pain in dressing and undressing, walking, running, climbing stairs, bending over a washbasin, sitting for extended periods, making the bed and so on; twelve such daily activities were specified. At each examination patients were asked to record their pain perception of each activity on a visual analogue scale, 0 on the scale denoting no pain and no restriction, and 100 as aggravated pain causing complete restriction of that activity. Outcomes were in the increase or decrease in the numbers of activities performed with <50 % pain compared to those numbers prior to treatment

Pain was subjectively assessed by presenting to patients 83 words describing its sensory intensity or affect, that is, in the quality of unpleasantness. The index was the numbers recorded at the preliminary examination, after treatment and at the final follow up. An additional subjective measure was in the assessment of pain after treatment and at follow-up recorded as 'improved', 'unchanged' or 'worse'.

Mobility was measured in degrees of flexion, extension, lateral flexion of the back and the straight leg raise at commencement, after treatments and at follow-up.

<u>Statistical analyses:</u> inter group comparisons of data for the treated and the control group were by the Student t-test used for two independent samples. ANOVA was used for multiple comparisons of outcomes. The numbers of patients for final analyses of responses to treatment were 27 treated and 10 of control group. From the original numbers 6 patients were excluded for not having satisfied or complied with the protocol.

Group Comparisons and Results

Demographic inclusion data of patients from the private clinic, research clinic and the control group showed no significant differences between them. Treated patients had a total of 6.8 ± 2.2 which included the three trials. Statistically significant improvement was seen on mobility, pain words and subjective pain. ADL did not show such improvement but the control group 6 weeks after the end of treatment had deteriorated on this measure. The treated group showed improvement on other measures.

7 patients chose to continue with MS, 9 with LF and 11 with HF acupuncture. For ADL and subjective pain assessments the LF group showed highly significant improvement, maintained into the follow-up. The details of the outcome between these modes are shown in the figures in the Thesis. It was evident that the LF mode of acupuncture showed the best outcomes for a small group of patients with Nociceptive Low Back pain on significantly more measures than those treated by manual or high frequency electrical stimulation.

The control group for this study, 10 patients on the waiting list, made a comparison with the natural history of low back pain patients, untreated as against those treated by acupuncture. No placebo control was attempted. In allowing patients to experience all modes of acupuncture and then to choose the mode to continue treatment possibly increased patient expectation—a major factor in the placebo effect. At a clinic a therapist would consider a change if a particular treatment was perceived as unhelpful and, to that extent, we retain in a study protocol a semblance of procedures of the clinic. Physician/patient contact and communication are maintained in delivering treatment and the need to evaluate progress from the trial protocols and in treatment. The evidence gathered from clinical studies must avoid bias on the one hand but at the same time retain an authenticity to the practice of the clinic, another point of divergence between medication and hands-on therapy. The therapeutic context here is not comparable to decisions about medication.

Clinical studies on acupuncture show a wide variation in results, and scrupulous replications of protocols understandably will not reproduce the variables involved in the separate studies. While there is consensus from meta analyses that acupuncture helps chronic Low Back Pain there are no studies that specify pain as Nociceptive. For musculo-skeletal problems Nociceptive pains when chronic may form a category that responds to acupuncture.

STUDY V

<u>Postoperative Dental Pain and Acupuncture</u> (Paper in Thesis) Treatment of post-inflammatory pain as a result of trauma is standard practice but, in spite of expending much research to managing pains after the controlled trauma of surgery, the older medication—non steroidal anti-inflammatory agents supplemented when necessary with opiates is still in widespread use. Suggestions that preoperative (pre-emptive) or intraoperative delivery of analgesics could reduce post-operative pain and consumption of analgesics have, to an extent, been followed up. Studies have shown that patients needed less post-operative analgesics if given opiates either pre-operatively or combined with the infiltration of a local anaesthetic at the operation site prior to a general anaesthetic. Another study has recorded significant reduction to phantom limb pain if epidural blockades are performed prior to amputations[xix]. Such interventions prior to surgery were thought to inhibit nociceptive afferent activity, the hyper excitability of cells resulting from surgery. These conclusions are not established, nor are the mechanisms for the reduction of post-operative pain very clear. Our hypothesis for the above study involved the possibility that acupuncture mechanisms could influence the reduction of the hyper excitability in central afferent cells of the pathway for pain. If that assumption was valid an indicator of such an effect clinically would be to reduce post-operative consumption of analgesics.

Patients undergoing extractions of impacted 3rd molar mandibular teeth were our subjects for the trial using acupuncture preoperatively in one group and post-operatively in another. 50 patients for surgery were randomly distributed to each group. Extractions in all groups were performed using the usual local anaesthetic. 60 patients who had a similar extraction using only local anaesthesia were the control group to those 50 (25 & 25) who had additional acupuncture intervention

Stress and tension, factors in postoperative pain were evaluated by standard questionnaires prior to surgery.

Three acupuncture points on meridians small intestine 19, Stomach 5 & 7 on the face and two distal points Sanjiao (Triple Burner) 5 and Large Intestine 4, were used for the groups subjected to acupuncture.

The Results

Details are available in Paper V of the Thesis. A summary is provided here. The results strongly suggest that the acute Nociceptive pain of patients subjected to this type of dental surgery and given acupuncture either before or after surgery is not reduced but, on the contrary, is increased post-operatively. Comparison to the control group made this evident. 15 out of 24 patients given acupuncture pre-operatively required additional local anaesthetic during the extraction, and the patients in both groups receiving acupuncture had a greater consumption of analgesic for their pain following surgery. The finding also correlated with patients' pain ratings on a visual analogue scale. Levels of both sensory and affective (unpleasantness) pain, were recorded hourly for 72 hours (except while asleep) after surgery. Patients were provided with 20 tablets, aspirin with codeine, and instructions to use 1 or 2 tablets 1-4 times/day.

Discussion

Compared to the control group post-operative pain was greater amongst patients given acupuncture both pre-, and post-operatively for extraction of a molar tooth. The presumed rationale for the use of acupuncture was to reduce postoperative pain for this type of nociceptive pain, acute rather than chronic; we hypothesised its possibility by using needles inserted either postoperatively or preoperatively. The preoperative rationale was to inhibit the impulses arising in the pain pathway after this surgical procedure and thus to reduce its intensity.

The reasons for an outcome contrary to the assumptions which initiated this study can be considered. The usual stress prior to any surgical procedure may increase endogenous opioids and could conceivably reduce the post-operative pain. Acupuncture is also known to reduce tension and stress, and in this instance effectually inhibited that mechanism with an impact on postoperatve pain. The patients *not* consuming analgesic tablets after their surgery were 21%, 28% respectively in the Pre and Post-surgical acupuncture groups and 47% in the control group who had their routine surgery with the usual local anaesthetic.

Another feature of acupuncture use is an increase of activity, sympatholytic vasodilatation, provoking the condition of 'dry socket' in these groups where the reduced blood flow into the socket and a diminished clot are factors that retards healing, a significantly greater occurrence in the groups given acupuncture than in the controls. The delay in healing could have been a factor in the increased pain in these groups in this particular study.

STUDY VI

<u>Pain and discomfort of Primary dysmenorrhea is reduced by the pre-emptive use of acupuncture and Low Frequency TENS</u> (Draft of the paper in thesis, since published[xx])

Altered hormonal metabolism disturbs the control and regulatory role of hormones in the patterns of the menstrual cyclical. Uterine mechanics change and are followed by myometrial ischaemia and uterine pain which trigger impulses from muscle afferents to maintain its central cells in a state of hypersensitivity. Excitation of sensitised central cells of the pain pathway has been postulated as the cause of the pain of dysmenorrhea. With the regulatory role of hormones disturbed, increases to prostaglandin levels are seen which also contribute to the hypersensitivity of these cells. The pain of primary dysmenorrhea could be characterised as a chronic nociceptive, cyclical visceral pain.

The usual schedules for treatment with acupuncture or Transcutaneous Electrical Nerve Stimulation (TENS) at Low or High Frequencies begin with the onset of pain. There have, however, been claims for the pre-emptive use of nerve blocks and epidural anaesthesia for the reduction of postoperative pain. It is thought that the procedures have an inhibitory effect on the excitability of large diameter afferents of the sensory pathway to pain and their terminal cells which, therefore, reduces pain even when the barrage of excitatory impulses from the operation site reaches those cells. The present study was designed to explore that possibility using acupuncture and TENS at specific times before the onset of the pain in dysmenorrhea. Premenstrual treatment is distinctly more comfortable for the patient than treatment during painful periods. Studies by other groups had demonstrated the benefits of TENS used during the pain of menstruation.

Patients and Methods

Thirty one patients with primary dysmenorrhea and a duration of longer than 5 years were recruited from the Dept. of Karolinska Hospital and a private Clinic. The trials were conducted at the Clinic and the Karolinska Institute. Nineteen patients were assigned to be treated by acupuncture modes. Two patients later were excluded from the study as they had not completed their treatment schedules. Twelve patients underwent the treatment schedules with the different modalities of TENS

All patients maintained records of a) perceived pain levels on visual analogue scales, marked thrice daily for 5 days commencing with their periods. b) blood loss recorded as 'scanty', 'moderate', or 'excessive'. c) records of nausea and/or vomiting. d) Hours of work lost. e) daily intake of analgesics. These records having been noted in the month previous to commencement of treatment, patients also made a subjective assessment of whether treatment had made them 'better', 'no change' or 'worse' at the end of their scheduled treatment.

Acupuncture modes and treatment schedules

The points for acupuncture were on the meridian of the bladder. The points are shown in the figures in the thesis. The points selected were in an area innervated by spinal segments, Thoracic 12 to Lumbar 2, and Sacral 1&2. They are convergence segments of the splanchnic and pelvic nerves, innervating, amongst other organs, the uterus. This segmental innervation also applies to those of the leg. The points were: Urinary Bladder (UB) 32, bilateral, a midline point Conception Vessel 4, midway between the umbilicus and the pubic symphysis, and Spleen 6 and 9 in proximity to the medial tibial border on the leg.

The modes of acupuncture used were, 1) manual stimulation after insertion of needles, back and forth rotary twists to the needles eliciting an additional sensation of soreness or heaviness at the site. (In comparison to the apprentice training of the traditional therapist, this is the only possible practical elicitation of the De Qi or Chhi equivilant). 2) Low Frequency (LF) stimulation at 2 Hz, by attaching the electrodes of an electric stimulator to 2 pairs of needles, on the leg and back. 3) similarly, High Frequency (HF), stimulation at 100 Hz. Electrical stimulation was never at intensities uncomfortable for the patient, LF was adjusted to mild muscle fibre contractions and HF for a local paraesthesia 4) Periosteal Stimulation (PS), momentarily intense stimulation for seconds over the periosteum of the 4 points which were in the vicinity of bone, i.e. excluding point CV 4.

Transcutaneous electrical nerve stimulation (TENS) for the group directed to that form of treatment. A pair of rubber electrodes were placed paraspinally roughly covering Thoracic 10 to Lumbar 1, to transmit current from the stimulator. Methods employed were: 1) Low Frequency TENS (LFT) at 2Hz. 2) High Frequency TENS (HFT) at 100 Hz and 3) Placebo TENS where electrodes did not transmit current, although patients were informed that the very high intensity of current might not be perceptible as sensation.

Entry of patients to each mode was randomised, though treatment mode sequences were of a serial order, independent of where in the series treatment commenced. In the final month, that is the 5th for the acupuncture group, and 4th for the TENS group treatment was carried out in the mode of the patient's choosing. Treatment times lasted for 20 minutes.

The Results of 17 patients in the acupuncture group and 12 in the group receiving TENS were analysed. The mean age of the former group was 30.4 ± 7.7, and the latter 27.8 ± 5.5. The groups did not differ significantly in the age of onset of their menstruation or pre-treatment assessment of pain.

Acupuncture groups showed improvement in comparison to pre-treatment values and was seen on several outcome measures. Pain values, subjective assessments and tablet consumption showed significant improvement varying between $p < 0.05$ to $p < 0.001$; nausea and vomiting, and work hours lost had also improved. Tablet consumption with LF acupuncture while showing a reduction was not statistically significant. There was no change to blood loss after treatment. The pattern to improvement was seen after the 5th treatment and significant improvement continued to be seen at the long term follow-up (3 months) in this group.

TENS Those treated with LF stimulation showed a similar outcome to the above but not with the HF or Placebo TENS. However, the improvement with LF did not measure up to statistical significance. After the chosen 4th treatment this continued as the outcome, but in the long term only the subjective assessment showed a positive outcome with LFT.

It is likely that the effective modes of treatment as used here for dysmenorrhoea had an effect on central sensitisation. The evidence of post parturition suggests that during the intervening months a reduction to this type of sensitisation occurs before the menstrual cycle recommences. Hence the benefit of pregnancy on dysmenorrhea. Provided there is a premenstrual awareness of the time of onset, timely intervention with acupuncture modes or Low Frequency TENS may be a therapeutic alternative from the evidence of this study, limited though it was in the patient numbers.

The Development of a Therapeutic Tradition

A biological approach to acupuncture treatment and research entails considerable modification to traditional precepts. Classical training for traditional medicine was a period of apprenticeship which cannot be sustained as the model for teaching in the medical culture of today. It may not be warranted. However, a country like India, with a wide-spread of Religious Systems of thought, faith-based Traditional systems of Healing, maintains its teaching and methods through institutional training, in its epistemological theories and practice. Traditional practices, without reference to modern medicine, as clinical practice have their draw backs and hazards. These have been indicated in Ch. IV. We, however, are not aware of evidence-based merit to their use for patient pathology as defined in science. The use for diseases is in another epistemology. A strict practice of traditional acupuncture is as yet to be systematically attempted in clinical studies and we can hardly evaluate the value of such a practice for patient pathology. What we have, as demonstrated in the above studies, are biological practices of acupuncture which have been better researched, and generally pass off as an acupuncture practice. Method and protocols of clinical study do not easily accommodate a traditional approach to treatment. As for research, discarding aspects of acupuncture's ancient epistemology is necessary to make some sense of its biology. But that does not preclude the systematic comparison of practices.

A protocol for study where acupuncture treatment is uniform for a patient cohort is anathema in tradition where each patient has to be individually considered. Traditional diagnosis is a shifting not a stable entity, which means that acupuncture modalities also change during the course of treatment By ignoring these concepts we may be losing out on the benefits of its use, although achieving clinical evidence is the necessary pursuit in the present climate of unsupervised healing methods.

Some caution is not out of place when discussing 'evidence'. We are inundated with 'studies' and reviews, called 'acupuncture' studies. Studies of acupuncture using convincing routines of tradition are comparatively few, and those conducted within protocols that include patients treated by traditional acupuncturists according to their lights, at least as controls, are rare. We cannot possibly come to any conclusions without including the entire gamut of Acupuncture's therapeutic possibilities—which will undoubtedly strain the ingenuity of clinical research entailing: controls, randomisation, blinding and the elimination of bias. Pronouncements and evidence about acupuncture protocols suggesting the traditional use of acupuncture can hardly entertain its regulatory essentials in those methods of study.

In clinical practice acupuncture is used for reducing pain, increasing joint mobility, controlling certain chronic inflammatory problems of organs, or for diseases relating to immuno-endocrine deficiencies. Its use has been, with varying therapeutic efficiency, a part of establishment clinical practices. Further conviction has been attempted through basic research or attested in clinical trials and, past much of the scepticism that is encountered in science, to interpret to some extent acupuncture effects within biology. There is evidence in human and animal biology of effects on the neuro-humoral-immune axis. There has been continual research interest in this area. Sizeable practices in tradition, beyond establishment control or based in the autonomy of an indigenous public need, is very much in vogue. For people, effective response is apparently obtained in a wide spectrum of ailments, spanning innumerable therapeutic modes well beyond the medicine of science.

Amongst the host of traditional therapies, acupuncture, at least, has entered the portals of research and provided some worthwhile evidence for possible use and neurophysiological explanations of the background for its effects. But many recent versions of the practices of acupuncture have their own self-sustaining theories, while a few of them have convincing research support. Theories about acupuncture routines for treatment in modern medicine generally lack evidence in clinical trials. The sizable work on the neural transmission involved in pain perception and its inhibition offers a general understanding of how acupuncture mechanisms may offset pain. But so far that evidence does not prescribe a set of regulations for its use in patient problems as have been prescribed in its traditional practice. In other areas extrapolative evidence from work on animals and healthy human volunteers are supportive of some of the further hypotheses on acupuncture, including those of endogenous opioid mediation (Basbaum and Fields, 1978; Pomeranz, 1981; Mayer 1988).

The research professional in this field reaching out to the Infallible Placebo, and the traditionalist adhering to the sufficiency of his Theory, each has his arbiter. In brief, many studies show evidence of substantial therapeutic effect. But the variety of methods used in different studies often lack the stringency expected of therapeutic research, undermining the validity of that evidence. Studies that gather data of the many clinical trials into a protocol of meta-analyses are ranked high in value for determining effectiveness. In the context of acupuncture, it is a steam roller; multiple data gathered from mutually incompatible study protocols and then graded for quality.

Individual studies use different but relevant protocols to elucidate, not merely outcome, but a diversity of parameters relating to its use. Acupuncture (unlike medication) cannot be a uniform and standardised input for the patient, nor can response to pathology override the individual's physiological response. Protocols attempt to overcome the issues in blinding and randomisation. It is not surprising that meta-analyses, which essentially focus on effective outcome, are seen to contradict those of well-designed individual studies. Protocols and methodology for assessing the effectiveness of pharmacological substances on patients do not easily transform to hands-on therapies. On the value scale for methodology, the evidence ranks high for studies with placebo controls. An acupuncture placebo control may be regarded as the claim for quality for the meta-analysis of acupuncture studies, but what is often dismissed or unaccounted for is that no inertness can be claimed or contrived for a sensory input; ergo its placebo does not exist. Most often it confounds the protocol, since its control is a modality of peripheral sensory stimulation rather than a placebo. A convincing placebo study is well-nigh impossible and outcomes claimed for 'placebo acupuncture' are, therefore, questionable. 'Sham' acupuncture, superficial acupuncture, or even contrivances offering non-penetration functions as a Peripheral Sensory Stimulus (PSS) and according to some searching for its Science PSS constitutes acupuncture. The subject of placebo gets some attention in the next chapter.

CHAPTER VIII

PLACEBO; BEECHER TO BENEDETTI

"Nothing in Biology Makes Sense Except in the Light of Evolution".
Theodosius Dobzhansky. The American Biology Teacher March 1973

"We are the D-Day dodgers, in sunny Italee" the cynical opening line to the song of the survivors of the Eighth Army who felt their combat contribution on the beaches of Southern Italy was belittled in comparison to the later definitive and more conclusive battles of the Allied armies which followed D-day and the war in Normandy. Many of the casualties on the bitterly fought Anzio beachheads of Italy in World War II were, indeed, permanently out of the war, but their contribution in retrospect is not diminished as the song suggests. Apart from the strategic merits of the war on the beaches of Italy, its injured soldiers provided the patient material for Beecher's work on pain in battle injuries. Their responses to often fearful injuries, and Beecher's observations and studies have helped carry aspects of pain research forward.

The study noted a paradox that patients were not unduly distressed by pain despite mutilating and extensive injuries, and this fact was objectively signalled in their minimal need of narcotics. Dupuytren, more than a hundred years previous to Beecher, had made similar observations on battlefront injury, but Beecher's was a systematic contribution made in the classic paper[i], where he recorded findings on 225 consecutive patients with five types of major injury. Their immediate responses to injury continued his interest in the phenomenon of the 'placebo'. Along with later studies, Beecher was able to stress the importance of the context in which the injury was sustained: war as compared with injury in civilian life, and the variable perception of human pain relating to its context.

From 225 battlefront casualties he excluded those in shock or where head injury had altered sensory responses, and was left with data on 215 patients. The injuries categorised were extensive soft tissue injury; compound fractures of long bones; penetrating trauma of thorax, abdomen, and head (cerebrum); with 50 patients each except the cerebral injury group, which had 15. Sixty-nine patients (32%) reported as being pain free on arrival at the forward hospital unit. That percentage repeats in his later study series with placebo controls for conditions of severe post-operative wound pain included with the figures from other placebo studies and reviewed by him. Placebo significance to therapeutic procedure was reiterated in that review and was stressed as a control for clinical trials.

Beecher deduced reasons for differences in opiate requirements in civilian post-surgical patients which were far higher compared to the wounded in combat, and he also noted its sometimes unwise use in treating the latter. Despite the magnitude of the injuries that soldiers suffered he surmised that their experience of less pain than expected was associated with their transfer from the immediate dangers of the battlefront to the sanctuary of a base hospital, and the immensity of relief in the further prospect of release from the war due to their injury. The patients in the civilian context had requirements of morphine generally far greater. The situation for them, on the other hand, was not relief, as experienced amongst the battlefront casualties, but the anxieties of prolonged hospitalisation after surgery, combined with uncertainty and the possibility of being permanently maimed with its implications for their, future, family, jobs and security[ii].

Beecher's original paper brought into focus the importance of pain following injury and the differing perception of that sensation depending on the circumstances of sustaining injury. An interesting footnote consists of a soldier maintaining that he had no wound pain but, like a normal patient, he could still vigorously protest at a 'venipuncture ineptly done'. Soldier casualties, it should be noted, on an average had already received 26 mgm of morphine before being transported from the front line to the time of their questioning at the base hospital 5-7 hours later. But the paper states that 36 patients received no morphine. 69 of the injured maintained that they had been pain free at the time of arrival at the hospital, but there is no record of whether or not there were soldiers amongst them who had not received morphine. Beecher's criticism of the pharmacological management of casualties by routine morphine administration for distressing conditions due to thirst, shock and agitation extends observations beyond that of just 'pain in men wounded in battle'.

Beecher's continuing studies were taken up with the issue of 'placebo' controls for clinical trials on Pain. The paper on the "The Powerful Placebo". (JAMA 1955) concludes with data from his own and other studies in civilian hospitals on the potency of placebo to command an impressive ± 30% of relief with therapy. Symptomatic relief is not the only expectation from placebo. It may extend to pathological manifestations of troublesome but real side effects with therapy or with placebo administration; weakness, palpitation and so on, and here he refers to the Wolf and Pinsky figures included in the paper. They note that after treatment one patient with placebo developed "a diffuse rash—itchy, erythematous and maculopapular—" descriptively sufficient and, as quoted by Beecher "it was diagnosed in referral to the skin specialist as 'dermatitis medicamentosa'. For the patient suffering this, it was a Panglossian diagnosis, having subsided on the withdrawal of the placebo!

Beecher insisted that placebo studies follow the methodology of two arms for a clinical trial, the one with patients receiving the drug, the other with 'placebo'. In their own patient series placebo provided 'satisfactory' relief of severe post-operative pain—50% or greater, checked at two intervals of 45 and 90 minutes after administration. In their studies over several years he states the figure was consistent, "—at an impressively high level, generally above the 30% mentioned.". His papers return *to the context of injury* in the need for analgesia. 87 % of his civilian post-surgical patients required more analgesia for pain, whereas only one third to one fourth of battlefield casualties requested it.

The patients assigned to a placebo group who demonstrate reduced pain in the protocol of a trial and combatants with relative lack of pain following injury in battle must mobilise inhibitory pathways modulating pain. What we know of placebo mechanisms and pain inhibition suggest the activation of common neural inhibitory networks at the level of the rostral anterior cingulate cortex (rACC), an area of CNS pathway involving endogenous opioids. Positron Emission Tomography (PET) shows the brain region to be activated by both the placebo as well as opioid agonists[iii]. Present research appears to favour 'expectation' as a cognitive factor mobilising analgesic mechanisms. However, the reactions following injuries in battle cannot be the expectation of benefit attributed to treatment. As acknowledged by Beecher, reduced pain in the injured is in the aftermath of pronounced relief at the prospect of permanent release from a battle situation. The soldier was for weeks or months under enemy fire, seeing fallen comrades and generally subject to the immense uncertainties of survival prior to being wounded himself. Less pain was a manifestation of the sudden termination of terror and overwhelming anxiety amongst personnel of a largely voluntary army. In battle he must accomplish yet survive, requiring an intense degree of attention. Injury pain may have been unperceived in the attention operative in the circumstance of battle, but injury finally obtained him a sanctuary from its anxieties.

Unlike 'placebo', a manipulated process in a clinical trial with expectation as the cue, the soldier contends with danger, with ongoing circumstances of uncertainty and fear, abstractions which culminate in a sudden reality. It is an unique context impossible to replicate. However different the context of battle injury and placebo cues are, a common neural mechanism is activated and directs pain inhibition. Cognitive-evaluative activation is an extension of the evolutionary features of organisms to human biological systems.

The placebo response is a conditioned response in the context of treatment to patient's concern, and hope of obtaining relief, and in present discussions, from pain. Beecher related the context as important. The perception of pain in injured soldiers differs from that felt by patients injured in civilian life and depends on their respective evaluation of their situation rather than the magnitude of injury. Both involve the somatic, excitatory and inhibitory neural pathways and the autonomic systems but responses vary to the context. Beecher's studies with similar systematic ones[iv] offered documentation of war, civilian injury and post-operative narcotic requirements. These were pioneering studies which helped establish special institutional organisation and management for the care of victims of accidents and trauma in present day societies.

Benedetti et al. The Placebo[v].

The civilian patient regards injury and its aftermath with considerable concern and insecurity in the future, and its immediacy has an impact very different from war injury. Patient pain has been considered in controlled post-operative studies, providing even more information on the subject of 'placebo'.

The routine introductions of placebo controls in randomised study trials are to quantify the efficacy of a drug or pharmaceutical ingredient from other factors in the therapeutic process. The methodology was needed to substantiate therapeutic efficacy in compliance with the mandatory requirements of the regulatory body before the pharmaceutical industry could introduce any new product into the market as effective and safe use for patients. However, the subject of placebo for clinical trials of therapeutic procedure has also raised a number of concerns and pertinent questions about the adequacy of method for its conclusions. The Benedetti group have studied the procedure extensively and made interesting observations on the subject. Amongst a list of problems encountered in the conduct of trials they refer to a principle originally stated in physics by Heisenberger: that any measurement is apt to change the dynamics of a system undergoing the measurement. While the principle applies to measurement of atomic or subatomic particles, their momentum or position, that value, in its determination by the observer is not a constant. The implication which they demonstrate in a well-designed trial using placebo controls in post-operative pain is that human response in measurements is subject to fluctuation. Other variables are the natural history of the condition that causes pain, regression to the mean etc., and allowance must be made for inconsistencies to measurements in patient trials, including those with the placebo as a control. Regression to the mean is the statistical assessment of the likely difference to patient's pain intensity at the outset of treatment when it had peaked as against its later measurement; a difference that could occur anyway and is not necessarily attributable to treatment benefit.

Of the dynamic biochemical systems of life those that respond to environmental stimuli have a specific organisation and carry its markings in biological and individual genetic variability. As such there is the likelihood of uniqueness to systemic adjustments amongst subjects or patients in the recruitment for experimental or clinical trial. Following explanations and, on their understanding of the experiment, consents to be signed, those ethical requirements in place for trials, patients and subjects form diverse awareness and expectations which, of course, differ from the expectations from a routine clinic attendance. The assumption that there is neutrality to a trial procedure, as made out by the bald statements of the protocol, is not the reality seen by the patient. Volunteer subjects and patients alike come to terms in their different ways in their understanding of trial procedures in situations quite unlike a visit to their physician for treatment. Clinical trials involving pain measures, further, depend on individual patient assessments of a sensation—subjective and necessarily related to its perceived intensity and quality. The placebo has been demonstrated in a number of related studies by the Benedetti group to be generally unreliable for the purpose of assessing drug effectiveness. The fluxes in experimental measurements of biological systems are considerable and increased by the uncertainties and differences of cognition and awareness in the individual.

The psychosocial context influences the individual's awareness of pain. Cognition bears on the variability, its perception mediated through a neural network for pain. The variability is dependent partly on biochemical balances, one of them between endogenously released cholecystokinin and opioid. Proglumide is an antagonist to cholecystokinin. Administered in the context of the patient's ordinary awareness of receiving treatment the balance will be tilted in favour of the endogenous opioid having blocked the cholecystokinin effect. Proglumide will thus function as an analgesic.

Within the setting of the therapeutic trial the use of 'hidden' delivery of medication provided substantiation of the proposition that stability in patient responses does not necessarily follow the dosages assumed to be effective for their pain. Using Proglumide the group were able to study this. Within trial strategies, with three patient arms conducted on classical lines, an analgesic effect of Proglumide was indeed seen. Administration of Proglumide proved a better analgesic than a placebo. The placebo, in turn, was better than no medication. These trials on postoperative patient pain went on to include a computer pump programmed to deliver proglumide *without patient awareness* of receiving it. In that event it was demonstrated that the patient felt no analgesic effect at all. Proglumide only acted as an analgesic within the cue provided to the conscious patient that the treatment he was receiving was the injection of a pain-killer. Proglumide in that context enhances opioid-mediated placebo effects.

Hidden delivery of medication was also used with morphine or non-opioid analgesics and again provided interesting results. With hidden delivery morphine dosages of 12 mg were required to achieve a level of analgesia which could be obtained with saline (as placebo) if injected and given to patients as the painkiller. The same level of analgesia could also be achieved by morphine in reduced dosages of 6-8 mgm provided they were administered with the patients' knowledge and in open view. These procedures of hidden and open injections of other commonly used analgesics—tramadol, ketorolac, etc. in a series of experiments conducted on patients in postoperative pain, generally led to discrepancies in dosage for effectiveness. A higher dosage was needed to obtain a 50% reduction of pain with hidden infusions than when the pain killer was given with the patients' knowledge. Another analysis found patients' postoperative pain to be of greater intensity when they were unaware of receiving the analgesic dose than when they were told that they were receiving an injection of the pain killer although given at the same dosage as the hidden delivery of the drug. These experiments provide reasonably conclusive evidence of the unreliability of drawing conclusions about trials with placebo control to establish the efficacy of drugs and dosages.

In the study it was shown that naloxone also could block the effect of the difference between 'openly' injected pain-killer substances and their hidden administration. Naloxone, the antagonist to opioids, blocks their pain reduction to the extent that they are involved in the placebo effect. The expectation involved in treatment procedures is also shown to be mediated by endogenous opioids. We can speculate about the expectation factor in general, the extent of patients' doubts and attitudes as to whether being administered treatment etc., in turn relating to placebo related analgesia an endogenous variable within the setting of a trial.

However, when interviewed in controlled trials, patients receiving placebo attributed improvement to their 'treatment'; presumably they 'hoped' past doubts that they were amongst those receiving the true drugs. Such imposed confusions in investigator explanation, may be circumvented for some patients, as candidates still entertain the possibility of therapeutic intervention to activate the endogenous mechanism toward pain relief. For these reasons, the Benedetti group suggest that, as an alternative in clinical trials, placebo might be replaced by hidden injections to obtain values attributable solely to the drug. The relevance of that value may not necessarily conform to the outcome experienced by an individual patient in his day-to-day negotiation of treatment in the clinic environment where contextual confusions of trial procedure are not contended with. The question of trial methodology within their alternatives has to be sufficient as evidence for regulatory bodies. For the clinician, the evidence is information, not the arbiter for determining his treatment for a patient.

Placebo activates biochemical mechanisms in patients or subjects and their responses depend on the context in which it is instituted. Placebo responses and the ones activated by the therapeutic ingredient on trial have some common pathways. The degree of the factual power of a therapy or a drug may always be supplemented since it functions like a conditioned stimulus in the context of a trial. Its value cannot be deduced in the simple resort to a separate placebo control. Endogenous opioid pathways may be activated by placebo, but placebo depends on the cues that provide the expectation of benefit. Expectation and the cues toward it are the highly relevant cognitive adjuncts to any therapeutic process. Hence, outcomes in classical trials on pain alter merely through changing the cue to the conditioned stimulus and can provide a benefit equivalent to that of the active therapeutic ingredient. Reverting to the Benedetti trials, 6-8 gms of either morphine given as hidden injection, or saline solution openly injected by the administrator, showed equal power in ameliorating pain in patients after oral surgery. A greater analgesic effect was recorded in these patients only when the morphine dosage was nearly doubled. Only hidden *administration of therapy* can overcome the cue of expectation, which the Benedetti experiments demonstrate well[vi],[vii].

Evolution and the placebo response

Nociception is a significant biological trait for the survival of species. Nociceptive responses manifest as patterns of behaviour, and in man that sensory perception, its quality and intensity, can be communicated as pain and also acknowledged in his behaviour. Nociceptive stimuli are likely to injure or, in the prospect of injury, initiate avoidance behaviour in the animal. Specific behavioural patterns are used experimentally to demonstrate nociception. The cue to a prospect of injury may also demonstrate patterns of similar behaviour.

Animals may use other cues which generate effective mechanisms to ease nociception. The lick of the tongue, a cue availed of by mammalian species, comes comparatively recently in evolution. The mother's 'kiss it better' is a likely extension of that cue to ease the hurt of a child. As the organism evolves in biological complexity its response to a nociceptive stimulus, frank injury or its likelihood (discernment of threat) will show appropriate nuances of behaviour learnt through or conditioned by the nature of environmental threat. Cognition at some level is essential to evaluating the threat as a cue. In a domesticated animal fear and fierce avoidance behaviour are usual when we attempt to inject an animal because it is seen as a threat or impending injury. For a patient, on the contrary, an injection is known to relieve pain, and therefore has a different cue value. An injectable is 'known' not merely to convey a pharmacological substance more rapidly than a swallowed tablet—some cultures insist that the needle—possibly in its associated perception—contains greater 'power' in therapeutic delivery than a drug by mouth. Conditioning and cues modulating pain are inputs that become complex as the organisms evaluative ability increases; the biological variables consequent to individual abstractions are additional capabilities in man. Despite the authority claimed for the protocol statistics can hardly iron out these patient variables in clinical trials with their small numbers.

Mechanisms built in to functional morphology increase in complexity in the evolution of species. The trait of nociception, while retaining primacy for rest as an aid to repair injury, demonstrates possibilities for behaviour other than rest. Evolution allows more than just the elemental manoeuvre required for the organism's survival. Nociception, per se, in enforcing rest may be a hindrance to staying alive in the threats posed by the environment but, if they are seen as cues, appropriate mechanisms are activated to minimise nociception, allowing the necessary behaviour against a predator. We have seen nociception or pain following injury to be at abeyance in attention and anxiety—a response of animal or man through recognition of environmental factors. Awareness of danger means that nociception must decrease following injury to negotiate the animal's survival either in 'flight or fight'. In his immediate responses, conditioning to threat is apparent, but an additional feature for man is that the response may modify within the groups' antecedent cultural experience.

Homo sapiens, possibly the lone survivor of the habiline tool-making species, continually enhance biological complexity even within a comparatively short evolutionary span. Finding sustenance and survival in his environment was easier, and food requirements less, as stature and muscle bulk reduced and foods became more digestible through the genetic novelty of his jaw, dentine structure and alimentary tract. Physique and functional morphology adjusted for his bipedal gait as he gained in terrestrial mobility, and allowed the human hand, particularly the thumb, unprecedented utility for better survival and fitness. The hand gained sentient qualities in evolution and its use implied evolving sensory and motor functions, and enhanced and improved mental capacity well beyond those of prior species. The hand made a considerable expanse in neural connectivity, interrelated to an increase in brain size of immense consequence to human cognition and the ability to learn. Tool-making coordinated brain and hand use with ever increasing sophistication, a corollary to newer CNS substrates. The hand and its neurology were the evolutionary contribution invaluable to the increase of man's mental capabilities and power to abstract concepts.

The skin of 'the hairless ape' is another development that reflected increased volume to the Central Nervous System. The features of fur-wrapped ancestral skin were revamped for sensory and reflex thermo-regulatory responses. As man converted to more permanent habitation, avoiding the constant wanderings, haphazard sustenance and danger, and discovering fire and its warmth, his skin adapted biologically to the environment. Skin morphology evolved to maintain homeostasis with an increase in that organ's dynamic qualities, vasculature and sensory modalities, and with greater amount and sensitivity of receptors to heat and cold, and numbers of sweat glands. Skin sensitivity to climatic change had evolutionary advantages and entailed increased neuronal connectivity as sensory and vascular autonomic motor reflex functions heightened responses to control heat gain and loss to maintain equitable body temperature. There was a simultaneous increase to the higher centres in connectivity from the neuronal cells of the dorsal horn where the reflexes for those controls were mediated. The changing morphology of human skin was a factor in quantitative and qualitative interneuronal increases, including those of brain tissue.

Groups form amongst species. Homo sapiens devolve activities for common social ends in tribal groups, having devised tools as means to achieve those ends. The means for negotiating a predatory, hostile and inclement environment lies in the awareness and perceptions obtained in his mental advance, and the ability to innovate, communicate and verbalise. A social structure commences in functional relationships—sub-groups making for the viability of the tribe and its common welfare in divisions of labour. The agency for healing may occupy only a few thousand years of man's history, but commenced in one such group activity. In transactions with the powers of the unknown by invocations and chants, fire and smoke, the incenses of burning herbs, these pristine sentient cues provided elementary forms of therapy. Initially therapeutics existed only in supportive socio-biological cues learnt and ingrained in the beginnings of human culture. Therapies emerged as cultural systems and practices for healing became more complex biological processes. We have noted that cognition plays a large and variable role in pain, its perception and self-generated healing. Physiological mechanisms may be more rapidly mobilised in the responses to pain in comparison with nociception and man's ability for abstraction. Culture and cues cast the process in the therapeutic mould.

Humans occupy but a small fraction of the evolutionary time-scale of life, but the variations in this species show sharp, random and unpredictable changes in gene mutation, selection and adaptation. On that scale simple organisms like bacteria formed a substantial part, with minimal increases in complexity over their billions of years. While the relative period of man's existence commencing from his hominid ancestor are measured only in millions of years, the evidence is that a few a genetic traits adapted from other mammalian species, and subject to rapid selection for their survival value, hasten his evolution. One example is considered below.

The trait of pain illustrates such genetic modifications. There are innumerable variables in the function and perception of pain as effected in man's evolution in response to environment and culture. Positive selection in some groups of mammalian genes appears to rapidly amplify possibilities offering features to adapt and modify the responses of the organism. The family of mas-related genes (MRG) expresses on specific nociceptive neurons and allows their ligand properties and protein expression to change. Rapid molecular evolution towards pain mechanisms yield the dynamism to this trait, allowing for species' survival and individual variability. Perceptual complexities within cognitive-evaluative social interaction (cultures) are immense and possibly the variables brought about through genetic modification allow the human species and their individuals to perceive pain in a complex and nuanced manner.

Mas-Related-Genes (MRG) are a family of genes that demonstrate positive selection and they are implicated in the modulation of nociception. As such, MRG encode a large group of receptors but are expressed only on highly specialised subset of sensory neurons at the dorsal roots and trigeminal ganglia, including the cytoplasm of C-fibre terminals. These restricted neurons and their particular opioid receptors manifest special features in their ligand properties by virtue of positive selection genes; while the general run of opioid receptors have a wider systemic distribution but show no evidence of positive selection. MRG encoded groups in the expression of genes enable rapid evolutionary features by creating novel receptor-ligand interactions, and offer variety and greater adaptability to the host's experience of pain or nociceptive properties, as can be noted in the human and mouse versions of MRG. Murine versions of MRG allow variations to the perception of nociceptive stimuli even within the same species of laboratory mice. For man and mouse, rapid change by positive selection to receptors on nociceptive sensory nerves provide pain responses which reflect a better survival value or adaptability and a better suited response to his environment[viii].

Variant Pain Response and Research Implications

The diversity of receptor-ligand properties created bears on intra-species pain. Man's responses to pain show great variability, but pain in its adaptability has a bearing on survival, for example, as seen in injuries sustained in different contexts. Rapid changes to genetic material have evolutionary significance in some species enabled with positive selection genes. But cues are triggered in culture, as in rituals: barefoot walkers over glowing coals, or spikes apparently inserted painlessly through cheeks, or in the group culture of warfare, are extreme examples of pain modulation. Cultural cues transmit their sustained imprint on human pain.

Patients who when treated show rapid improvement the 'Responders' have been posed as a group within the context of treatment with acupuncture[ix]. It is uncertain whether their response is due to individual biological variability to the stimulus of the needle as suggested by Felix Mann, or whether it lies in the power of that particular cue. We have noted with regard to the perception of pain, its relative absence or unimportance following battle injury, however gross, but which shows an intense awareness in civilian injury of a similar calibre. The importance of the cue in culture and environment is considerable. Venesection, for instance, was perceived as painful amongst some of Beecher's soldiers while their gross battle injuries caused comparatively little concern! Post-operative pain amongst injured soldiers of different ethnicity and cultures, treated for identical injury but in the military hospitals of their respective countries, demonstrate significant differences in the post-surgical requirement of morphine for their pain.

A patient in pain, therefore, in response to therapy reveals state-related variation in his requirement of analgesic to offset pain, and demonstrating that requirement as placebo may only partly answer for the value of therapy. In a clinical trial, patients after oral surgery had shown equal analgesic benefit with either a particular dose of morphine or to saline, the placebo in this context, but more effective analgesia was obtained when the morphine dosage was doubled. This is in contrast to the soldiers sustaining the grossest injury in battle, where pain hardly presented as a problem. While positive selection genes may account for a part of individual variability, we are only aware of an importance to the thread of cultures and cognition-related individual evaluations to modulating pain.

Pain, the placebo and specific treatment effects may also be viewed as developments to nociceptive modulation. Man responds to various cues, either social or uniquely individual, to deal with pain and decrease its perception. Cues can be effectively demonstrated in other species, but the outstanding complexities of placebo are noteworthy and demonstrable in human pain. The placebo, conceived as the conditioned stimuli for clinical research, is used on the patient to distinguish between the activity of a specific therapeutic ingredient, or a drug, and the biological capacity to enhance or mimic the effect of the drug. But pain and nociception are initiated in neural mechanisms, and inhibition can be an endogenously mediated function within that circuitry.

Agency regulates respective therapeutic procedures, whether in the delivery of drugs, hands-on therapy or surgical procedure, enhancing potency or its cue effectiveness. The attempts to negotiate them separately, to insulate the effects of one from the other, are difficult to achieve, as we have seen from the series of Benedetti trials. Experimental flux is amply demonstrated in the placebo and biological response measurements, making the evidence of a clinical trial by the placebo methodology never as stable as is assumed.

It is of some concern that clinical trial research uses a unique window to find standardised evidence for therapies. It relegates the biological variance of a patient response to therapeutic procedure to a factor to be separated from the evidence. In this discussion we note a few reasons for the heterogeneity of patient responses to pain. The pharmaceutical industry has to adhere to evidence of effect for standard dosages of their products before they can be promoted for public consumption. That is an issue of substantiating evidence for the use of a drug. But extensions of that method as are used to measure effectual response of patients seeking forms of therapy that find acceptance for the public contend with that appreciation in the evidence. The method only confirms, in the evidence of separate trials, that patient cohorts are not consistent in their responses to the same therapeutic procedure. We need to reconsider methods that convey the evidence of effectual response or otherwise. For much of therapeutics, the agency mediating its delivery to a patient and individual response to delivery are inductively related factors in the outcome. There is little reason to question that equation when the method presently most favoured has not provided sufficient stability to a concept that therapies have delineable values, one for the therapeutic ingredient, and another relating to the agency for its delivery or related factors, conceived as the artefact to treatment.

In evaluating hands-on therapies we are left with the proposition that methods for investigation must even out variables or biological individuality. Those studies with randomised protocols can only cast a pale statistical shadow across individual variability, but do not serve the purpose of overcoming them. The attempt to even out variability is possible if large patient numbers are involved, and that too only for the diagnostic cohort of the particular study. It is reasonable to assume that in replicating the study with another group with a similar diagnosis, the responses of the patients will not correspond to the original study. For therapies like acupuncture there is the further variable of individual response to acupuncture, dichotomised broadly in the term 'responders' and 'non-responders', which may in the future be resolved in further information relating to genetic variance. Again, individual response tends to vary with progressive treatment; an initial non-responder may show effective responses in the course of later treatment[x].

There are many contending factors and variables when patients in chronic pain are brought under a diagnostic category in these studies. With acupuncture for chronic 'back' or 'head and neck' pain, shortcomings to patient treatment may reflect in a diagnosis conceived as a problem of regional anatomy rather than the more specific pathophysiology of pain. Some patients may have a distinct neurogenic element to their back ache, others inflammatory and nociceptive pain following degenerative change, and yet others may have complex regional pain syndromes (CRPS) following surgery on their spine. Such pathophysiology cannot be ignored when treating chronic back ache or head and neck pain where the response to treatment differs and all the more so with acupuncture. Protocols with groups of patients with better definition in pain pathophysiology as above appear to respond more consistently to peripheral stimulatory techniques[xi].

Using acupuncture for pain or for any other diagnostic category, the therapist generally considers a few apparent features of the individual patient in deciding his stimulus inputs. Traditional medicine insists on patient individuality in treatment. But we have no evidence that the claim for individual therapy is factual or merely a nod to the epistemology of traditional therapeutics. Investigation of hands-on therapies conducted within the context of clinic and therapist, the latter's examination of the patient and recognition of specific therapeutic needs, and her confidence in his evaluative explanation are invariably a therapeutic input which are offset or denied by trial methodology.

Evidence for therapeutic efficacy can yet be confirmed or negated if arrived at by comparisons of routine treatment, conducted in their respective clinics with differing acupuncture practices. They would function as controls for one another. Detailed documentation should be maintained, and requisite patient data kept as predetermined by a protocol but without recourse to changes to the usual clinical procedures. Specific therapy and differing contextual factors can possibly be weighted and analysed as statistical outcomes of the results. But the clinic is the determinant of treatment. Any modifications and streamlining data should only be in further collaborative studies between clinics in their respective settings. They will eventually provide a data base of large patient numbers from which diagnostic categories could be reviewed for specific evidence. Obviously the short duration RCT clinical trials and protocols for a hands-on therapy like acupuncture could be pursued, but the format for such therapies should ultimately provide a data base from which more stable conclusions may emerge.

Reflections on the studies of Benedetti and Beecher

In the context of a clinical trial, randomised and conducted with controls like the placebo, there are inherent conflicts for the patient which he attempts to resolve. In accepting recruitment for a trial, individual patient reaction and apprehension bear on overall response and reflect in its measurement. Patient volunteers are subjects who accept their role to the solution of the problem by clinical trial and have its hypothesis explained by the investigator. They face uncertainties in the methodology of the trial, and one that they try to resolve, if possible, is whether they are receiving placebo or treatment. Past the confusions of assessing their subjective response they may be required to measure that response, and the subject (now hardly a patient) tends to relate experience to uncertainty in the blind trial protocol. The quandary for each patient will differ but will affect the response in clinical trials where hope for amelioration must persist. Trials are not conducive to an expectation of benefit compared to the reality in approaching his/her clinic for treatment. Patients obtain it without facing the predicaments of a clinical trial. Trials are contextually skewed and may suggest insufficiency to therapy, and reflect in the outcome to the extent that they deviate from the routines of a clinic.

Assessments of patients in a clinical trial where the methodology is directed toward avoiding patient/investigator bias leads to doubts and apprehensions for patient and therapist to a degree not encountered when treatment is ordinarily instituted. The contextual difference between the clinic and the disorientating circumstances of a clinical trial is ignored, but must reflect in the data. The occasional post trial questionnaires obviously cannot cover patient predicaments in their categories. Kaptchuk et al are on valuable record detailing the confusions and uncertainties of patients in such trials, and even the symptom relief they experience is questioned as to its reality or whether it is hope. Qualitative and comprehensive in depth interviews underline the unreality of clinical trials. The Kaptchuk[xii] et al interviews were conducted on a smaller group of patients amongst those recruited for a large placebo controlled study on irritable bowel syndrome. As compared with the measurement disturbance of the Heisenberger proposition for physical systems proposed by Beneditti as extending to measuring human response, we have maintained that measurement entails manifold biological and cultural variations in individual perception to pain; Kaptchuk demonstrates further imponderables of cognition confusing a patient's ability to make an assessment of treatment response when he is part of of an experiment.

In the method for achieving valid evidence, the Randomised Placebo Controlled trial, the separation of artefact—which includes therapist and other clinical cues ordinarily, present—retains the currently conceived essence of the biochemical ingredient of therapy. Separation involves a change to the value of therapy and placebo controlled investigations have been repeatedly questioned for the value thus obtained even for pharmaco-dynamic products. The Benedetti trials confirm this regarding pain when patients are unaware of the product delivery. Placebo controlled trials of drugs for pain offer a value, an effective dose for a drug, but that value is unstable if shorn of normally prevalent cues.

There are other sources of inconsistency that further confound answers from the classic trial design. Drug effectiveness for pain is generally accepted as the extent it exceeds the quantified relief shown in the outcomes of the placebo arm of the trial. Clinical trials of pain contend with profound variables, individual patient differences, notably the responders and the non-responders in the group. In the routine protocol of a trial we are unaware of patients who may be more or less responsive to the drug. Methodological changes to trials have been suggested in recognition of this[xiii].

In the immediate commencement of the effect of a drug in trials on pain, a responder may enhance relief of pain. It may be drug efficacy. The efficacy of the drug may also be a cue allowing the 'responder' to mobilise endogenous neural response in greater measure than would a non-responder patient. In other words, within the treatment group receiving the drug, there may well continue to be varying degrees of placebo function, which is a variable but a hidden factor in the outcome of the trial. Benefit manifest in the aftermath of drug action may reinforce the psycho-somatic networks and further the placebo response. Therefore, while a control group measures placebo (environmental conditioning), the group that is subject to the active pharmacological ingredient may continue the innate responses which could be placebo reinforcement and not directly or entirely attributable to drug efficacy. That value, though, is concealed in the final measurement of drug efficacy.

The two arm formula, a therapy cohort and a placebo control group, is never an absolute predictor of the result, effectiveness or its lack, with any particular therapeutic modality. Trials of placebo show widely varying rates of placebo response, and conclusions from them increasingly reveal inconsistencies that open up the discussion. The medical scientist is deeply bound to the role of placebo meant to answer virtual therapeutic efficacy. The placebo often unravels as putative therapy without necessarily designating value for the drug on trial. From the abstract of the paper above Colloca and Benedetti state, "The mental events induced by placebo administration can activate mechanisms that are similar to those activated by drugs, which indicates a similarity between psychosocial and pharmacodynamic effects". The attempt at drug and placebo delivery have come some way to deciding pharmacodynamic evidence for the drug or medication used for the trial, but as yet may only apply to the subjects of that particular context.

As placebo studies recognise complementarity to individual response, further innovations to study protocols have established that a program to screen patients before the definitive placebo two arm formula is applied could improve the evidence of dosage related response. The screening involves finding the levels by response titration, minimal to optimal drug efficacy, and with the least side effects amongst patients over a trial period before the more definitive trial protocol with placebo is started. The initial trial period helps stratify the patients in groups of 'responders', and is seen as an 'enrichment' program to the commencement of the trial. It is understood to provide more stable data[xiv].

The placebo trial in general poses considerable challenges to design. We are aware that the straightforward two arm formula to extract valid evidence has drawbacks even for drugs. To reduce certain other therapeutic modes to the RCT and control by placebo can evince evidence more confounding. The surmises from the trials are varied, ranging from reasonably conclusive outcomes through to less dependable ones, and to those where the demonstrated validity is questionable because the controls used for acupuncture were indeed 'sham' but hardly placebo.

There is increasing cause for concern in the ethics pertaining to experiments which demonstrate marked variability to placebo response. Within the established ethical norms for conducting trials it has been possible to slant protocols introducing surrogate treatment and manipulations, unknown to the patient. Manipulating a patient's response may appear legitimate for the purpose of assessing the worth of a product, there should, however, be little doubt or confusion regarding a social benefit as opposed to a commercial one. Patients unable to appreciate the purpose of an investigation or, worse, completely in the dark about the trial being conducted, have been used—for science. Clarifications of the science and biology of the placebo responses are valuable answers toward treatment, but investigations must rest within the ethics of medicine. Research has repeatedly controverted a medical tenet—the trust placed in his physician by a patient—on a global scale today.

The Benedetti group conducting the experiments referred to here are aware of the implications which they duly consider. It is difficult to draw a line about trials which have patient consent. Even so, those that are manipulative of patient confidence or trust should loom as an ethical issue. Wider acknowledgement, discussion and debate of procedures to understand the science behind placebo appears to take us uncomfortably beyond a methodology for evaluation of therapy into media exploitation. The history of medical science has more than a few unsavoury legacies to warrant a constant wariness to drug related research. Patient confidence in the system, already somewhat frayed, must not be further undermined by unawareness about the treatment and its control protocol on the part of the patient in agreeing to clinical trial, nor its implications of likely hazards.

This chapter deals with acute pain, its perception and relationship to the placebo. The pioneering work of Beecher on soldiers and their injuries at war, and that of the Benedetti group on patients with post-operative pain where the dimension of injury is minimised in the operative procedure, are a contrast in pain perception attributable to respective context and situation. Amongst the latter, reparative mechanisms, acute inflammatory and immune responses are already in place and the medication offered is in the context of expectation and confidence in treatment to minimise pain. Medication and therapies are designed to improve upon or aid the on-going mechanisms of healing which come into play from the time of injury.

Many more variables may need to be accounted for in clinical trials for patients in chronic pain, and a few relating to valorisation of evidence following treatment with acupuncture have been considered in previous chapters. Much of therapy hinges on the placebo enigma that is far from resolution; while there is little need for medication for pain amongst subjects of gross war injury, medication requirements and its 'placebo' component for patients with post-operative pain show great variations and uncertain values in clinical trial.

Treating pain with acupuncture is another instance where the available evidence obtained in similar method may well be contested. The 'evidence' for and against does not appear to have much relationship to the popular appeal of the therapy. One must assume the patient sees a benefit, despite research being inconclusive. Recommendation by a physician may be the background to acupuncture treatment; despite a lack of conviction in its merits there is awareness of the nature of its appeal. Educational support from health establishments in developed and developing countries is increasingly visible. The results of clinical trials have not substantiated its use yet it continues to be held as a therapeutic utility in spite of academic scepticism.

The clinical scientist should note that the passage of an outsider therapy like acupuncture into mainstream medicine has not needed the aids of marketing and other expensive promotions of the pharmaceutical industry for its products. That aspect of a therapy gaining access into the public domain should be part of the debate within the medical community. The question of evidence for acupuncture must be formulated for a subject's response to a therapeutic procedure which has not the simplicity to delivery of a pharmacodynamic product. A clinical trial for acupuncture poses the problem of deriving evidence from the procedure of inserting a needle and evoking a response from the subject's sensory attributes itself with qualitative potential that is apparent and claimed as being systematically manipulated for improved therapeutic effect.

Clinical trial methodology requires appropriate adaptation to a procedure of treatment before assessing patient responses and outcomes of the trial. The fact that the benefit obtained for patients must rest in a range of sensory responses to the manipulation of the needle after insertion obviates a convincing placebo control to account for numerous subjective sensory attributes. That is beyond clinical trial ingenuity, and obviously there is a lack of conviction to trials which necessitate the previous placebo control to be superseded by the next variant on the scene. It does suggest that the ultimate placebo for acupuncture has not arrived; finding a suitable 'placebo' control for an acupuncture trial is to negotiate the additional hurdle of numerous sensory variables amongst subjects or patients. The placebo was fashioned for a simpler mode of treatment delivery. The volunteer subject may ponder whether an effect derives from consuming the pill or its placebo, but their respective appearance and delivery being indistinguishable makes placebo control far more plausible.

Contextual studies like Beecher's mark the importance of systematic evidence for medicine but go further to understanding characteristic biological responses of a human group, soldiers at war, a social unit taught to function together when facing danger to themselves and comrades in the immense stress of battle. His study and its particular hypotheses is well supported in the recorded detail of observations, and in the documentation and data of features in the context of battle. Their implications have led beyond the original hypothesis to further understanding of pain and the reasons for its modulation and perception. Applications for research based in the concept of placebo are now routine controls for determining therapeutic evidence. Beecher's findings were in a context that obviously cannot be replicated or even simulated. The importance of understanding the evidence of reduced pain is only viable in its context. The evidence extracted from systematic data is partly empirical, but applications

287

enhance its validity. The evidence obtained in the original Beecher study is restricted and though its hypothesis was limited to to the context it has since stimulated invaluable applications of that powerful response; but the 'placebo' has also assumed a connotation in medical research such that it distracts from an essential value of a therapeutic ingredient. The biology of placebo to human well-being, since it is not a therapeutic contribution, must be considered an artefact. The concept brings therapeutic innovation into a slight conflict with evolutionary biological processes for self-limiting pain and disease.

In conclusion

Self-regulated healing is an evolutionary attribute with additional features which are developed and utilised in the history of human culture from the beginnings of man's social being. We have mentioned in other chapters some of the ancient rituals that promoted healing, diminished pain and dealt with mental disorder. These were cues initiating neural reflexes and biological responses conditioned by a communal culture for the individual's well-being and survival. Man's evolutionary history and the ability to mitigate pain from injury or to enhance his survival, extend through his social being. Pain symptoms and self-limiting illness are eased and healing hastened in numerous cultural cues that promote reflex neural and bio-endogenous responses. The responses are enhanced through cues including therapeutic ones and, while that contribution to therapy must be accepted, appropriately designed methodology should be used to validate and differentiate respective contributions of a therapeutic procedure.

Certain features of science may be detrimental, if not antagonistic, to the development of biological responses that are mobilised against disease. One example lies in the looming prevalence of bacterial resistance to medication. Understanding and improving human immunity and related mechanisms is invaluable to resisting diseases, especially those with a viral, bacterial or parasitic etiology. Immunity is yet another in-built feature of human response to disease. Pharmaceutical innovations generally threaten bacterial survival, while human immune responses resist bacterial ravages without necessarily eliminating the bacteria. Consolidating disease resistance by improved immunity is presently pursued with less vigour than the search for drugs to combat bacteria and bacterial resistance. Bacteria necessarily evolve in their hosts despite threats to it. But man's ingenuity with drugs has fostered resistant bacterial strains and thus increased their ability to transmit vigorously across hosts.

Transmittable diseases manifest in humans not merely in the presence of bacteria, but when inadequate nutrition reduces host immunity to their ubiquitous presence. Medical science and research attempt the pharmaceutical options to eliminate bacteria, to overcome their resistance to existing drugs. This, of course, is a medical imperative once a disease is manifest. But there are options open to promotion as ancillary aids to medication, if not of direct benefit to the patient. Greater attention needs be paid toward those well-worn possibilities. It is likely that bacteria will find methods to survive as we know they have done past the battery of antibiotics that were created for their elimination. The immense benefit of antibiotic development has also led to variant disease problems, while research ingenuity tries to re-establish the original promise and enthusiasm in the discovery of penicillin and other specific bactericidal agents. But after a few successful decades we face almost intractable problems. The recommended multi-pronged medication with drugs has not met with sufficient success to warrant that approach as an answer to the problem of bacterial resistance to single drugs in certain diseases. It is also a hedge to dealing with the indiscriminate use of antibiotics by the medical community, and the drug industry has obliged by the production of newer and more powerful antibiotics. In some parts of the world there was an indiscriminate, unwarranted use, and often over-the-counter sale of antibiotics: a windfall for the commerce in drugs but one which reinforces the survival and staying power of bacteria.

Improving human resistance by better nutrition and education must play a far larger role in combating disease, and developing that aspect requires better institutional funding—part of the process to constant development of immune research. The possibilities of specific immune responses, vaccines etc. are primarily important as an evolutionary choice for humans, but an approach that understandably finds less pharmacological enthusiasm.

The older therapeutic epistemologies stressed in their systems concepts to combating disease by building and improving the innate health capabilities of the subject. In present research and in the language of modern medicine we may attempt to rediscover such offerings, should they in fact exist. Every therapeutic system in any past civilisation, starting with herbal potions and concoctions, stressed dietary values and products to build resistance to disease. In the present pharmaceutical advances, if there is specific potential in TCM, Ayurveda, Siddha or Unanni towards boosting immunity, there are prospects to be explored but unlikely to enthuse commercial research.

Acupuncture epistemology has more direct reference to points with specific potency and some modern research is directed at those possibilities[xv]. Epistemological practices have empirical content sufficient to warrant investigation. There is a growing market and unsound media promotions for 'alternate therapies' but at the same time a marked disinclination by the institutional authorities responsible to the public for obtaining essential supervision over health care to confront their organisation. That need is replaced by a denigration of possible therapy like acupuncture after some generally inappropriate studies, but where others have suggested a degree of validity. There is a long way to go before the sceptics will concede that research does not lie in the search for the placebo for acupuncture or the insistence that acupuncture amounts to the placebo, and hence is not therapeutically valid.

I quote, "from Chapter titled 'The Remarkably Powerful Highly Underrated Placebo Response' in the book referenced below:

"Researchers have spent a lot of time and money studying acupuncture in people who claim it works. First they compared outcomes by inserting needles into correct or incorrect acupuncture points. No difference. Then they used both standard and retractable needles; patients felt the sting but did not know whether it had entered the skin. Again no difference.—"[xvi].

It is difficult to resist a comparison to the methods of G K Chesterton and Hillaire Belloc to discover the reason for inebriation "—by applying principles of pure Logic. They met one night and drank nothing but whisky and water, and they got drunk. They met the next evening and drank nothing but brandy and water and again they got drunk. They met the the third night and drank nothing but gin and water, and, they got drunk once again. They decided that as the constant factor was water it was obviously responsible—a conclusion which was probably most agreeable to Bacchic circles". This was related by Aneurin Bevan while countering the British Medical Associations assertion that it was his personal qualification—a Welshman to boot, that prevented them from reaching an accommodation over the National Health Service, whereas he was at pains to inform them that their problem was with every Minister of Health they negotiated with prior to his taking over the Ministry[xvii].

NOTES

Introduction

i   Celestial Lancets. A History & Rationale of Acupuncture & Moxa: Lu Gwei—Djen and Joseph Needham. Cambridge University Press 1980

ii   Porkett M. The Theoretical Foundations of Chinese Medicine. MIT Press, Cambridge. Mass. 1982

iii   *Secrets of the Silk Road* an exhibition at the Bowers Museum, Santa Anna, California. 2011, March 28-July 25 and Catalogue edited by Victor Mair, Bowers Museum.

iv   Science A Four Thousand Year History. Patricia Fara. Ch II, Interactions. Oxford University Press 2009

v   Al-Dabbagh SA. Ibn Al-Nafis and the pulmonary circulation. Lancet 1 978;1:1148

vi   Black Athena: The Afroasiatic Roots of Ancient Civilisation. Martin Bernal. Vintage 1991.

vii   Bull N Y Acad Med. 1936 July; 12(7): 446-462. Role of the Nestorians as the Connecting Link between Greek and Arabic Medicine Allen O. Whipple

viii   Notes from: Science and Medicine by Max Meyerhof In: The Legacy of Islam Eds: Sir Thomas Arnold & Alfred GOxford University Press Reprints from sheets of first edition, 1941, 1942, 1945

ix   Now, Let Me Tell You About My Appendectomy in Peking . . . By James Reston New York Times, Monday July 26, 1971

x   Compendium of Acupuncture

xi   Pain Mechanisms. a new theory R Melzack and P D Wall in Science, 150 (1965) 971-979.

xii   Pain. Problems pertaining to the transmission of nerve impulses which give rise to pain. W Noordenbos. Elsevier Publishing Company 1959

xiii   Complex Regional Pain Syndrome. Chapter 12, A Prospective Clinical Model for Investigating the Development of CRPS S P Stanos Jr et al. Progress in Pain Research and Management Vol.22 IASP Press

xiv   S Arnèr. Diffrentiation of Pain and Treatment Efficiency. Thesis (1991). Karolinska Institute, Stockholm, Sweden

xv   Moolamanil Thomas. Treatment of Pain with Acupuncture. Factors Influencing Outcome. Karolinska Institute. Thesis. 1995

xvi   Review in Pain 2009 3:15 Damien G Finniss, Michael K Nicholas and Fabrizzio Beneditti

xvii   See, Karl Popper. Vol. II, The Open Society and Its Enemies; Chapter 11, p 12.

xviii   The Placebo and the Placebo Response. Chapter 71. Patrick Wall in Textbook of Pain 3rd Edition 1994

xix   PAIN: vol 144 (1-2) Jly 2009 ref. editorial and Beneditti art

xx   Choi SS and Lahn BT, 2003 Adaptive evolution of MRG, a neuron dpecific ene famaily implicated in nociception. Genome Research 13, 2252-2259.

xxi   The structure of Scientific Revolutions. Thomas S Kuhn. 3rd Ed.1996

xxii   ebars, Dickensson and Besson. Diffuse noxious inhibitory controls (DNIC) I. Pain 6 (1979a) 283-304

xxiii   Acupuncture. Felix Mann Second Edition 1983 William Heinemann Medical Books Ltd, London.

xxiv   The Role of Traditional and Alternative Health Systems in Providing Health Care Options: Evidence from Kerala. Deepa Sankar. Health Policy Research Unit, Institute of Economic Growth. University Enclave Delhi 110007, India.

xxv   Aneurin Bevan. Volume II: by Michael Foot. Mcgibbon and Kee, 1962.

CHAPTER I

REDISCOVERING TRADITIONAL KNOWLEDGE IN SCIENTIFIC DISCIPLINES

i   *Han JS. The Neuro-chemical Basis of Pain Control by Acupuncture. Beijing, China: Hu Bei* Technical and Science Press; 1998.

ii   *Amoenitatum exoticarum politico-physico-medicarum fasciculi v, quibus continentur variae relationes, observationes & descriptiones rerum Persicarum & ulterioris Asiae, multâ attentione, in peregrinationibus per universum Orientum, collecta, ab auctore Engelberto Kaempfero. Lemgoviae, Typis & impensis* H.W. Meyeri, 1712.

iii   *Celestial Lancets,* Lu Gwei Djen and Joseph Needham. CH 6. *Influences on other cultures*

iv   *PAIN* Vol 6 Issue 3, Pages

v   Dickenson in Felix Mann

vi   see, Notes in CH. VII & VIII for a few studies published in Sweden.

vii   Amartya Sen, *History and the Enterprise of Knowledge. New Humanist: Volume 116 Issue 2 Summer* 2001,

viii   *Randomized controlled versus naturalistic studies: A new research agenda* Falk Leichsenring, PhD. Bulletin of the Menninger Clinic. Vol. 68. No 2 (Spring 2004)

ix   Bernal, Martin Black Athena: *Afroasiatic Roots of Classical Civilisations* Rutgers University Press 1987.

x   M Kline: *Mathematics: A Cultural Approach.* Reading, MA, Addison-Wesley.1962).

xi   Santillana, G. de 'on *forgotten sources in the history of Science'.* In A C Crombie, ed *Scientific Change: Historical Studies on the Intellectual, Social and Technical Conditions for Scientific Discovery and Technical Invention, from Antiquity to the Present.* pp 813-828. London 1963).

xxii   Ibid, IX

xxiii   *The Grand Titration. Science and Society in East and West.* Joseph Needham. George Allen and Unwin. 2nd Ed. 1976.

xxiv   C D Darlington. *The Evolution of Man and Society*, Simon & Schuster 1970

xv   Braudel, Fernand. *Civilization and Capitalism*. Vol!

xvi   Steven Fuller. *Prolegomena to a World History of Science in, Situating the History of Science*. Eds. Irfan Habib and Dhruv Raina, OUP 1999.

xvii   Josè Bové: *The Guardian Weekly*, June 28-July 4 2001;p 30

xviii   G G Joseph. Crest of the Peacock. Non-European Roots of Mathematics. Penguin. 1992

xix   Ibid xiv

xx   *History of Science and the Oikumene* by Romila Thapar: in, *Situating the History of Science*. Ed. Irfan Habib and Dhruv Raina. Oxford University Press, New Delhi, 1999.

xxi   *From the Ruins of Empire*. Pankaj Mishra

xxii   *Discovery of India*. Jawaharlal Nehru

xxiii   *Health Medicine and Empire*. Eds. Biswanath Pati and Mark Harrison. Orient Longman. Ltd., 2001

xxiv   (ref *From the Introduction to Colonialism and its Forms of Knowledge, The British in India*. Bernard S Cohn. Oxford University Press 1997),

xxv   Ramchandra Guha., *Savaging the Civilized—Verrier Elwin, his tribals and India*, University of Chicago Press; OUP.

xxvi   Bundgaard, H, *Indian Art Worlds in Contention*. Fischer Taschenbuch Verlag-Forum Wissenschaft Hochschule;, Surrey. Nordic Institute of Asian Studies, vol. 80

CHAPTER II

THERAPEUTIC SYSTEMS, KNOWLEDGE EXCHANGE AND ENHANCEMENT

i   J Weatherfield. *Early Andean experimental agriculture.*

ii   Steve Fuller in. *Situating the History of Science*. Eds. Irfan Habib & Dhruv Raina. OUP. 1999

iii   Norman Davies: *Europe. A History* Pimlico 1997, and Ibid xxiv

iv   *Frontline. A Tale of Two Horses*. Vol. 17, No 23, Nov. 11-24, 2000

v   A K Ramanujam. *Collected Essays. 'A hundred Ramayanas'* 1999.

vi   *Celestial Lancets*, Lu Gwei Djen and Joseph Needham.

vii   Bernard S Cohn. *Colonialism and its Forms of Knowledge*. O U P.

viii   Martin Bernal. *Black Athena*. Rutgers University Press. 1987.

ix   Ibid

x   Sir Steven Runciman: *'A History of the Crusades*, Volme 3, *The Kingdom of Acre'*; p 480. Cambridge University Press, 1955)

xi   *The Rise of Scientific Europe.* Ed, Goodman and Russell; Hodder and Stoughton 1991

xii   A L Basham. *The Wonder that was India*. Sidgwick and Jackson, London 1954.

xiii   Ibid XI

xiv   D Guthrie. A History of Medicine. J B Lippincot 1946

xv   Fernand Braudel, A History of Civilizations (1963), Penguin Books, 1995

xvi   *History of Science and the Oikumene* by Romila Thapar: in, *Situating the History of Science.* Ed. Irfan Habib and Dhruv Raina. Oxford University Press, New Delhi, 1999.

xvii   D J de Solla Price. *Science since Babylon.* New Haven, Connecticut, 1961

xviii   *The Structure of Scientific Revolutions.* Thomas S Kuhn 3rd Ed. University of Chicago Press

xix   *The Grand Titration. Science and Society in East and West.* Allen and Unwin, 1979

xx   *Situating the History of Science.* Ed. Irfan Habib and Dhruv Raina. Oxford University Press, New Delhi, 1999.

xxi   Fernand Braudel. *A History of Civilisations.* Penguin. (1995)

xxii   See, Oxford English Dictionary.

xxiii   Neshat Quaiser. Ch. in, *Health, Medicine &Empire.* Eds Biswamoy Patti and Mark Harrison Orient Longmans Ltd. New Delhi. 2001.

xxiv   *The Legacy of Islam* edited by Thomas Arnold and Alfred Guillaume. Oxford University Press 1931. See Science and Medicine. Max Meyerhof

xxv   *The Rise of Scientific Europe.* Ed, Goodman and Russell; Hodder and Stoughton 1991.

xxvi   Ibid, *The Legacy of Islam.*

xxvii   *The Crest of The Peacock.* George Gheverghese Joseph. Penguin Books. 1990

xxviii   A LBasham. *The Wonder That was India*, Reprint London Picador 2004.

xxix   Amartya Sen. 'Passage to China' NYR of Books Vol L1, Number 19

xxx   Ibid, xxiv.

xxxi   *A History of Science* Alexander Hellemans and Bryan Bunch; Simon and Schuster. Library of

xxxii   *The Birmingham Accident Hospital*, see Wikipedia, the free encyclopedia

xxxiii   Barbara Tuchman. *A Distant Mirror*: reprint Papermac 1995

xxxiv   Rosemary Fitzgerald *'Clinical Christianity'* in HM&E

xxxv   Joshua S Horn: *Away with all Pests: An English Surgeon in Peoples China.* Monthly Review Press 1971

xxxvi   *Two years without polio.* T Jacob John. The Hindu. Jan 14, 2013

xxxvii   Jean Dreze. Amartya Sen,: *An Uncertain Glory.* See, Statistical Appendices. Allen Lane. Penguin Publication. 2013.

xxxviii Ganapthy Mudhur. BMJ., 2001 Nov. 10, 323(7321) 1090

xxxix   Hookyas, in David Goodman *SCIENCE IN EUROPE* 1500-1800 VOLUME 2 A SECONDARY SOURCE ANTHOLOGY. Paperback—January 1, 1991

CHAPTER III

EPISTEMOLOGIES AND THERAPEUTIC ENHANCEMENT

i   *Lokāyata: Debiprasad Chattopadhyaya*, Peoples Publishing House; 1959

ii   G Thompson: *Aeschylus and Athens*. London 1941.—Religion. 1950

iii   Basham A L. *The wonder that was India.*, New York: Grove Press, 1959

iv   *Meyerhoff: in the Legacy of Islam*. eds Sir Thomas Arnold & Alfred Guillauame. OUP 1945.

v   S Radhakrishnan. *Eastern Religions and Western Thought*. OUP. 1959.

vi   Manfred Porkert *The Theoretical Foundations of Chinese Medicine*. MIT Press 1982.

vii   *The Crest of The Peacock. Non-European Roots of Mathematics* by George Gheverghese Joseph. Penguin Books 2000

viii   *The Essentials of Chinese Acupuncture*. Foreign Languages Press, Beijing. 1980,

ix   Yo San University, 13315 W. Washington Blvd. Los Angeles CA 90066

x   A J R MacDonald et al., *Superficial Acupuncture in the relief of Low Back Pain*. Annals of the Royal College of Surgeons of England. 65. 1983

xi   *The Business of ADHD.*, see in Frontline, PBS

CHAPTER IV

DICHOTOMISED MEDICINE AND SOCIAL IMPLICATIONS

i   *Textbook of Pain*. Eds P D Wall & R Melzack. Churchill Livingstone, 1994

ii   Chas Bountra. Rajesh Munglani. William K. Schmidt. editors, *Current Understanding, Emerging Therapies, and Novel Approaches to Drug Discovery* edited Marcel Dekker AG 2003.

iii   R Moynihan. '*Who pays for the Pizza*'. BMJ. 326: 1189-92. 5

iv   Arnèr, S. *Differentiation of Pain and Treatment Efficiency*. Thesis (1991). Karolinska Institute, Stockholm, Sweden

v   *A Prospective Clinical Model for Investigating the Development of CRPS*. S P Stanos, R N Harden, L Wagner-Raphael, S L Saltz. in *Complex Regional Pain Syndrome*. Eds. R N Harden, R Baron, W Janig *Progress in pain Research and Management* Volume 22, International Association for the Study of Pain. 2001

vi   Groopman, Jerome. *How Doctors Think*. Houghton Mifflin Company, New York 2007

vii   ePorkert M. *The Theoretical Foundations of Chinese Medicine. Systems of Correspondence*. MIT Press, Cambridge, Mass., (1982)

viii   Lu Gwei-Djen & Jospeph Needham. *Celestial Lancet*. Cambridge University Press 1980.

ix   Ibid. p202

x   Ibid. p141

xi   *The Role of Traditional and Alternative Health SystemsIn Providing Health Care Options: Evidence from Kerala.* Deepa Sankar* Health Policy Research Unit. Institute of Economic Growth. University Enclave Delhi 110007, INDIA. *Address for Correspondence

xii   1986 British Medical Association. *A Report 'Alternative Therapy',*

xiii   *Complementary Medicine. New Approaches to Good Practice.* British Medical Association 1991

xiv   Felix Mann. *Scientific Aspects of Acupuncture.* William Heinemann, London 1983

xv   AJR Macdonald et al. *Superficial Acupuncture in the Relief of Chronic Low Back Pain.* Ann. Royal Coll. of Surg. Engl. 65, 1983

xvi   R. A. Mashelkar, CSIR, Director General, quoted in, Hindu, Oct 27 '03)

xvii   Catherine Abbo. *Traditional Healing Practices for Severe Mental illnesses in two Districts of Eastern Uganda.* Karolinska Institutet, Stockholm, Sweden & Makarere University, Kampala, Uganda. Doctoral Thesis 2009.

xviii   *Kompendium i Akupunktur.* Akab Utbildning. Kungälv, Sweden. 1992

CHAPTER V

ACUPUNCTURE MECHANISMS

i   *Does Acupuncture Work?* Pain Clinical Updates: International Association for the Study of Pain. November 1996 Vol VI, Issue 4.

ii   Long Term—Head & Neck pain:

iii   S A Andersson, E Holmgren. *On acupuncture analgesia and the mechanism of pain.* Am J Chin Med 3 (1975) 311-334

iv   *Scientific Aspects of Acupuncture.* Felix Mann 1983 II Edition. William Heinemann Medical Books Ltd London

v   Karl Popper. *The Logic of Scientific Discovery.* Routledge Classics 2002

vi   P D Wall in *The Gate Control Theory of Pain mechanisms. A re-examination and restatement:* BRAIN (1978) 101, 1:18.

vii   Y Wan, S G Wilson, J-S Han, J S Mogil. *The effect of genotype on sensitivity to electroacupuncture analgesia. Pain* 91 (2001) 5-13.

viii   Macdonald, A.J.R et al, *Superficial acupuncture for the relief of chronic lowback pain.* Annals of the Royal College of Surgeons of England, 65 (1983) 44-46.

ix   Editorial, Berman & Bausell. Pain 85:2000, 313-315

x   (Kolmodin, G.M. and Skoglund, C.R. *Analysis of spinal interneurons activated by tactile nociceptive stimulation.* Acta Physiol. Scand., 50 (1960)

xi   Reynolds DV (1969) *Surgery in the rat during electrical analgesia induced by focal brain stimulation*. Science (Wash DC) 164:444-445

xii   B. Pomeranz, D. Chiu, *Naloxone blocks acupuncture analgesia and causes hyperalgesia: endorphin is implicated*, Life Sci. 19 (1976) 1757-1762.

xiii   W. Noordenbos. *PAIN*. Preliminary Statement. Elsevier 1959

xiv   P D Wall in *The Gate Control Theory of Pain mechanisms. A re-examination and restatement: BRAIN* (1978) 101, 1:18.

xv   *Culture and Pain*. Pain Clinical Updates. Kathryn E Lasch. Vol X, No 5. Dec.2002.

xvi   Kathleen K.S. Hui et al. *The integrated response of the human cerebro-cerebellar and limbic systems to acupuncture stimulation at ST 36 as evidenced by fMRI*. NeuroImage 27 (2005) 479-496.

xvii   *Kompendium i Akupunctur*. Akab utbildning.

xviii   Pomeranz B (1986) *Acupuncture neurophysiology*. In Adelman G (ed) *Encyclopedia of Neuroscience*. Birkhauser, Boston.

xix   Kawakita et al. in. *Japanese Acupuncture and Moxibustion* M 2005,1,16-26

xx   Ruda M A Opiates and pain pathways: demonstration of enkephalin synapses on dorsal horn projection neurons. Science (1982) 215: 1523-25.

xxi   Jacqueline Filshie and Adrian White. *Medical Acupuncture*. Churchill Livingstone

xxii   Andersson S A. *The Functional Background of Acupuncture Effects*. In (Ed) O Hook. Acupuncture. Scand. J. Rehab. Med. Suppl. 29 (1993) 31-60.

xxiii   LeBars D, Dickensson A H, Besson J M,. *Opiate anaesthesia and descending control systems*. In (Eds) J J Bonica, U Lindblom and A. Iggo. *Advances in Pain Research and Therapy*. Raven Press, New York (1983) 341-372

xxiv   *Diffuse Noxious Inhibitory Control*. Anthony Dickenson. Chapter 11. See, Felix Mann. *Scientific Aspects of Acupuncture*. 1983 II Edition. William Heinemann Medical Books Ltd London.

xxv   Ref. *American Journal of Chinese Medicine*. Vol. VIII, No. 4, pp 331-348. 1980 *Central Neurotransmitters and Acupuncture Analgesia*. J S Han, J Tang, M F Ren, S G Fan and X C Qiu. Dept. of Physiology. Peking Medical College, Peking, China.

CHAPTER VI

PAIN PHYSIOLOGY

i   *Gender, Pain and the Brain*. Pain, Clinical Updates, Vol. XVI, Issue 3. April 2008

ii   Clifford J. Woolf. *Pain: Moving from Symptom Control toward Mechanism—Specific Pharmacologic Management.*, Ann Intern Med 2004; 140: 441-451

iii   (Jänig W. CRPS-I and CRPS-II: *A strategic view. In: Complex regional Pain Syndrome, Progress in Pain Research and Management*. 2001:3-15.

iv   Pain Clinical Update. *Molecular Biology of Pain: Should Clinicians Care?* Issue, Vol. VIII, No 2, March 2000

v   *Peripheral mechanisms of opioid analgesia. Stein* C, Lang LJ. Curr Opin Pharmacol. 2009 Feb;9(1):3-8.

vi   Irene Lund. *Pain, its assesment and treatment using sensory stimulation techniques Methodological considerations.* Thesis, Karolinska Institutet, 2006.

vii   Howard L Fields. *Pain.* McGraw-Hill Book Company 1987.

viii   Wall and Melzack. *Text Book of Pain.* 3rd. Ed. Churchill Livingstone

ix   Baba H, Doubell TP, Woolf CJ. *Peripheral Inflammation facilitates Aβ fibre—mediated synaptic input to the substantia gelatinosa of the adult rat spinal cord.* J. Neurosci. 1999; 19: 859-869.

x   P.W Nathan. *The Gate Control Theory of Pain. A Critical Review.* Brain, 1976; Mar; 99 (1): 123-58.

xi   E. Haker *Lateral Epicondylalagia.* Thesis 1991

xii   P D Wall *The Gate Control Theory of Pain Mechanisms. A Re-examination and Restatement.* Brain, 1978, 101, 1-18.

xiii   Woolf C J, in *Pain.* Vol. 62: 1995, 1-128.

xiv   Willis. Volume 308, Issue 1136 of *Philosophical transactions of the Royal Society of London: Biological sciences*

xv   Treede RD et al. in *Pain.* 79. 1999:105-111

xvi   Greenspan, J D et al in Treede RD et al. *Pain.* 79. 1999:105-111

xvii   *Nature Medicine* 9, 1003-1008. 2003. Christoph Stein, Michael Schäfer & Halina Machelska Klinik für Anaesthesiologie und Operative Intensivmedizin, Freie Universität Berlin, Klinikum Benjamin Franklin, Hindenburgdamm 30, 12200 Berlin, Germany

xviii   Woolf C J. Pain: *Moving from Symptom Control toward Mechanism-Specific Pharmacologic Management: Physiology In Medicine.* Ed. Dennis A. Annals of Internal Medicine. 2004; 140: 441-451

xix   Bowsher, D. *The physiology of acupuncture.* J. Intractable Pain Society of GB and Ireland. 1987

xx   Makota Tsuda, Kazuhide Inoue and Michael W. Salter. *Neuropathic pain and spinal microglia: a big problem from molecules in 'small' glia.* In Trends in Neurosciences Vol 28 No 2 Feb 2005.

xxi   J D French. *The reticular formation,* J Neurosurg. 15. 1958

xxii   Kolmodin G M. Skoglund G R. *Analysis of spinal interneurons activated by tactile nociceptive stimulation* Acta Physiol. scand., 50 (1960) 337-355.

xxiii   Patrick Wall. *Introduction.* Melzack and Wall., *Text Book of Pain* 3rd Ed,. Churchill Livingstone. 1994

CHAPTER VII

TRADITION TO BIOLOGY

i   Lars-Erik Dryberg. *Effects of Somatic Stimulation in Chronic Musculoskeletal Pain.* Thesis. Department of Physiology and Pharmacology. Göteborg University, Sweden. 1998

ii   Gunilla Brodda Jansen. *Contributions of Calcitonin Gene Related Peptide in Ischaemia, Inflammation and Nociception.* Department of Physiology and Pharmacology, Karolinska Institute, Stockholm, Sweden. 1996

iii   Maria Blom. *Studies on Acupuncture Treatment of Xerostomia. Department of Physiology and Pharmacology,* Karolinska Institute, Stockholm, Sweden. 1999.

iv   Elisabet Stenner-Victorin. *Acupuncture in Reproductive Medicine. Departments of Obstetrics and Gynaecology.* Göteborg University, Sweden. 2000.

v   Pagel, Walter (2nd ed. 1982). Paracelsus: *An Introduction to Philosophical Medicine in the Era of the Renaissance.* Karger Publishers, Switzerland

vi   Karl Popper: *The Logic of Scientific Discovery.* Routledge Classics. London and New York. 2002

vii   *British Journal of Surgery* Volume 91, Issue 2, 146-150, February 2004

viii Andersson S A. *Pain Control by Sensory Stimulation.* In (Eds) J J Bonica, J C Liebeskind and D G Albe-Fessard. *Advances in Pain Research and Therapy.* Vol 3, Raven Press, New York 1979.

ix   Paul Offit. *Killing Us Softly.* Fourth Estate, London. 2013.

x   *Essentials of Chinese Acupuncture.* Foreign Languages Press, Beijing. First Ed. 1980

xi   Howard L Fields. *PAIN.* McGraw-Hill Book Company. 1987

xii   Han J S et al. *High and Low frequency elecrto-acupuncture Analgesia are mediated by different opioid peptides.* Pain (Suppl. 1984 a).

xiii Sjolund and Eriksson. In Vol 3. *Advances in Pain Research and Therapy* (Eds) Bonica, Albe-Fessard and Liebeskund

xiv   Moolamanil Thomas. *Treatment of Pain with Acupuncture.* Department of Physiology and Pharmacology, Thesis. Karolinska Hospital & Karolinska Institute. 1995

xv   Williams JBW and Spitzer RL. *Idiopathic Pain Disorder. A critique of Pain Prone Disorder.* J. Nerv. Ment. Dis. 170. 1982. 415-419.

xvi   Felix Mann. *Acupuncture.* William Heineman. 1983.

xvii *Health Care: Who Knows 'Best'?.* Jerome Groopman The New York Review of Books Feb 11, 2010 Andersson S A et al. *Electro-acupuncture. Effect on pain threshold measured with electrical stimulation of teeth.* Brain Res.63, (1973) 393-396.

xviii Bach S, Noreng M F and Tjellden N U. *Phantom limb pain in amputees during the first twelve months following limb amputaion after pre-operative lumbat epidural blockade.* Pain 33 (1988) 297-301.

xix   Bach. S. et al. Phantom limb pain in amputees during the first 12 months following amputation after preoperative lumbar epidural blockade. PAIN 33 (1988) 297-301.

xx   *Pain and discomfort of Primary dysmenorrhea is reduced by the pre-emptive use of acupuncture and Low Frequency TENS* (Thomas M, Lundeberg T, Bjork G, Lundstrom-Lindstet V. Eur J Phys Med Rehabil.1995;4:71-6.)

CHAPTER VIII

PLACEBO; BEECHER TO BENEDETTI

i   H K Beecher. *Pain in men wounded in battle.* The Annals of Surgery, 1946.

ii   H K Beecher "*The Powerful Placebo*" (J:A:M:A., Dec 24, 1955.

iii   Predrag Petrovic, Eija Kalso, Karl Magnus Petersson, Martin Ingvar. *Placebo and Opioid Analgesia. Imaging a Shared Neuronal Network.* Science Vol. 295 March 2002.

iv   Nicholas Coni., *Medicine and The Spanish Civil War.* J.R. Soc. M: 2002, **95**

v   Luana Colloca, Fabrizio Benedetti., *Nature Reviews.* Neuroscience Vol 6 July 2005: 545-552

vi   Editorial, in PAIN: vol 144 (1-2) July 2009.

vii   Luana Colloca, Fabrizio Benedetti. *Placebo analgesia induced by social observational learning.* PAIN: vol. 144 (1-2) July 2009 p. 28-34

viii Sun Shim Choi and Bruce T. Lahn. *Adaptive Evolution of MRG, a Neuron-Specific Gene Family.* Genome Research. 2003 13: 2252-2259.

ix   Felix Mann. *Acupuncture.* William Heinemann. 1983.

x   Ibid

xi   Moolamanil Thomas, *Acupuncture for the Treatment of Pain. Factors Influencing Outcome*; Thesis, Karolinska Institutet. Stockholm 1995.

xii   Kaptchuk et al. *Cult Med* Psychiatry (2009) 33:382-411.

xiii R A Moore et al., *Responder analysis for pain relief and numbers needed to treat in a meta-analysis of etoricoxib osteoarthritis trials: bridging a gap between clinical trials and clinical practice.* Ann Rheum Dis. 2010. 69(2): 374-379.

xiv   Sebastian Straube, Sheena Derry, Henry J McQuay, and R Andrew Moore. *Enriched enrolment: definition and effects of enrichment and dose in trials of pregabalin and gabapentin in neuropathic pain. A systematic review.* Br J Clin Pharmacol. 2008 August; 66(2): 266-275.

xv   T Lundeberg in *Scandinavian Journal of Rehabilitation Medicine* (ed O Höök) 1993

xvi   Dr Paul Offit. *Killing Us Softly.* p 224. Fourth Estate, London. 2013.

xvii Michael Foot. *Aneuran Bevan. A Biography.* p 178 Volume Two. David Poynter. London 1973.